MENTAL ILLNESS AND SOCIAL POLICY

THE AMERICAN EXPERIENCE

MENTAL ILLNESS AND SOCIAL POLICY

THE AMERICAN EXPERIENCE

A

TREATISE

ON

INSANITY

AND

Other Disorders

AFFECTING THE MIND

BY JAMES COWLES PRICHARD

ARNO PRESS

A NEW YORK TIMES COMPANY

New York • 1973

Reprint Edition 1973 by Arno Press Inc.

MENTAL ILLNESS AND SOCIAL POLICY:
  The American Experience
ISBN for complete set: 0-405-05190-5
See last pages of this volume for titles.

Manufactured in the United States of America

———◆———

Library of Congress Cataloging in Publication Data

Prichard, James Cowles, 1786-1848.
    A treatise on insanity and other disorders affecting
the mind.

    (Mental illness and social policy: the American
experience)
    Reprint of the 1837 ed. published by Haswell,
Barrington, and Haswell, Philadelphia.
    1. Psychiatry--Early works to 1900.   I. Title.
II. Series.   [DNLM: WM P947t 1837F]
RC340.P83 1973   616.8'9   73-2412
ISBN 0-405-05222-7

A

TREATISE

ON

INSANITY

AND

Other Disorders

AFFECTING THE MIND.

———◆———

BY JAMES COWLES PRICHARD, M.D. F.R.S.

CORRESPONDING MEMBER OF THE INSTITUTE OF FRANCE;
MEMBER OF THE ROYAL ACADEMY OF MEDICINE OF PARIS, AND OF THE
PHILOSOPHICAL SOCIETY OF SIENNA;
SENIOR PHYSICIAN TO THE BRISTOL INFIRMARY.

———◆———

" Usqueadeo res humanas vis abdita quædam
Obterit ———
Quid mirum si se temnant mortalia sæcla !"

———◆———

PHILADELPHIA:
HASWELL, BARRINGTON, AND HASWELL.
1837.

PREFATORY OBSERVATIONS.

ALTHOUGH the subject of mental derangement is one to which for more than twenty years I have been led to devote much study and reflection, I should probably never have undertaken the work now laid before the public, if I had not been requested to contribute to the Cyclopædia of Practical Medicine. While employed in preparing for that compilation an article on Insanity, and some others more or less connected with it, I became more fully convinced than I had before been, that, although many excellent treatises exist on various matters connected with mental derangement in the English, French, and German languages, there is yet not one work extant in either of them which exhibits the *present state* of knowledge and opinion on the whole subject of diseases affecting the mind. To supply this want was found not to be within the limits which propriety seemed to mark out for an article in the Cyclopædia, but having become fully interested in the undertaking, I felt desirous, after the publication of my papers in that work, of finishing what I had begun, and of drawing up, in a deliberate manner and with unconfined space, a more complete treatise on the same subject. In this design I was greatly encouraged by the spontaneous and kind advice of some of my friends, and particularly by that of Dr. Tweedie, one of the editors of the Cyclopædia. The task was further recommended to me by the opportunity which it offered of stating in a more convincing manner my opinions on some important questions connected with the nature of Insanity, with respect to which I believe the notions generally prevalent, and sanctioned by the highest medical and legal authorities in this country, to be not only erroneous, but the sources of great practical evils. On this subject I have no need to explain myself at present more fully than by referring my readers to the first and second sections of the second chapter, and to the third and following sections of the eleventh chapter, in the following treatise.

ANALYSIS OF THE CONTENTS.

INTRODUCTORY CHAPTER—I.

PRELIMINARY REMARKS ON THE DEFINITION OF INSANITY : NOSOGRAPHY
OF THE DISEASE AND OF ITS VARIOUS FORMS.

Notes on the preceding Chapter.

CHAPTER II.

PHENOMENA OF INSANITY DESCRIBED AS THEY ARE MANIFESTED IN THE
DIFFERENT FORMS OF THE DISEASE.

1*

CHAPTER III.

OF THE TERMINATIONS OF INSANITY.

CHAPTER IV.

OF THE CAUSES OF INSANITY.

CHAPTER V.

RESULTS OF NECROSCOPICAL RESEARCHES INTO THE CHANGES OF STRUCTURE CONNECTED WITH INSANITY.

CHAPTER VIII.

OF PUERPERAL MADNESS.

CHAPTER IX.

OF IDIOTISM AND MENTAL DEFICIENCY.

CHAPTER X.

STATISTICS OF INSANITY.

CHAPTER XI.

OF UNSOUNDNESS OF MIND IN RELATION TO JURISPRUDENCE.

CHAPTER XII.

OF ECSTATIC AFFECTIONS.

A
TREATISE ON INSANITY

AND

OTHER DISORDERS OF THE MIND.

INTRODUCTORY CHAPTER.

PRELIMINARY REMARKS ON THE DEFINITION OF INSANITY: NOSOGRAPHY OF THE DISEASE: ITS DIFFERENT FORMS.

WRITERS on disorders of the mind have frequently remarked that it is difficult to furnish a definition of insanity, which may enable us at once to recognise it when it exists, and to distinguish it from all other conditions whether of health or disease. So great, indeed, has this difficulty appeared to some authors, that by them it has been thought better to lay aside such an attempt. It is, however, requisite, at the commencement of a treatise on any subject of extensive relations, that the writer should make known to his readers in as clear and definite a manner as possible what is the precise nature of the objects to which their attention is to be directed. On this consideration I find it to be incumbent upon me to take some notice of the attempts which have been made to define or characterise insanity ; and if these attempts should be found, on examination, unsuccessful, to supply the defect if not by a new definition, at least by some brief description that may answer the same purpose.

It has been said, with perfect accuracy, that insanity is a disorder of the system by which the sound and healthy exercise of the mental faculties is impeded or disturbed. The definitions adopted by several modern writers have nearly this meaning, though expressed in various terms.* Yet this statement cannot be considered as a

---

* See MM. Heinroth, Fodéré, Georget, Guislain, Broussais, Jacobi.

APRIL, 1837.　　　　2

sufficient definition of insanity, for while it probably comprises every form of that disorder, it includes also many other morbid affections. Among the latter may be mentioned the varieties of delirium which occur in phrenitis, typhus, and other febrile and inflammatory diseases, and which ought not to be confounded with insanity, though they are comprehended within the definition above proposed. On this account it becomes necessary to introduce some express limitations. For a similar reason it appears requisite to exclude the disordered state of the mental faculties, consisting chiefly in stupor and diminished capability of sensation and perception, which accompanies lethargy, apoplexy, and other comatose diseases. There are some other morbid conditions of the brain and of the faculties dependent for their exercise on the functions of that organ, which must in like manner be excluded by particular restrictions. Such are congenital idiotism and the mental weakness of old age. Now it is obvious that a definition loses all its utility, when it is found necessary to encumber it with so many additional circumstances. Thus the endeavour to define insanity in the most simple and obvious terms which suggest themselves, is found to afford no satisfactory result, and a like disappointment has ensued on every similar attempt.

It appears that the practical advantages of a definition can, in this instance, only be attained by stating what are in reality those disturbances which the mental operations sustain in cases of insanity. These disturbances, however, present very different phenomena in different forms of the disease, and we cannot attempt to enumerate them or describe them in a collective statement, till we have taken notice of their principal varieties.

It has generally been supposed that the chief, if not the sole disorder of persons labouring under insanity consists in some particular false conviction, or in some erroneous notion indelibly impressed upon the belief. Mr. Locke made a remark which has often been cited, that " madmen do not appear to have lost the faculty of reasoning ; but having joined together some ideas very wrongly, they mistake them for truths, and they err, as men do that argue right from wrong principles." From Mr. Locke's time it has been customary to observe that insane persons reason correctly from erroneous premises; and some instance of illusion, or some particular erroneous impression has been looked for as the characteristic of the disease, or an essential circumstance in it. Dr. Cullen seems to have had Mr. Locke's observation in his mind when he laid down the definition of insanity, which occurs in his ' First Lines.' He describes this disease to be, " in a person awake, a false or mistaken judgment of those relations of things which, as occurring most frequently in life, are those about which the generality of men form the same judgment, and particularly when the judgment is very different from what the person himself had before usually formed." Cullen attempted to draw even this description within narrower limits, by observing that " there is generally some false perception

of external objects, and that such false perception necessarily occasions a *delirium* or *erroneous judgment,* which is to be considered
as *the disease.''* That this is by far too limited an account of insanity, and only comprises one among various forms of mental
derangement, every person must be aware who has had opportunities of extensive observation.

An attentive consideration of the phenomena which present themselves in different cases of insanity, enables us to observe several
forms of varieties, which are distinguishable from each other by well-
marked lines. To one division of cases,—namely, to those which
are referrible to the form of madness termed *melancholia, monomania,* or *partial insanity,*—the preceding remarks of Mr. Locke
and Dr. Cullen are alone applicable. These are instances in which
the illusion of the understanding is connected with some particular
subject, and leaves the judgment comparatively clear in other respects. The phenomena of such cases are very different from those
of *mania* or *raving madness,* in which the mind is totally deranged, and the individual affected talks nonsense, or expresses himself wildly and absurdly on every subject. There is, in the third
place, a class of persons generally reckoned among lunatics, but
consisting chiefly, though not entirely, of individuals whose disorder has already reached an advanced or protracted stage. In these
the condition of the faculties is such as to preclude the possibility
of any mental effort or voluntary direction of thought. The most
striking characteristics in this state are the rapid succession of ideas,
and the unconnected manner in which they enter into the mind,
without order or coherence, or, at least, without following their ordinary and natural arrangement and association. *Incoherence* is
the characteristic of this morbid condition.

The modifications of insanity already mentioned are affections of
the understanding or rational powers, but there is likewise a form
of mental derangement in which the intellectual faculties appear to
have sustained little or no injury, while the disorder is manifested
principally or alone, in the state of the feelings, temper, or habits.
In cases of this description the moral and active principles of the
mind are strangely perverted and depraved; the power of self-
government is lost or greatly impaired; and the individual is found
to be incapable, not of talking or reasoning upon any subject proposed to him, for this he will often do with great shrewdness and
volubility, but of conducting himself with decency and propriety
in the business of life. His wishes and inclinations, his attachments,
his likings and dislikings, have all undergone a morbid change, and
this change appears to be the originating cause, or to lie at the
foundation of any disturbance which the understanding itself may
seem to have sustained, and even in some instances to form throughout the sole manifestation of the disease. The older nosologists,
Sauvages, Sagar, and Linnæus, were not wholly unaware of these
distinctions, for in their distributions of mental disorders, we find,
besides an order of *Vesaniæ* or *Hallucinationes,* in which errone-

ous impressions were supposed to affect the understanding, another department, styled *Morositates,* or *Morbi Pathetici,* consisting of depraved appetites and other morbid changes in the feelings and propensities. The disordered states, however, which are classed under these heads, are not, all of them at least, strictly forms of insanity ; and Pinel appears to have been the first writer who, with a clear conception of the subject, distinguished a class of mental disorders under the term of "madness without delirium." Pinel, who was an acute and original observer, and whose opinions carry much weight on account of his extensive opportunities of investigating the history of madness, has made the following remark in reference to the sentiments of Mr. Locke:—"We may justly admire," he says, "the writings of this philosopher, without admitting his authority upon subjects not necessarily connected with his inquiries. On resuming, at Bicêtre, my researches into this disorder, I thought, with the above author, that it was inseparable from delirium or delusion, and I was not a little surprised to find many maniacs who at *no period gave evidence of any lesion of the understanding,* but who were under the dominion of instinctive and abstract fury, as if the active faculties alone had sustained injury."

The examples given by Pinel in illustration of this remark were not fortunately chosen, and they are all of one kind, namely, of that in which the principal manifestations of insanity were violent fits of anger or rage. The general observation which the author has so clearly expressed, that insanity consists, in certain cases, in a morbid perversion of the affections and moral feelings exclusively, and without any perceptible lesion of the intellectual faculties, is a fact of the highest importance, pathologically and practically, and the opinion of the author above cited, in this particular, deserves the most attentive consideration. In the following pages I hope to confirm this opinion, and to show that the facts which I shall adduce are sufficient to authorise a more general statement than the particular instances hitherto related would lead us to adopt.

If the preceding observations are well founded, we shall be enabled to distinguish the principal forms or varieties of insanity under the following terms:—

1. *Moral Insanity,* or madness consisting in a morbid perversion of the natural feelings, affections, inclinations, temper, habits, moral dispositions, and natural impulses, without any remarkable disorder or defect of the intellect or knowing and reasoning faculties, and particularly without any insane illusion or hallucination.

The three following modifications of the disease may be termed *Intellectual Insanity* in contradistinction to the preceding form. They are severally :—

2. *Monomania,* or partial insanity, in which the understanding is partially disordered or under the influence of some particular illusion, referring to one subject, and involving one train of ideas, while the intellectual powers appear, when exercised on other subjects, to be in a great measure unimpaired.

3. *Mania*, or raving madness, in which the understanding is generally deranged ; the reasoning faculty, if not lost, is confused and disturbed in its exercise ; the mind is in a state of morbid excitement, and the individual talks absurdly on every subject to which his thoughts are momentarily directed.

4. *Incoherence*, or dementia. By some persons it may be thought scarcely correct to term this a form of insanity, as it has been generally considered as a result and sequel of that disease. In some instances, however, mental derangement has nearly this character from the commencement, or at least assumes it at a very early period. I am therefore justified in stating it, after Pinel, to be a fourth and distinct form of madness. It is thus characterised by that justly celebrated writer :—" Rapid succession or uninterrupted alternation of insulated ideas, and evanescent and unconnected emotions ; continually repeated acts of extravagance ; complete forgetfulness of every previous state ; diminished sensibility to external impressions ; abolition of the faculty of judgment; perpetual activity."

If I am correct in assuming that all the varieties of madness may find their place under one of the descriptions thus marked out, a short nosography of the disease, which will answer many of the purposes of a definition, will be furnished by summing up the characteristics of the different forms. We may, then, describe insanity as a chronic disease, manifested by deviations from the healthy and natural state of the mind, such deviations consisting either in a *moral perversion*, or a disorder of the feelings, affections, and habits of the individual, or in *intellectual derangement*, which last is sometimes partial, namely, in *monomania*, affecting the understanding only in particular trains of thought ; or general, and accompanied with excitement, namely, in *mania*, or *raving madness ;* or, lastly, confounding or destroying the connections or associations of ideas, and producing a state of *incoherence*.

I shall now endeavour to draw an accurate and tolerably complete description of the phenomena of insanity, containing a statement generalized from a multitude of particular examples. In this description, while I avail myself of the aid afforded by the best practical writers of different countries, it will be my aim to avoid the admission of any circumstance or feature of disease which I have not in more or fewer instances actually observed. The reader will find, if I am not mistaken in the evidence of facts which I shall lay before him, enough to confirm and illustrate the preceding remarks, and to show how far the distinctions laid down are sufficient and complete.

NOTES ON THE PRECEDING CHAPTER.

The division of the forms of insanity pointed out in the preceding chapter is the most simple that is admissible, or adapted to the

existing varieties of the disease ; it is entirely practical, and founded
on observation.   A more extensive arrangement has been laid down
by Professor Heinroth, in his celebrated Treatise on Derangement
of the Mental Faculties, a work which, though singular and absurd
in some of its fundamental principles, is, perhaps, of all treatises on
disorders of the mind, the most elaborate and comprehensive.
Heinroth's distribution is rather theoretical or speculative than the
result of actual observation and experience ; yet it will be found
worthy of consideration.

The disorders of the mind, according to this writer, are only
limited in number and in kind by the diversities which exist in the
operations of the mental faculties.   The mental operations are of
three distinct kinds, and are referred on the testimony of consciousness to three different departments in our inward nature, viz. to
those of the feeling or sentiment (des gemüths), the understanding,
and the will.   The emotions of joy, grief, pleasure and pain, the
mental processes of reflection and contemplation, and the voluntary
act of self-determination, are three kinds of mental phenomena,
which, as they present themselves to our inward consciousness, are
so clearly and strongly distinguished from each other, that it is
impossible to confound them.   " If the cause of derangement is in
relation to one of these manifestations of mental existence—and to
one or another it must belong, since the mind is ever occupied with
phenomena related to one out of the three classes—we have only to
inquire to which modification the disorder actually refers itself, or
whether it affects the feelings, the understanding, or the will.   Since
one of these has' possession of our consciousness, or is at least
predominant at every point of time, whichever function of the mind
happens to be that which is falling into disorder, by it the form of
insanity is determined."   Thus we have, continues Heinroth, three
classes of mental diseases corresponding to the three departments
of our minds.   A second distinction is founded on the character of
the disturbance which is experienced ; whether it is of the nature
of exaltation or depression, of increased or diminished excitement.

It would be superfluous to follow Herr Heinroth closely through
the particulars with which he has filled up the preceding outline.
It appears, indeed, to me that he has inadvertently lost sight of his
original principle of discrimination, and has confounded essentially
separate forms of mental disorder, for which he had provided distinct places in his system.   I shall simply enumerate the principal
modifications of derangement of the mind, or of its diseases and
defects, according to the principles of Heinroth's method.

First kind of mental disorder.—Disorders of the moral dispositions.

The first division consists, as above stated, in disorders of passion,
feeling, or affection, of the *gemüth*, or moral disposition.   This has
two forms.

First form :—*Exaltation or excessive intensity.*
            Undue vehemence of feeling.
            Morbid violence of passions and emotions.

Second form :—*Depression.*

Simple melancholy, dejection without illusion of the understanding.

Second kind of mental disorders.

The second division consists of disorders affecting the understanding or the intellectual faculties.

First form :—*Exaltation.*

Undue intensity of the imagination, producing mental illusions.

To this head belong all the varieties of monomania.

Second form :—*Depression.*

Feebleness of conception ; of ideas.   Imbecility of the understanding.

Third kind of mental disorders.

The third division comprises disorders of the voluntary powers, or of propensities, and of will.

First form :—*Exaltation.*

Violence of will and of propensities.-

Tollheit, or madness without lesion of the understanding.

Second form :—*Depression.*

Weakness or incapacity of willing.

Moral imbecility.

To these annexed forms others are added under each division, displaying combinations of several simple varieties.   Thus, exaltation of feeling with an exalted state of the imagination constitutes derangement of the understanding with violent excitement or raving madness.   Delusion with depression of feeling or melancholy constitutes insanity with sorrowful dejection.   In one of these divisions every variety of mental disorder finds its appropriate place.

No systematic arrangement of mental disorders can be contrived more complete than that of Professor Heinroth.   Although founded on abstract views rather than on observation, it may furnish some useful suggestions.   Instances of mental derangement really exist of which the characteristic is a morbid state of the feelings and affections.   Nor is there any uncertainty as to the existence of disorders which refer themselves to Heinroth's third division: in this the voluntary powers and propensities are the department of our mental constitution which betrays the symptoms of a disordered state.   Propensities, however, are so nearly allied to passions and emotions, that they are generally referred to the same division of the faculties or of mental phenomena : both are included by metaphysicians in the ethical or moral department of the mind, as contradistinguished from the intellectual.   A multiplicity of subdivisions is inconvenient and burdensome, and it appears, on the whole, better to adhere, in describing mental disorders, to the more simple classification adopted in the preceding section.   In this, the disorders of affection or feeling, as well as those of the active powers or propensities, are comprehended under one head, to which the desig-

nation of Moral Insanity is given. If it were desirable to affix a
single compound epithet to this class of mental disorders, the most
appropriate would be Parapathia, or, perhaps, Pathomania, in coincidence with the Monomania of M. Esquirol. The subdivisions of
this department may comprise all the modifications or disordered
feeling or affection which belong to the fiist division of Heinroth,
as well as the disorders of will or propensity, which constitute the
third department of that writer. The second division, that of disorders of the intellectual faculties, are, in the arrangement which I have
selected, distributed into general and partial, termed Mania and
Monomania, to which Incoherency or Dementia is added in the
third place : and this division is more in accordance with actual
phenomena than that of exaltation and depression adopted by Heinroth.   On the whole, I do not discover any reason for changing the
distribution already selected, and which, in fact, I had adopted before the work of Professor Heinroth came into my hands.   His
scheme is, however, the most complete system that can be formed,
and I have laid the outline of it before my readers, as it may tend
to render more distinct their conception of the relations of the different forms of insanity to each other.

CHAPTER II.

PHENOMENA OF INSANITY DESCRIBED AS THEY ARE MANIFESTED
IN THE DIFFERENT FORMS OF THE DISEASE.

Section I.—*Moral Insanity.*

This form of mental derangement has been described as consisting in a morbid perversion of the feelings, affections, and active
powers, without any illusion or eroneous conviction impressed upon
the understanding : it sometimes co-exists with an apparently unimpaired state of the intellectual faculties.
    There are many individuals living at large, and not entirely sepa-
rated from society, who are affected in a certain degree with this
modification of insanity.   They are reputed persons of a singular,
wayward, and eccentric character. An attentive observer will often
recognize something remarkable in their manners and habits, which
may lead him to entertain doubts as to their entire sanity ; and
circumstances are sometimes discovered, on inquiry, which add
strength to his suspicion. In many instances it has been found that
an hereditary tendency to madness has existed in the family, or that
several relatives of the person affected have laboured under other
diseases of the brain. The individual himself has been discovered
to have suffered, in a former period of life, an attack of madness of

a decided character. His temper and dispositions are found to have undergone a change ; to be not what they were previously to a certain time : he has become an altered man, and the difference has, perhaps, been noted from the period when he sustained some reverse of fortune, which deeply affected him, or the loss of some beloved relative. In other instances, an alteration in the character of the individual has ensued immediately on some severe shock which his bodily constitution has undergone. This has been either a disorder affecting the head, a slight attack of paralysis, a fit of epilepsy, or some febrile or inflammatory disorder, which has produced a perceptible change in the habitual state of the constitution. In some cases the alteration in temper and habits has been gradual and imperceptible, and it seems only to have consisted in an exaltation and increase of peculiarities, which were always more or less natural and habitual.

In a state like that above described, many persons have continued for years to be the sources of apprehension and solicitude to their friends and relatives. The latter, in many instances, cannot bring themselves to admit the real nature of the case. The individual follows the bent of his inclinations ; he is continually engaging in new pursuits, and soon relinquishing them without any other inducement than mere caprice and fickleness. At length the total perversion of his affections, the dislike, and perhaps even enmity, manifested towards his dearest friends, excite greater alarm. When it happens that the head of a family labours under this ambiguous modification of insanity, it is sometimes thought necessary, from prudential motives, and to prevent absolute ruin from thoughtless and absurd extravagance, or from the results of wild projects and speculations, in the pursuit of which the individual has always a plausible reason to offer for his conduct, to make some attempt with a view to take the management of his affairs out of his hands. The laws have made inadequate provision for such contingencies, and the endeavor is often unsuccessful. If the matter is brought before a jury, and the individual gives pertinent replies to the questions that are put to him, and displays no particular mental illusion,—a feature which is commonly looked upon as essential to madness,—it is most probable that the suit will be rejected.

Persons labouring under this disorder are capable of reasoning or supporting an argument upon any subject within their sphere of knowledge that may be presented to them ; and they often display great ingenuity in giving reasons for the eccentricities of their conduct, and in accounting for and justifying the state of moral feeling under which they appear to exist. In one sense, indeed, their intellectual faculties may be termed unsound ; they think and act under the influence of strongly excited feelings, and persons accounted sane are, under such circumstances, proverbially liable to error both in judgment and conduct.

I have already had occasion to observe that the existence of moral insanity as a distinct form of derangement has been recognized by

3*

Pinel ; the following example recorded by that writer is a characteristic one. Pinel terms this affection " emportement maniaque sans délire."*

" An only son of a weak and indulgent mother gave himself up habitually to the gratification of every caprice and passion of which an untutored and violent temper was susceptible. The impetuosity of his disposition increased with his years. The money with which he was lavishly supplied removed every obstacle to the indulgence of his wild desires. Every instance of opposition or resistance roused him to acts of fury. He assaulted his adversary with the audacity of a savage; sought to reign by force, and was perpetually embroiled in disputes and quarrels. If a dog, a horse, or any other animal offended him, he instantly put it to death. If ever he went to a fête or any other public meeting, he was sure to excite such tumults and quarrels as terminated in actual pugilistic rencontres, and he generally left the scene with a bloody nose. This wayward youth, however, when unmoved by passion, possessed a perfectly sound judgment. When he became of age, he succeeded to the possession of an extensive domain. He proved himself fully competent to the management of his estate, as well as the discharge of his relative duties, and he ever distinguished himself by acts of beneficence and compassion. Wounds, lawsuits, and pecuniary compensations, were generally the consequences of his unhappy propensity to quarrel. But an act of notoriety put an end to his career of violence. Enraged with a woman who had used offensive language to him, he threw her into a well. Prosecution was commenced against him ; and on the deposition of a great many witnesses, who gave evidence to his furious deportment, he was condemned to perpetual confinement in Bicêtre."

Several other practical writers have given a testimony which is sufficiently conclusive as to the existence of moral insanity, though they have not designedly and in set terms marked it as a distinct form of mental derangement.

The following remarks by M. Esquirol, expressed as they appear to have been without the design of supporting any system or theory, prove that the writer was led by his ample experience to adopt an opinion similar to that of Pinel. He regards at least the perverted state of the moral feelings as not less essential to insanity than that of the intellectual faculties, and even as furnishing in some instances the whole manifestation of the disorder.

" The insane conceive an aversion for those persons who are most dear to them, revile them, ill-treat them, anxiously shun them, in consequence of their mistrust, their suspicions, and their fears. Prejudiced against every thing, they are afraid of every thing. A few appear to form an exception to this general rule, in preserving a sort of affection for their relatives and friends ; but this feeling of attachment, which is sometimes excessive, subsists without confi-

* Traité Médico-Philosophique sur l'aliénation mentale: 2de edit. Paris, 1809, p. 156.

dence in those persons who before the attack of disease had been the directors of the thoughts and actions of the patient. A melancholic, who is devotedly attached to his wife, is deaf to her counsels and advice. A son would sacrifice his life for his father, but will not make the slightest attempt, in compliance with the entreaties of the latter, to overcome the morbid impressions which occasions him so much grief.

" This moral alienation is so constant," says M. Esquirol, " that it appears to me to be the proper characteristics of mental derangement. There are madmen in whom it is difficult to discover any trace of hallucination, but there are none in whom the passions and moral affections are not disordered, perverted, or destroyed. I have in this particular met with no exceptions."

" A return to the proper and natural state of the moral affections," says the same writer, " the desire of seeing once more children or friends ; the tears of sensibility ; the wish manifested by the individual to open his heart and return into the bosom of his family, to resume his former habits, afford a certain indication of cure, while the contrary dispositions had been a mark of approaching insanity, or the symptom of a threatened relapse. This is not the case when there is merely a disappearance of the hallucination, which then only is a certain sign of convalescence, when the patients return to their natural and original affections."*

I shall have occasion in the sequel to cite the opinion of this excellent observer, expressed in still stronger terms as to the existence of a form of mental derangement, which comes under the definition of moral insanity.

M. Georget has described a morbid state of the feelings and active principles of the mind, or of the propensities and habits, as a particular modification of madness. He observes " that individuals predisposed to mental disease by a faulty education or by previous attacks, have often continued for a long time, or perhaps even during their whole lives, to attract observation by caprices in their deportment, by something eccentric in their manner and habits of life, by an ill-regulated fondness for pursuits of the fancy, and the mere productions of the imagination, combined with a striking inaptitude in the study of the exact sciences." The last-mentioned particular will scarcely be sufficient to excite a suspicion of madness in this country, whatever may be the case in France. " These persons are noted," continues the same writer, " for singularity of opinions, of conduct, for transitory fits of intelligence, or sallies of wit, which are too strongly contrasted with their habitual state of nullity or monotony ; for a levity in thoughts, a weakness in judgment, a want of connexion in their attempts at reasoning. Some individuals are presumptuous, desirous of undertaking every thing, and capable of applying themselves to nothing; others are extravagant and mobile in the utmost degree in their opinions and sentiments;

* *Esquirol*, Dict. des Sc. Méd. tom. xvi.

many are susceptible, irritable, choleric, and passionate ; some are
governed by pride and haughtiness without bound ; a few are
subject to vague anxieties or to panic terrors.

It must be remarked that, although M. Georget has described this
state of disease as a first stage, or as what he terms, with M. Esquirol, the *incubation* of madness, yet as he says that it often lasts
through the life of the individual, we may consider his testimony
as given, in point of fact, in favour of the real existence of the disorder here described, as a particular modification of insanity. There
are, indeed, numerous instances in which phenomena, similar to
those of the previous stage, last for many years, perhaps to the end
of life ; sometimes maintaining their ambiguous and undefined character, in others becoming aggravated in degree, but without undergoing a transition into that form of madness which is attended with
illusions and strongly-marked disturbances of the intellectual faculties.

The term which I have adopted as designating this disease, must
not be limited in its use to cases which are characterised merely
by preternatural excitement of the temper and spirits. There are
many other disordered states of the mind which come under the
same general division. In fact, the varieties of moral insanity are
perhaps as numerous as the modifications of feeling or passion in
the human mind. The most frequent forms, however, of the disease are those which are characterised either by the kind of excitement already described, or by the opposite state of melancholy
dejection. One of these is, in many instances, a permanent state ;
but there are cases in which they alternate or supersede each other ;
one morbid condition often lasting for a time, and giving way, without any perceptible cause, to an opposite state of the temper and
feelings. The prevalent character of the disorder is sometimes
derived from the constitutional disposition of the individual ; but
there are instances in which it is strikingly different from his natural temperament : lively and cheerful persons become dejected and
melancholy, while the gloomy and taciturn change their disposition
for one that is sanguine and excitable.

A considerable proportion among the most striking instances of
moral insanity are those in which a tendency to gloom or sorrow is
the predominant feature. When this habitude of mind is natural
to the individual and comparatively slight, it does not constitute
madness ; and it is perhaps impossible to determine the line which
marks a transition from predisposition to disease ; but there is a degree of this affection which certainly constitutes disease of mind,
and that disease exists without any illusion impressed upon the understanding. The faculty of reason is not manifestly impaired, but
a constant feeling of gloom and sadness clouds all the prospects of
life : the individual, though surrounded with all the comforts of existence, and even, exclusively of his disease, suffering under no
internal source of disquiet, at peace with himself, with his own conscience, with his God, yet becomes sorrowful and desponding. All

things present and future are to his view involved in dreary and hopeless gloom. This tendency to morbid sorrow and melancholy, as it does not destroy the understanding, is often subject to control when it first arises, and probably receives a peculiar character from the previous mental state of the individual, from his education, and his religious or irreligious character. Persons of well-regulated minds, when thus affected, express grief and distress at the inaptitude of which they are conscious to go through the active duties of life: frequently they feel a horror of being driven to commit an act of suicide or some other dreadful crime. This idea haunts them, and renders them fearful of being a moment alone. It, however, subsides, and such cases often terminate in recovery. Persons of an opposite character give themselves up to *tædium vitæ*, to morose disgust; they loathe their very existence, and at length, unless prevented, put an end to it.

A state of gloom and melancholy depression occasionally gives way after an uncertain period to an opposite condition of preternatural excitement: in other cases this last is the primary character of the disease. Individuals thus affected are always in high spirits, active and boisterous, full of projects and enterprises. Such a habit of mind within a certain degree is natural to many persons; but in those instances which form cases of moral insanity, it is beyond the limit that belongs to natural variety of character, and has besides peculiar features. In some cases it appears in persons whose temperament is the very reverse of the state described; and in such examples it is so much the more striking. In this form of moral derangement the disordered condition of the mind displays itself in a want of self-government, in continual excitement, an unusual expression of strong feelings, in thoughtless and extravagant conduct. A female modest and circumspect becomes violent and abrupt in her manners, loquacious, impetuous, talks loudly and abusively against her relations and guardians, before perfect strangers. Sometimes she uses indecent expressions, and betrays without reserve unbecoming feelings and trains of thought. Not unfrequently persons affected with this form of disease become drunkards; they have an incontrollable desire for intoxicating liquors, and a debauch is followed by a period of raving madness, during which it becomes absolutely necessary to keep them in confinement. Individuals are occasionally seen in lunatic asylums who under such circumstances have been placed under control. After the raving fit has passed off, they demand their release; and when they obtain it, at the first opportunity resort to their former excesses, though perfectly aware of the consequences which await them.

In examples of a different description the mental excitement which constitutes this disease is connected with religious feelings, and this is often the case when the period of excitement has been preceded by one of melancholy, during which the individual affected has laboured under depression and gloom, mixed with appre-

hensions as to his religious state. A person who has long suffered
under a sense of condemnation and abandonment, when all the
springs of hope and comfort have appeared to be dried up, and ro-
thing has been for a long time felt to mitigate the gloom and sorrow
of the present time and the dark and fearful anticipations of futurity,
has passed all at once from one extreme to another: his feelings
have become of a sudden entirely changed ; he has a sense of lively
joy in contemplating the designs of Providence towards him, amounting sometimes to rapture and ecstacy. Such a change has been
hailed by the relatives of the individual thus affected, when they
have happened to be pious and devout persons, as a happy transition from a state of religious destitution to one of acceptance and
mental peace; but the strain of excitement is too high, the expressions of happiness too ecstatic to be long mistaken : signs of pride
and haughtiness are betrayed, and of a wild and boisterous deportment, which are quite unlike the effects of a religious influence,
and soon unfold the real nature of the case ; or it is clearly displayed
by the selfishness, the want of natural affection, the variableness of
spirits, the irregular mental habits of the individual. In the cases
to which I have now referred, there has been no erroneous fact impressed upon the understanding; no illusion or belief of a particular
message or sentence of condemnation or acceptance specifically revealed : a disorder so characterised would not fall under the head of
moral insanity. The morbid phenomena in the cases of disease
which I am now attempting to describe extend only to the state of
the feelings and spirits, the temper, the preternaturally excited sentiments of hope and fear, and the results which these influences are
calculated to produce in the mental constitution.

Besides the more usual aspects of moral insanity which refer
themselves to morbid depression and excitement, particular cases
are marked by the prevalence of certain passions and mental habits
when displayed under modifications of which the human mind in a
sane state appears scarcely to be susceptible.

One of the most striking of these forms is distinguished by an
unusual prevalence of angry and malicious feelings, which arise
without provocation or any of the ordinary incitements. All the
examples of madness without delirium reported by Pinel belong to
this class of disorders. On this account the cases described by Pinel
failed for a long time to produce conviction on my mind, as to the
existence of what he terms *manie sans délire,* or *folie raisonnante.*
I am now persuaded that he was correct in his opinion, and I have
even been led to generalise his treatment. M. Esquirol has assured
me that his impression on this subject was similar. He considered
Pinel's cases as inconclusive, and for a time was disposed to entertain strong doubts as to the existence of insanity without intellectual error or delusion. M. Esquirol has expressed his conviction of
the reality of this form of mental derangement. Medical writers,
as well as other reporters, have generally endeavoured to reconcile

these phenomena with the established opinion respecting the nature
of insanity, by assuming, on conjecture, the existence of some
undetected illusion. These conjectures have their foundation in
attachment to system ; they are not supported by facts. There are
instances of insanity in which the whole disease, or at least the
whole of its manifestations, has consisted in a liability to violent fits
of anger breaking out without cause, and leading to the danger or
actual commission of serious injury to surrounding persons. The
characteristic feature of this malady is extreme irascibility depending on a physical morbid cause. There are other instances in which
malignity has a deeper die. The individual, as if actually possessed
by the demon of evil, is continually indulging enmity and plotting
mischief, and even murder, against some unfortunate object of his
malice. When this is connected with the false belief of some personal injury actually sustained, the case does not fall under the head
of moral insanity. It involves hallucination or erroneous conviction
of the understanding ; but when the morbid phenomena include
merely the expressions of intense malevolence, without ground or
provocation actual or supposed, the case is strictly one of the nature
above described.

In many instances the impulses or propensities to which the individual is subject, rather than his feelings or habitual temper and
disposition, give the principal or sole manifestations of insanity.
This is the form of madness to which, when accompanied with excitement, Reil, Hoffbauer, and other German writers, who, however, have written since the observations of Pinel, have termed
reine tollhiet. Many instances are well known in which a sudden
impulse to commit some atrocious act has arisen in the mind of a
person otherwise apparently sane, and certainly in full possession of
his intellectual powers. The impulse has often been resisted by
reason and voluntary effort ; it has been confessed with grief and
alarm to physicians or other persons, who have been entreated to
adopt precautions of safety in order to prevent some lamentable
catastrophe. In other cases crimes have been perpetrated without
any fixed object or motive, and the punishment of the law has fallen
upon the unfortunate victim of disease.

Some insane persons display their condition by a propensity to
commit every species of mischief, though devoid of any feeling of
malevolence. A case of this description, strongly marked, was
lately pointed out to me in the York Lunatic Asylum, by Dr. Wake,
the able and intelligent physician to that institution. The individual is a youth of good temper, cheerful and active, having no defect of understanding that could be discovered, even after long
observation. He is continually prone to commit every kind of mischief in his power, and not long ago escaped from his confinement
and made his way to Bishopthrope Palace, with the design to set it
on fire. Dr. Wake has assured me that several cases have occurred
precisely similar to that above related in all essential symptoms,

during his superintendence of York Asylum, which has continued eighteen years.*

A propensity to theft is often a feature of moral insanity, and sometimes it is its leading if not the sole characteristic. I have lately seen a lunatic, confined in an asylum, who would only eat when he had stolen food, and his keeper made it a constant practice to put into some corner within his reach various articles destined for his sustenance, in order that he might discover and take them furtively. Many instances are upon record of individuals noted for a propensity to steal, without the desire of subsequent possession, though in other respects of sound mind, or at least not generally looked upon as deranged. Probably some of these would afford, if accurately scrutinized, examples of moral insanity, while others might be found referrible to eccentricity of character. The discrimination—if indeed the two things are essentially different—could only be made in particular instances by taking into the account a variety of circumstances, such as the hereditary history of the individual and his consanguinity with persons decidedly insane, his former character and habits, and the inquiry whether he has undergone a change in these respects at some particular period of his life.

Eccentricity of conduct, singular and absurd habits, a propensity to perform the common actions of life in a different way from that usually practised, is a feature in many cases of moral insanity, but can hardly be said to constitute sufficient evidence of its existence. When, however, such phenomena are observed in connexion with a wayward and intractable temper, with a decay of social affections, an aversion to the nearest relatives and friends formerly beloved,—in short, with a change in the moral character of the individual, the case becomes tolerably well marked. With some of the traits above described, it happens not unfrequently that extreme penury is combined, and the aggregate of peculiarities makes up a character which is generally the laughing-stock of the neighbourhood or of the whole circle of acquaintance by which the individual is surrounded.

A variety of instances are mentioned by systematical writers in which the unusual intensity of particular passions or emotions has been thought to constitute mental disease, and a series of compound epithets has been invented for the purpose of affording names to such states of the mind and its affections. Nostalgia and erotomania have been considered as disorders of sentiment; satyriasis and

---

* Dr. Joseph Frank saw, at Bedlam, a child ten years of age, who was constantly under the influence of an irresistible impulse to break and destroy every thing that came in his way. This child appeared in other respects as reasonable as one could desire; he even seldom failed to demand, of his own accord, the punishment allotted to the mischief which he had committed. M. Guislain, Traité sur l'Aliénation, tom. i. p. 217. Some other cases of moral insanity occurring in children will be mentioned in the sequel. See chap. iv. sect. 2. On Predisponent Causes, article *Age.*

nymphomania of the physical feelings. The excessive intensity of any passion is disorder in a moral sense ; it may depend physically on certain states of the constitution ; but this does not so clearly constitute madness as the irregular and perverted manifestation of desires and aversions. There is reason to believe that this species of insanity has been the real source of moral phenomena of an anomalous and unusual kind, and of certain perversions of natural inclination which excite the greatest disgust and abhorrence.

Facts have occurred within my knowledge which afford proof and illustration of this remark. A young man, previously of most respectable character, became subject to severe epileptic fits, which were the prelude to attacks of violent mania, lasting, as it generally happens in this form of the disease, but a few days, and recurring at uncertain intervals. These complaints after a time disappeared in a great measure, but they left the individual excessively irritable in temper, irascible, and impetuous, liable to sudden bursts of anger or rage, during which he became dangerous to persons who were near to him. Of symptoms of this description, a state approximating to the satyriasis of medical writers is no unusual accompaniment, but in the present instance the diseased propensities of the individual were displayed in such a manner as to render confinement in a lunatic asylum the only preservative against criminal accusations.

A form of mental derangement has been described by some writers which is peculiar to old age. It is not of frequent occurrence, but certainly exists as a particular modification of madness. It has been termed *delirium senile,* but more properly by Dr. Burrows, who has accurately distinguished it, *senile insanity.* It constitutes a variety of moral insanity.

This disordered state makes its appearance in old men who have never before been insane or suspected of any tendency to mental derangement. It consists, like other forms of moral insanity, in a morbid excitement of passions and a remarkable perversion of the temper and propensities. The whole moral character of the person is changed. " The pious," says Dr. Burrows, " become impious, the content and happy discontented and miserable, the prudent and economical imprudent and ridiculously profuse, the liberal penurious, the sober drunken." In some elderly persons impulses which had long been effete become of a sudden excited, and a strong tendency to vicious habits is displayed. " In fact the reverence which age and the conduct suited to it always command, is converted into shame and pity at the perversion of those moral and social qualities which, perhaps, have hitherto adorned the patient's declining days." This description coincides accurately with the character of moral insanity. There are instances, though rare, of the appearance of hallucinative madness in old persons, but the case we have now described is of a different character, and consists in a disordered condition of the moral or active powers alone.

The prognosis in cases of moral insanity is often more unfavourable than in other forms of mental derangement. When the disorder is connected with a strong natural predisposition, it can scarcely be expected to terminate in recovery. Such we must conclude to be the case in those instances in which the phenomena bear the appearance of an increase or exaltation of peculiarities natural to the individual, and noted as remarkable traits in his previous habits. When, likewise, this disease has supervened on some physical change in the constitution, it is likely to be permanent, unless the circumstances under which it arose can be reversed ; and for bringing about such a salutary result, we have too often to regret that the art of medicine affords very inadequate resources. If, however, this morbid state of the mind has been the effect of any external and accidental cause, which admits of removal, or if the individual can be abstracted from its influence or defended against it, there is reason to hope that the disorder may gradually subside. Such recoveries have in fact taken place within the sphere of my own personal observation. But unless the desired change has been made at an early period, the disease is likely either to be permanent, or to terminate in another form of insanity.

Section II.—*Of Monomania, or Partial Derangement of the Understanding.*

This form of insanity is characterized by some particular illusion or erroneous conviction impressed upon the understanding, and giving rise to a partial aberration of judgment. The individual affected is rendered incapable of thinking correctly on subjects connected with the particular illusion, while in other respects he betrays no palpable disorder of mind.

Melancholia is the term by which this species of insanity was distinguished by medical writers from the age of Hippocrates until within a few years. This expression, as it was well observed by M. Esquirol, suggested the idea, not always consistent with facts, that partial derangement of the understanding is essentially of a gloomy character, or connected with sadness and despondency. The illusions which possess the mind are not constantly, in individuals partially insane, indicative of grief or melancholy. Some patients of this description are proud and elated, and fancy themselves kings or emperors, but on ordinary subjects are capable of talking coherently if not rationally ; they appear to be happy in their delusions. Others are insane upon some metaphysical or abstract notion, on which they talk absurdly, but without any predisposition to grief or mental dejection. Melancholia seemed to be an improper designation for cases of this kind ; and the term monomania, which was happily suggested by M. Esquirol, has been universally adopted in its place.* The meaning attached by former

---

* The term *melancholia* has, however, only become improper, in modern times ; for anciently this word, in ordinary language at least, conveyed no idea of gloom

writers to *melancholia* was, however, precisely the same as that
which is now expressed by monomania. It is thus laid down in
the most explicit terms by Van Swieten. " A maniâ distinguitur
melancholia, quod nondum adsit sævus ille furor, qui in maniacis
observatur. Præterea et illud signum diagnosticum melancholiæ
est, quod uni et eidam cogitationi pertinacissimè inhæreant tales
ægri, et ferè circa hanc illamve opinionem delirant tantùm; in reli-
quis omnibus sanam ostendunt mentem et sæpè accutissimum inge-
nium."

The notion, however, which many persons entertain as to the
nature of this disease, is far from being correct in its full extent. It
is supposed that the mind of the monomaniac is perfectly sound
when its faculties are exercised on any subject unconnected with a
particular impression, which in itself constitutes the entire disease.
Cases are indeed on record, which, if faithfully related, fully come
up to this description. In general the real character of monomania
is very different. The individual affected is, under ordinary circumstances, calm, and exhibits no symptom of that perturbation and
constant excitement which are observed in raving madness. But
on careful inquiry it will be found that his mind is in many
respects in a different condition from that of perfect health. The
habits and disposition have, perhaps, been long, in a greater or less
degree, in the state which characterizes moral insanity. If we
advert to the order and connection of morbid phenomena, we often
learn that on a settled and habitual melancholy, or on a morose and
sullen misanthropy, long growing and indulged, or on some other
disordered and perverted state of the feelings and affections, a particular illusion has more recently supervened. An individual of
melancholic temperament, who has long been under the influence
of circumstances calculated to impair his health and call into play
the morbid tendencies of his constitution, sustains some unexpected
misfortune, or is subjected to causes of anxiety; he becomes dejected
in spirits, desponds, broods over his feelings till all the prospects of
life appear to him dark and comfortless. His inclinations are now
so altered that no motive has sufficient influence over him to rouse
him to voluntary and cheerful exertion. During this period, if
questioned as to the causes of his mental dejection, he will probably
assign no particular reason for it. At length his gloom and despondency becoming more and more intense, his imagination fixes upon
some particular circumstance of a distressing nature, and this
becomes afterwards the focus round which the feelings which harass
him concentrate themselves. This circumstance is often some real,

---

or dejection. *Melagcholan* meant simply to be mad, to be out of one's mind. In
that sense exactly the word is often used by Aristophanes, without any reference
to lowness of spirits; see Plutus, v. 366, 904. Birds, v. 14. A distinction,
however, was made by medical writers, though it was by no means constantly
observed. Hippocrates, speaking of the case of Timocrates, says, " *Mainomenos
de upo cheles melaines epie to pharmakon.*" Here *mania* includes melancholy as a
particular variety. (Epidem. 5.)

occasionally some trifling act of delinquency for which the individual expresses the strongest and perhaps disproportionate self-con-
demnation. In other instances an unreal phantom suggests itself, in
harmony with the prevalent tone of the feelings, which at first
haunts the mind as possible, and is at length admitted as reality.
Other individuals begin by indulging morose and unfriendly sentiments towards all their acquaintance, magnifying in imagination every
trifling neglect into a grievous contumely. They fancy, at length,
that they find in some casual occurrence glaring proofs of premeditated designs to ruin them and expose them to the contempt and
derision of society. The disease in these cases has its real commencement long before the period when the particular illusion,
which is only an accessory symptom, is discovered, and even before
it became impressed on the imagination; but it is not until that
impression has taken place that the case assumes the proper character
of monomania.

The illusion which torments the monomaniac is generally something bearing a near relation to his former habits of business, or to
the usual occupation of his thoughts. I was consulted some years
ago on the case of a youth who had become insane, as his friends
supposed, through unusual excitement and exertion of mind. He
had been attending the sermons of a preacher noted for the vehemence of his language, and at the same time had devoted himself to
studies for which he was unprepared, to the neglect of sleep and
bodily exercise. He became depressed in spirits, and disordered
both in body and mind. The morbid feelings which afflicted him
at length conjured up for themselves an imaginary cause, which
soon became indelibly impressed upon his belief. He fancied himself to be suspected of some horrible crime, for which a process
had commenced against him ; and whenever the door of his room
was opened, he supposed that officers of justice were coming to
apprehend him. This youth was the son of an attorney in a county
town, who was frequently employed in criminal prosecutions.

That the order and succession of morbid phenomena in the
development of this disease is really such as I have described it to
be, I shall prove, in the following section, by the statement of some
cases in which the actual supervention of erroneous belief or illusion
on a previously existing moral insanity was clearly marked, and
admitted of no doubt.*

Medical writers have distributed the forms of monomania into

* This account of the nature and succession of symptoms in monomania
exactly coincides with the observations of Jacobi. " Das verstandesleiden
entsteht bei diesen Seelenstörungen durchaus nur in Folge des Gemüthsleidens,
wird durch dasselbe unterhalten, und verschwindet nicht nur mit demselben,
sondern wird auch durch, auf das Gemüth gerichtete, Einwirkungen gehoben.
Der melancholische wird nicht durch diese oder jene traurige Idee in seine
Krankheit gestürzt, sondern die Idee entsteht weil er an solcher Krankheit leidet.
Eben so wenig machen die lächerlichen Absurditäten, in denen sich der Narr
gefällt, diesen zum Narren, sondern er muss sich darin gefallen, weil er an einer
Krankheit leidet die dieses bedingt."

many classes or divisions. The subdivision would be endless if we were to constitute as many different kinds as there are modes and varieties of hallucination ; but the most proper and useful distribution is founded on the prevailing passions or feelings which give origin and impart their peculiar character to the disease.

Mental dejection or melancholy, which extinguishes hope and gives the mind up to fear and the anticipation of evils, lays the foundation for many kinds or varieties of monomania. The most numerous and the worst instances are those in which the thoughts are directed towards the evils of a future life. The unseen state opens the most ample scope to the dark and gloomy anticipations of melancholy and remorse, and hence it is selected by the desponding monomaniac as a field for the exercise of his self-torturing imagination. If the habits of his mind lead him to fix by preference on scenes connected with the present life, he still finds imaginary objects of terror and disquietude. Two centuries ago persons were every where to be found who fancied themselves possessed by demons, just as the ancients were pursued and agitated by the furies. Dæmonomania occupies an important place among the forms of insanity described by the old writers, and we are informed by Jacobi that this is still the character which, in some catholic countries, insanity connected with superstition frequently assumes. " In modern times," says M. Esquirol, " the punishments which the priest denounces have ceased to influence the minds and conduct of men, and governments have recourse to restraints of a different kind. Many lunatics express now as much dread of the tribunals of justice as they formerly entertained of the influence of stars and demons." " C'est toujours la pusillanimité, l'inquiétude, la crainte qui aggissent sur ces infortunés, comme elles étaient la cause des maladies des possédés. Tel individu est aux Petites-Maisons, parcequ'il craint la police, qui eût été brulé autrefois parcequ'il aurait eu peur du diable."

When fear and apprehension subside into a confirmed and settled despondency, as the latter state of feeling is less agitating than the former, the mind displays more the appearance of tranquillity, but it is a deceitful calm, concealing profound grief and misery. Of this description, however, are some of the most remarkable cases of intellect apparently sound in all other respects, but labouring under one delusion, on which, as on certain data, individuals reason correctly and acutely. Such illusions turn always on some circumstance connected with the person of the lunatic, his treatment by his relatives or by society in this world, or his destiny hereafter. Many religious persons, labouring under a predisposition to grief and despondency, have conceived the opinion that they are doomed to future perdition, their own cases forming particular exceptions to the otherwise merciful dispensations of Providence. A singular modification of this result of despondency is related in the striking ease of Samuel Brown, who, at a time when all the powers of his mind subsisted in full vigour, conceived that his rational soul had gradually perished under the displeasure of God, and that an animal life merely was left to him, in common with the brutes.

A great number and variety of cases coming under the same head, of monomania associated with fear and despondency, are instances in which the apprehensions of the individual are concentrated on his bodily feelings, or relate to some diseased or preternatural state in which he conceives himself to exist. In the first stage this disease is hypochondriasis ; the patient dwells constantly on some trifling ailments, which he magnifies in apprehension, broods over, and on account of which he makes himself miserable. In this form hypochondriasis constitutes a variety of moral insanity, and a hundred cases of this description are to be found for one which actually makes the transition into erroneous belief. When this change has taken place, the disorder is accounted a decided one of insanity, as when a man fancies that his head has grown larger than his body, that his legs are made of glass, that he has a wolf or a fish in his stomach. The absurd ideas which the diseased imagination frames in order to account for trifling bodily suffering are as numerous as they are strange and surprising. I well remember a lunatic who laboured apparently under neuralgic pains. He fancied that the physician to whose care he was confided had the power of torturing him by electricity, and that invisible wires were spread through every part of the house as conductors of the fluid, which was used at night as the instrument of cruel and tyrannical persecution. Many a flatulent hypochondriac has fancied the existence of a goblin or demon in his stomach ; and the association between his internal feelings and the idea by which it was accounted for, has become so firm that nothing in future has been capable of changing it. A case exemplifying this remark is related by Dr. Jacobi, which is so curious that I have determined to extract it.*

" A man, confined in the lunatic asylum at Würtzburg, in other respects rational, of quiet, discreet habits, so that he was employed in the domestic business of the house, laboured under the impression that there was a person concealed within his belly, with whom he held frequent conversations. He often perceived the absurdity of this idea, and grieved in acknowledging and reflecting that he was under the influence of so groundless a persuasion, but could never get rid of it. It was very curious to observe," says Jacobi, " how, when he had but an instant before cried, ' What nonsense ! is it not intolerable to be so deluded?' and while the tears which accompanied these exclamations were yet in his eyes, he again began to talk, apparently with entire conviction, about the whisperings of the person in his belly, who told him that he was to marry a great princess. An attempt was made to cure this man by putting a large blister on his abdomen, and at the instant when it was dressed and the vesicated skin snipped, throwing from behind him a dressed-up figure, as if just extracted from his body. The exper-

* Dr. Max. Jacobi's Sammlungen für die Heilkunde der Gemüthskrankheiten.

iment so far succeeded that the patient believed in the performance, and his joy was at first boundless in the full persuasion that he was cured, but some morbid feeling about the bowels, which he had associated with the insane impression, still continuing, or being again experienced, he took up the idea that another person similar to the first was still left within him, and under that persuasion he continued to labour."*

Dejection of spirits combined with malevolent feelings gives rise to misanthropical monomania, which is a very frequent form of the disease. The individual who labours under it is almost as miserable as the melancholic or hypochondriac. He fancies himself the object of hatred and persecution, of secret machinations, of plots of all descriptions, sees enemies in his dearest friends, suspects poison in his food, and imagines that injuries of every kind are perpetrated or at least designed against him. A case very descriptive of this variety of monomania will be related in the next section, in which its supervention or moral insanity is clearly evident.

Excess of self-love is an ingredient in every modification of monomania, and when this is combined with an elate and sanguine disposition instead of depressed spirits and a morose temper, it produces cheerful illusions, which always maintain their relation to the person of the lunatic. A monomaniac fancies himself a king, the pope, a favourite of heaven. This, however, does not constitute a single delusion, leaving the mind perfectly sane in other respects: the same individual magnifies himself in other relations. I saw lately a lunatic at Bicêtre who fancies himself a monarch. Perceiving me, as I suppose, to be a stranger, he accosted me with the words, " Je parle toutes les langues." Most gay and cheerful monomaniacs display a degree of this insane vanity. A characteristic case of the same kind was given by Bonetus, which Dr. Arnold has extracted in his work on insanity.

I believe that the remarks which I have made on the varieties of partial insanity above mentioned, and the mode of its origin, will be found to apply to every instance of monomania, properly so termed. The illusion is always some notion as to the powers, property, dignity, or destination of the individual affected, which is engrafted upon his habitual state of desire or aversion, passion and feeling.

There is another class of illusions, which belong not to insanity, but to extasis. They constitute, not a simple erronenous notion, impressed on the belief like the hallucinations of the monomaniac, but an entire imaginary scene displayed to his view like a series of real transactions, or a continuous dream. When the individual perseveres in believing their reality, a species of derangement ensues, but it is so peculiar and so unlike any of the ordinary forms

* Sammlungen für die heilkunde der Gemüthskrankheiten, herausgeg-von Dr. Max. Jacobi, Elberfeld, 1822, l. b, p. 21.

of madness, as to require a separate consideration under the head of
ecstatic affections, to which I have referred it.

Before I proceed to describe the remaining forms of mental derangement, I purpose to lay before my reader the statements of a
few select cases exemplifying the character of moral insanity, as
well as that of monomania, and likewise of some which tend to
illustrate the connexion between these two forms of disease, and the
transition from one into the other.

SECTION III.—*Cases exemplifying the Description of Moral
Insanity and that of Monomania, or illustrating the Relation
between these Forms of Disease, and the Transition from one
into the other.*

The first case that I shall relate, is one which for some years bore
precisely the character attributed to moral insanity. During this
period many of the friends of the individual affected supposed him
to be only *very eccentric;* while some, who had opportunities of
observing him closely, were convinced that he was deranged. His
disorder at length broke out in a form which admitted of no doubt,
viz., that of monomania accompanied with great distress of mind,
and it terminated in suicide. I give the details of this case as I received them from an intimate friend of the individual affected.

Case 1.—A. B., a gentleman remarkable for the warmth of his
affections, and the amiable simplicity of his character, possessed of
great intellectual capacity, strong powers of reasoning, and a lively
imagination, married a lady of high mental endowments, and who
was long well known in the literary world. He was devotedly
attached to her, but entertained the greatest jealousy lest the world
should suppose that, in consequence of her talents, she exercised an
undue influence over his judgment, or dictated his compositions.
He accordingly set out with a determination of never consulting
her, or yielding to her influence, and was always careful, when engaged in writing, that she should be ignorant of the subject which
occupied his thoughts. His wife has been often heard to lament
that want of sympathy and union of mind which are so desirable in
married life. This peculiarity, however, in the husband so much
increased, that in after years the most trifling proposition on her
part was canvassed and discussed by every kind of argument. In
the mean time he acquired strange peculiarities of habits. His love
of order, or placing things in what he considered order or regularity,
was remarkable. He was continually putting chairs, &c. in their
places ; and if articles of ladies' work or books were left upon a
table, he would take an opportunity *unobserved* of putting them in
order, generally spreading the work smooth, and putting the other
articles in rows. He would steal into rooms belonging to other
persons for the purpose of arranging the various articles. So much

time did he consume in trifles, placing and replacing, and running from one room to another, that he was rarely dressed by dinner-time, and often apologised for dining in his dressing-gown, when it was well known that he had done nothing the whole morning but dress. And he would often take a walk in a winter's evening with a lanthorn, because he had not been able to get ready earlier in the day. He would run up and down the garden a certain number of times, rinsing his mouth with water, and spitting alternately on one side and then on the other in regular succession. He employed a good deal of time in rolling up little pieces of writing-paper which he used for cleaning his nose. In short his peculiarities were innumerable, but he concealed them as much as possible from the observation of his wife, whom he knew to be vexed at his habits, and to whom he always behaved with the most respectful and affectionate attention, although she could not influence him in the slightest degree. He would, however, occasionally break through these habits ; as on Sundays, though he rose early for the purpose, he was always ready to perform service at a chapel a mile and a half distant from his house. It was a mystery to his intimate friends when and how he prepared these services. It did not at all suprise those who were best acquainted with his peculiarities, to hear that in a short time he became notoriously insane. He fancied his wife's affections were alienated from him, continually affirming that it was quite impossible she could have any regard for a person who had rendered himself so contemptible. He committed several acts of violence, argued vehemently in favour of suicide, and was shortly afterwards found drowned in a canal near his house. It must not be omitted that this individual derived a predisposition to madness by hereditary transmission : his father had been insane.

Case 2.—The second case is one which had likewise for a considerable period the character of moral insanity, and degenerated into, or assumed that of monomania. The details which 1 relate are such as I collected from the friends of the individual, and from his own communications.

C. D., a gentleman about thirty years of age, has laboured for several years under symptoms of moral insanity. He has been long dejected in spirits and morose in temper, dissatisfied with himself, and suspicious of all that surrounded him. He was capricious and unsteady in his pursuits, frequently engaging in some new study in the most sanguine manner, and soon abandoning it in despair of making any progress, though possessed of good talents and considerable acquirements of knowledge. He passed the requisite period of time at one of the universities, but could not be prevailed upon to go in for his degree, either through timidity and want of resolution, or, as it was conjectured by his friends, from a morbid apprehension that the examiners would not deal fairly with him, and award him the station to which he aspired and believed himself entitled. He applied himself afterwards to the study of medicine, and then to that of metaphysics, and speedily relinquished both.

He frequently changed his residence, but soon began to fancy himself the object of dislike to every person in the house of which he became the inmate. His peculiarities appearing to increase, he was visited by two physicians, who were desired to investigate the nature of his case. On being questioned narrowly as to the ground of the persuasion expressed by him, that he was disliked by the family with which he then resided, he replied that he heard whispers uttered in distant apartments of the house indicative of malevolence and abhorrence. An observation was made to him that it was impossible for sounds so uttered to be heard by him. He then asked if the sense of hearing could not, by some physical change in the organ, be occasionally so increased in intensity as to become capable of affording distinct perception at an unusual distance, as the eyes of mariners are well known to be accommodated by long effort to very distant vision. This was the only instance of what might be termed hallucination discovered in the case after a minute scrutiny. It seemed to be a late suggestion. The individual had been for years labouring under a gradually increasing moral insanity. His judgment had become at length perverted by the intensity of his morbid feelings, and admitted as real an erroneous impression, suggested by his fancy, which happened to be in harmony with his feelings, and served to account for them.

Case 3.—This case was strictly one of moral insanity for some years after its commencement, and it maintained that character throughout its duration, except that at one period, under great excitement, the patient began to display signs of an approach of monomania, in the groundless suspicions which she expressed respecting the persons who were about her. These symptoms, however, continued but for a very short time, and have never recurred. At the period when this individual came under my observation, her disorder had precisely the character of moral insanity.

E. F———— is a maiden lady, aged about forty-eight, of short stature, and somewhat deformed. " Her natural disposition was steady and industrious ; she accomplished her undertakings by dint of application rather than by energetic or sudden efforts. She was constant rather than ardent in her attachments, free from resentment, never the subject of lively emotions ; a great respecter of truth, just and very exact in all that she said or did. Her charitable acts were commensurate with her means, deliberate, and the result of principle rather than arising from the mere impulse of compassionate feeling. She was cautious and reserved in her communications, and scarcely if ever formed any familiar and particular intimacies with young persons of her own sex. Being debarred by her infirmities from associating with the young and active, she seemed more like an adult member of the family than a child. She was very clever in arithmetic and in all matters of business, and was fond of regulating and controlling the little affairs of those who formed the domestic circle surrounding her. Young persons and servants, finding that they derived advantage from her advice, generally gave her an opportunity of gratifying her inclination. Her dress, which was always plain and in good taste, was to her an object of greater attention than it often is to persons of fashion."

In March 1822 she was attacked by severe inflammation in the lungs, attended by expectoration of bloody mucus. This was the first time in her life when it was necessary to confine her to bed. She submitted with great reluctance to the restrictions that were needful for her recovery, and would not be persuaded, until she had heard the opinion of an old friend of her family, who is a medical practitioner, that the means adopted were proper and required by her case. She was then, however, in a great measure reconciled, and after seven or eight weeks was so far recovered as to bear a removal into her native county. At this period nobody believed that she would survive another winter. Her restoration to her usual state of health was very slow, and her sister, who was her constant companion, perceived with sorrow that her temper was now much changed. She appeared restless, always wishing to go somewhere, or to do something to which she was unequal ; becoming unjustly irritated when she could not urge her sister, whose health and spirits were declining, to fall in with her ideas, and occasionally giving way to her reproaches which were keenly felt. She tried every method of persuasion to induce her sister to go to the neighbourhood of London, though for the preservation of her life the latter had been obliged to give up the custom of spending the winter there, and the attempt was considered dangerous to her. Every inducement, every argument was suggested to promote this favourite object : other towns were too warm and too cold, too hilly, too much intersected with water, too *foggy*. In 1827 she determined to go without her sister to H———, near London. She went, and from her letters her sister perceived that she was living in a state of excitement far surpassing that of her former habits ; paying short visits to her friends in the surrounding villages, going out in the common short stages, without so much regard to weather as was usual to her even in the summer ; receiving small parties at home, attending a very crowded church, writing a great many letters, &c. &c. She used to write to her sister in rather a boastful style, frequently mentioning her good health and high spirits, as if to justify her choice of a residence near the metropolis. When the sisters met during the summer at their house in ———shire, her high spirits were gone, she looked more aged than the time elapsed would have led any one to expect, took less interest in her garden, appeared exhausted, and, without contributing her share to the conversation, used frequently to sleep in her chair. She lay much in bed, nursed herself up, and in October went again to H———, as much agog as ever. Another winter passed much as the preceding one had done. She spoke much again of her high spirits, visited much, was observed to be unusually liberal in her presents to most of her acquaintances. A second summer of inertness was succeeded by a winter at H———. She was now weak, indisposed for visiting, and, in fact so much worse as to be unable to follow her inclinations. In the spring of 1830 she had an attack of the same nature as that in 1822, but not so severe or lasting. In the summer she was nearly as before, and quite as eager to resume her plans, as enthusiastic in her commendations of every body and every thing at H——.

About this time some riots took place in London, and more were apprehended. She now expressed herself as apprehensive that "very awful times were at hand," and wrote frequent letters to her sister full of indecision, and expressive of distrust in her servants, her host and his family. A friend who called upon her "was shocked to find her in so low a way." He thought her unfit to be alone, and she was unwilling to adopt any plan for leaving her lodgings, or having any one with her. She said she should be happy with her sister, and knew that she should be taken care of by the latter, but dreaded becoming a burden to her and making her ill ; yet feared that if she did not go to her sister, "some one would put her where no one would know, and cause her to sign papers which she ought not to sign." She was evidently apprehensive of being sent to a lunatic asylum. She thought her host was a writer of "Swing letters,"* and dreaded that he might fill the house with combustibles and blow it up with her in it. A medical man who was taken to see her, said that she was in a state of great mental excitement, and ought to be taken to her sister as soon as possible. The frost was severe when she was escorted to her sister, who was then settled at Bristol, yet she took no cold, experienced no injury from fatigue, and lost that feeling of terror to which she had for some time been subject. Since she has been with her sister, she has been increasingly obstinate, suspicious, undecided, restless, parsimonious even to meanness, indisposed to any employment bodily or mental, except as far as relates to a most troublesome interference with the most minute actions of others. Could she have her own way, she would control the food, dress, and employment of every one near her. She has become negligent in dress, and comparatively dirty in her habits, yet has an insatiable desire for new clothes, which she never finds the right time to wear. She is constantly predicting her utter ruin, is sure she will not have money enough to live until such and such a time ; knows that enough will not be found to pay Dr. ——; knows he will not let any one of so shabby an appearance be long in his house ; does not know where she shall go when he is tired of her ; thinks that "it is the devil that makes her behave as she does;" "that her heart is hardened to do what she ought not to do ;" "she is like the man spoken of in the Gospel, who could not be bound even with fetters." She sees people look at her ; hopes they do'nt think she drinks too much ; is quite sure she never did. These impressions are continually varying ; but no sooner is her mind tran-

---

* It may hereafter require to be explained that, about the period above mentioned, the threatening letters of incendiaries in various parts of the country frequently bore the signature of *Swing*.

quilized on one subject than another source of disquietude arises, so that she exhausts every person who is long with her. Her bodily health is better than it was for years previous to her mental derangement. A constitutional asthma, to which she has been subject from the age of six or seven years, has nearly subsided, and the habitual profuse expectoration has considerably diminished. She wears less clothing, and appears less sensible to cold or damp than heretofore."

I had several interviews with the subject of the foregoing relation, during some of which she gave replies to a variety of questions referring to the past and actual state of her health, both bodily and mental. No impression could be traced in her mind that bore the character of insane hallucination. The circumstances most observable in her condition was a perpetual disposition to find fault with every action, even the most trivial, that was witnessed by her. When asked if she was not aware of this propensity, she seemed to give an unwilling affirmative to the question, and she was plainly aware of the fact, for on the inquiry being made whether the habit had only existed of late years, or had been a part of her natural character, she steadily averred that such was not her natural disposition, " that she was formerly very different."

Case 4.—This case is one of moral insanity with high excitement, which never displayed any of the signs of intellectual madness, and terminated in recovery.

G. H., a farmer, several of whose relatives had been the subjects of mental derangement, was a man of sober and domestic habits, and frugal and steady in his conduct, until about his forty-fifth year, when his disposition appeared to have become suddenly changed, in a manner which excited the surprise of his friends and neighbours, and occasioned grief and vexation in his family. He became wild, excitable, thoughtless, full of schemes and absurd projects. He would set out and make long journeys into distant parts of the country to purchase cattle and farming-stock, of which he had no means of disposing ; he bought a number of carriages, hired an expensive house ready furnished, which had been inhabited by a person much above his rank, and was unsuitable to his condition. The following incident was related as an instance of his capricious conduct. He had expressed a desire to survey an estate belonging to a gentleman in the neighbourhood, with a view of becoming his tenant, and had been told that he should be conducted over the ground whenever he chose to call upon the steward. The time which he selected for this purpose was the middle of a dark night. The steward was awakened, and listened with surprise and suspicion to the proposal. He remonstrated for some time, but finding G. H. determined on his purpose, and pleading a positive promise from the landlord of the estate, he at length acquiesced, and accompanied the farmer, with a lantern, over the fields. G. H. made remarks on the trees which denoted the quality of the soil, the thickness of the hedges, and the usual signs which distinguish good

from sterile land. He had gone over the estate, and took his leave
just as the morning light began to dawn. G. H. was irascible and
impetuous, quarrelled with his neighbours, and committed an assault
upon the clergyman of the parish, for which he was indicted and
bound to take his trial. At length his wife became convinced that
he was mad, and made application for his confinement in a lunatic
asylum, which was consequently effected. The medical practitioners who examined him were convinced of his insanity by comparing his late wild habits and unaccountable conduct with the
former tenor of his life, taking into consideration the tendency to
disease which was known to prevail in his family. The change in
his character alone had produced a full conviction of his madness in
his friends and relatives. When questioned as to the motives
which had induced him to some of his late proceedings, he gave
clear and distinct replies, and assigned, with great ingenuity, some
plausible reason for almost every part of his conduct. After a period
of time passed in quiet seclusion, his mind became gradually tran-
quilized ; the morbid excitement of his temper and feelings disappeared, he was set at liberty, and has since conducted himself with
propriety.

A brother of the above patient has been at two different times
confined in the same asylum, labouring under symptoms of derangement in all essential particulars resembling those above detailed.
His disorder has consisted chiefly in morbid excitement, wildness
and irregularity of conduct, differing from his usual habits and
character, without any hallucination or disturbance of the intellectual faculties. He has, on both occasions, remained in the asylum
until he was fully convalescent, and after his departure has ackow-
ledged his conviction that he had been deranged, and in a state
requiring control and seclusion from society.

Case 5.—It may be doubted whether this case may be set down
as one of moral insanity or of intellectual derangement. The individual had, probably, by nature a very weak understanding ; yet I
think it probable that the impressions which had fixed themselves
on his mind were modified by disease.

I. K. had been for many years confined in a lunatic asylum,
when, an estate having devolved upon him by inheritance, it became
necessary to subject him anew to an investigation. He was examined by several physicians, who were unanimous in the opinion
that he was a lunatic ; but a jury considered him to be of sound
understanding, attributing his peculiarities to eccentricity, and be
was consequently set at liberty.

The conduct of this individual was the most eccentric that can
be imagined : he scarcely performed any action in the same manner
as other men ; and some of his habits, in which he obstinately per-
sisted, were singularly filthy and disgusting. For every peculiar
custom he had a quaint and often ludicrous reason to allege, which
indicated a strange mixture of shrewdness and absurdity. Among
other singular customs, he made it a regular practice to open his

window at a certain hour every night, and cry out *murder* exactly twelve times, and to go every day after dinner into the middle of the quadrangle near his room, and throw up his hat into the air a precise number of times, vociferating at each throw. It was discovered that his motive for acting thus was a notion that by consistency and uniformity of conduct he afforded a proof of his sanity. When a person whom he understood to be a physician attempted to approach him, he recoiled with horror, and exclaimed, "If you were to feel my pulse, you would be lord paramount over me the rest of my life !"

This individual was set at liberty, and has lived for many years on his estate, where his conduct, though eccentric, and not that of a sane man, has been without injury to himself or others.

Case 6.—L. M., a working tradesman, of industrious and sober habits, conducted himself with propriety until about forty-six years of age, and had accumulated a considerable property from the fruits of his exertions. About that period he lost his wife, and after her death become more and more penurious. At length he denied himself the comforts, and in a great measure even the necessaries of life, and became half-starved and diseased ; his body was emaciated and beset with a scaly eruption. Mr. S————, a gentleman who had long known him, hearing of the condition into which he had sunk, sent a medical practitioner to visit him, by whose advice L. M. was removed from a miserable dirty lodging to a lunatic asylum. Mr. S————, who was present on the occasion, observed that L. M., previously to his quitting the room in which he had immured himself, kept his eyes fixed on an old trunk in the corner of the apartment. This was afterwards emptied of its contents, and in it were found, in the midst of various articles, dirty bank notes, which had been thrown into it apparently at different times, to the value of more than a thousand pounds. L. M., after his removal to an asylum, where he had wholesome food and exercise, soon began to recover from his bodily infirmities, and at length became anxious to be at large. At this time I was requested to visit him. I conversed with him for some time, in order to ascertain his mental condition. He betrayed no sign of intellectual delusion, nor did it appear that any thing of that description had ever been a part of his complaint. His replies to questions were rational according to the extent of his natural capacity. He was determined to go and manage his property, and get a wife who should take care of him. In a few days after his release he was married to a servant belonging to the lunatic asylum where he had been confined. His new wife found after some months that it was impossible to endure the strange conduct of her husband, and after trying various expedients, brought him back to the asylum, with a certificate from a medical man, who had examined him and declared him to be insane. He still remains in confinement, and his derangement is now more complete than formerly, as it plainly involves his intellect, which is under the influence of various illusions.

L. M.'s disorder consisted, at the period of his first confinement, in a perversion of moral habits, in which was a penury so extreme as to prevent ordinary care for self-preservation. His disorder had greatly increased at the period of his second confinement.

Case 7.—N. O., aged about fifty-five, was subject some years ago to epileptic fits, which were not frequent, nor were they supposed to affect his intellect. They were attributed to his manner of living. He used but little exercise, was in the habit of dining often in company, and drank daily too much port wine. His countenance was florid, and his body was evidently plethoric. Some years ago events occurred which overwhelmed him with grief and despondency : the occupations in which his mind had been engaged were entirely broken off, and nothing remained on which he could attach hope or interest. Without sustaining the least injury in the powers of his understanding, still fully capable of reasoning in the most correct manner on the circumstances of his state, as acute and intelligent as ever he had been, he underwent a total change in his manners and habits. He took to his bed, and would never rise from it unless compelled ; and he would scarcely ever dress himself. I saw him on two or three occasions after the interval of some years from the time when his change of habits had taken place, and once when it was requisite for him to transact some business. To this he was perfectly competent. He could not be prevailed upon to put on his clothes ; he was dirty, and negligent of his person ; irascible to such a degree that he would sometimes strike the persons who had the care of him, and who often took him out for the benefit of air and exercise, on which occasions it was found necessary to put on him a straight waistcoat. I found, on inquiry, that the state of his mind was that of constant despondency, and that he was without any power of rousing himself to the most trifling exertion. In the same state he continued, and though not in a lunatic asylum, he was considered by his relatives to require the constant superintendence of a physician, who devotes his time chiefly to the cure of the insane, and whose assiduous management supplied, in some degree, the total want of self-control. I advised confinement in a lunatic asylum, but this was perseveringly declined ; and the event was calamitous.

The preceding cases, with one exception, were published in the article ' *Insanity*' contributed by me to the "Cyclopædia of Practical Medicine." Since that paper was printed, I have had opportunities of making inquiries at different lunatic asylums and among medical correspondents interested in the subject of mental disorders ; and from many whose abilities and opportunities of observation led me to place a particular value on their judgment, I have solicited an opinion as to the existence of moral insanity as a distinct form of mental derangement. In these inquiries I have scarcely, if ever, failed to obtain some strong evidence in confirmation of my previous opinion. Dr. Wake of York assured me that many instances have occurred in the York Asylum precisely coinciding with the description I have given of this disorder, and that he considers no point relating to the history of mental derangement better established than its existence. Dr. Bompas has shown me several examples precisely of similar character, and has communicated other information to the same effect, either from the records of cases kept by his predecessor Dr. Cox or from his own notes. The house-steward of Bethlem pointed out some examples of a similar description, and assured me that there are always instances of insanity in that hospital in which the conduct, temper, and habits of the patient are alone disordered, while the reasoning faculty remains unaffected. I am under great obligations to Mr. Hitch, the resident medical officer of the Gloucester Lunatic Asylum, for communications with which he has favoured me on this and other subjects, and particularly for a series of most interesting examples, which I shall presently insert, and which, with the notes of another case kindly given me by Dr. Symonds, will, as I trust, leave nothing deficient in the history of moral insanity. I shall first insert Dr. Symond's case, which is characteristic of some peculiar features of moral madness, and shall conclude with the communication from Mr. Hitch, which will be given entire as I derived it from him, or with a very trifling abridgement.

Case 8.—" Some time ago I was requested to visit a gentleman, in order that I might give my opinion on the propriety of placing him under control, as one incapable of conducting his affairs. I was previously put in possession of the following facts. Several years ago he laboured under an attack of acute mania, from which, although it subsided sufficiently to allow his being set at liberty, it was the opinion of those who had closely observed him, that he had never completely recovered. In his social relations he had become fickle, suspicious, and irascible; he was reckless in his expenditure, and uncertain in his projects, while his general behaviour was such as to impress almost every one who came in contact with him, that he was what is commonly designated 'flighty' or 'cracked;' yet there was no evidence that he entertained any belief in things morally or physically impossible, or in opposition to the general opinion of mankind. It was true that among other absurd acts he had published a volume containing a history of family grievances, described in hyperbolical language; and although the statements were false, it was difficult to say whether they emanated from a diseased imagination, or were wilfully feigned for a malicious purpose. A few months before I visited him, he had suffered a severe concussion of the brain, and since his recovery had conducted himself more extravagantly than ever. He advertised for sale property which he knew to be entailed; after a little increase of income by the death of a near relative, he commenced great alterations in his residence, and before they were finished suddenly left his family, together with a large establishment, under the care of a youth, his son, who was provided with no other means of supplying the wants of the household than a power of attorney for collecting rents.

5*

Soon after his departure, for which he had assigned no reason, he despatched orders for the removal of every kind of property that admitted of conveyance, such as furniture, cattle, &c., from his estate to a distant place where he was then sojourning. If his directions were not immediately attended to by his son, he was in the habit of writing letters to him of the most violent and abusive description. Some of these productions were shown to me, and I found not only the expressions most ridiculously disproportionate to the subjects, but the whole style so confused and incoherent, and the external superscription so absurd, that it seemed impossible to believe that any person of sound mind could have indited them. Many other strange practices were mentioned, but there was one fact that made a very strong impression on my mind. Having heard that certain individuals, strangers to himself, but deeply interested in the welfare of his family, had made inquiries respecting his movements, he printed a pamphlet, professedly for their instruction in his domestic history. A more insane document than this I scarcely ever perused. The sentences were so involved and undistinguished, that, although the ideas were not absolutely incongruous with each other, it was impossible to collect more than the general tenor of a long passage. The greater part consisted of allusions to events, persons, and places, without any names or other clue being afforded, and of appeals to the reader, as if the latter were in possession of facts that seemed known only to the writer.

" I was able to learn very little of his personal condition, excepting that he was extremely irregular, and dirty in his habits, and this very important circumstance, that he was in the constant habit of passing his evacuations in bed.

" He had latterly committed so great injury to property in which he had only a life-interest, had involved himself so deeply in debt, and was, notwithstanding, so lavish and absurd in his expenditure, that it became a very desirable object to enforce some restraint upon his actions. Having with some difficulty obtained an interview with him under the pretext of conversing with him concerning certain members of his family, towards whom he had conceived a most unfounded hostility, I endeavoured, by a variety of expedients, to discover any latent hallucination, but failed in my attempts. He manifested a morbid emotion of enmity for certain persons, and addressed one of them who was present in coarse and indecent language ; but on my questioning him as to the cause of his aversion, he was ready enough to vindicate his feelings by means of stories and allegations that I knew to be groundless, but which did not necessarily involve any insane conviction on his part, and might, therefore, have been fabricated with an intention to deceive. Although, while conversing on these subjects, he manifested intense earnestness, and accompanied his discourse with theatrical gesticulations, he very easily, on my leading the way, passed off to a discussion of matters quite foreign and indifferent, and returned with equal facility to his domestic wrongs. Interrogations as to the motives of his conduct on various occasions produced answers by no means unplausible. The most extravagant notion that he betrayed was in an avowal of his resolution to change his name, for no other reason than that he might not be disgraced by bearing the same name as his wife.

"After due deliberation I came to the conclusion, that, although I had been unable to trace any positive intellectual error, there was such a morbid condition of the feelings, habits, and motives, as to constitute a case of what has been correctly designated by Dr. Prichard as moral insanity. I therefore did not hesitate to sign the usual certificate."

I shall conclude this section with the before-mentioned communication from Mr. Hitch.

"I could easily furnish a great number of instances coinciding with your description of *moral insanity*. We have recognised them here for a very considerable time, and term individuals so affected, '*insane in conduct and not in ideas*,' a distinction which has often led us into a difficulty of explanation and a still greater difficulty of producing conviction, when justifying our detention of a patient who has made a plausible and very reasonable tale to the visiting magistrates. Your discrimination of this disease from intellectual insanity, and the further separation of the latter from actual madness or mania, has much gratified me : it accords with my own observations, and tends to support a belief, which I have long indulged, that many who have been convicted of crimes ought to have been pronounced insane. I do not imagine that you desire to have a long series of cases, resembling each other in general character, and differing only in some particular features, but presume that you are rather desirous of ascertaining how far others, whose opportunities of observation entitle them to hold an opinion on the subject, have been led to form conclusions similar to your own. I shall send you an extract from my note-book, containing the outlines of a few cases which have excited a strong feeling of interest in my own mind.

"*Case* 1.—Mr. W., aged about forty, was a corn-dealer and baker, and a man of mild and retiring disposition ; steady in business, regular and domestic in his habits, highly conscientious, religious without ostentation, correct and cautious in his conversation, and kind and benevolent to all persons. His health was considered to be delicate, but he was never ill ; and he avoided great exertion, feeling himself not equal to it. He was a married man and had several children, of whom he was extremely fond. He experienced some severe losses in his business which weighed heavily upon his mind, and he became exceedingly depressed. He made a great effort to rouse himself from his despondency, and exerted himself with the view of recovering for his family what he had unavoidably lost. He was, to a great extent, very soon rewarded for his efforts. It was shortly afterwards observed by his friends that his increased exertions had improved his spirits, which, it was remarked, had become much more elevated than they were previously to his depression. He now began to extend his business, in which he was become more keen ; at market he displayed more acuteness in buying and selling, and seldom trusted to others any thing he could accomplish himself ; and he was ever watchful of an opportunity to make purchases or to effect sales to his advantage. These changes in his habits went on until the character of industry appeared to his friends to be over-performed, and they feared that he indulged something like unnecessary exertion and anxiety, and that his excessive activity of mind and body would destroy his health. His journeys became longer and more frequent, and his nights were greatly shortened ; and he was often absent from his accustomed place of worship on Sundays. After some months had passed, and while these changes were going on, his family ventured to remark to him that such extended journeys to transact uncertain business withdrew his attention from that at home, which was regular and profitable. For the first time he was then observed to speak in a tone of voice, and with an expression of feeling, which had never belonged to him. Still his family and friends had no fear of madness, but entertained a dread lest he should overstep the line of security in business, or undermine his bodily health by excessive exertion. His temper, which was naturally so mild, from this time grew hasty and irascible ; he became incapable of hearing an opinion opposed to his own, and was irritated if a check was offered to his present proceedings. Still he prosecuted the same scheme of business without as yet deviating from his course ; he extended but did not alter his plans ; and thus were more than ten months disposed of. A change now became manifest in his feelings towards his family ; he frequently spent his evenings in the society of others rather than in that of his wife and children, to which practice he had ever been habituated. He spoke in approbation of all he saw elsewhere, and found innumerable faults and objections to what was done at home : his children were less engaging and intellectual than those of his neighbours ; and his wife's domestic arrangements were less complete, and he was evidently less attached to her. He was at this time in the habit of taking freely of stimulating drinks, to which he had never been accustomed, and excused himself under the plea that his great exertions required support. He became addicted to strange women ; and the fact being brought home to him by his wife, brought on the crisis which had been long approaching. Having given vent to the most passionate expressions, and threatened violence of the most serious character, he quitted his home, forsook his family and his business, wandered about the country, sleeping in the open air, and subsisting by the meanest artifices. His friends at length found him, and consigned him to my care. Twelve months had fully elapsed from the time when they perceived a change in his natural habits.

" When I received him, the expression of his countenance was animated and lively ; great activity was indicated by the quickness of his eye ; but the unsteadiness of his looks, together with a quivering smile playing about his lips, marked it as an activity without object or motive. His face was pallid, the conjunctiva finely injected, the pupil contracted, the head was hotter than the rest of the body, and the hair, which was thin, felt crisp ; the tongue was foul and the bowels constipated ; the hands and feet were colder than the rest of the body ; and the former had that soft feel peculiar to the highly nervous: the pulse was slower than natural, feeling full and bounding, but it could be compressed, and the current of blood checked by the slightest pressure ; the respiration was tranquil and regular, slow, and scarcely perceptible by looking at the chest. In conduct and manner he was anxious, eager to be doing something; moving from place to place without any apparent object; removing every article of furniture that was moveable ; abounding in speculations and new projects ; proposing long journeys to be executed in haste ; talking incessantly, but coherently, and for the most part rationally, upon a great variety of subjects ; he used no expressions of antipathy against his family, nor indeed against any person ; but it was evident that the mention of his wife or children greatly increased his agitation. He had no fixed notion which influenced his conduct, and *no delusive ideas.* When addressed on the subject of his situation, he was fully aware of the place he was in, and knew the reason of his confinement; he attached no blame to any one for placing him under my care, and admitted that he had felt unlike himself for some months, but had flattered himself that his health was improved, and that his increased spirits were the legitimate consequences of this and of his improved finances : he was conscious of his conduct to his family, but neither blamed himself nor extenuated it. On business he would converse most rationally: but if the opportunity had presented itself, would have expended his money in the most useless purchases. He was capable of making the nicest calculations connected with his own affairs, and was correct in all his data when speaking to a second person ; but when left to himself, his conduct and language were ridiculous in the extreme.

" This individual perfectly recovered in about three months.

" I copy this case as one in which the deviation from healthful and natural habits were complete, and brought about in the most gradual manner. It is worthy of remark, from the momentary conviction which the individual obtained of his state when he ceased to direct his own movements and to be his own master. He often told us, on his recovery, that the idea that he had been mad for some time, and was then so, flashed across his mind at the moment when he entered the establishment.

" Simple as this case is, and it is one of the most simple we meet with, we yet find associated all the forms of moral debasement. Simple over-excitement was the commencement of the disorder ; but a change in the habits of life and temper, a perversion of the natural feelings and affections, a loss of the sense of moral rectitude, and a complete deprivation of self-control, gradually followed.

" Of this description of cases I have met with very many instances, not in those who have fortunately been treated as insane, but who, remaining at large, have gone on from one misfortune to another, till they have become beggared in estate and reputation, and sunk at length into a loathsome jail or a wretched workhouse.

" *Case 2.*—The following case is not a common one. In the spring of 1827 I was requested to visit the daughter of a farmer, in some branches of whose family insanity existed. The little girl was only *seven* years old. She was reported by her parents to have been a quick, lively child, of ready apprehension, mild disposition, affectionately fond of the members of her family, and capable of quite as much application to her school duties as children usually are. She had been sent home from school in consequence of a great change which had taken place in her conduct. She had become rude, abrupt, vulgar, and perfectly unmanageable ; neglecting her school duties, running wildly about the fields and gardens, and making use of the most abusive language, when chidden for her misdemeanours. I found her in this state, with the addition of having become extremely passionate, in consequence of corrections to which she had been subject, and to escape which she was prone to invent falsehoods. She was also changed in her appetite, preferring raw vegetables to her ordinary food ; and she would sleep on the cold and wet ground rather than in her ordinary bed. Her parents had no control over her; indeed she appeared to despise them in proportion as they kindly remonstrated with her. She was cruel to her younger sisters ; taking every opportunity to pinch or otherwise hurt them, when she thought she could escape observation. She could not apply herself to any thing, but had yet a perfect knowledge of persons and things, and a complete recollection of all that had occurred and of all she had learned previously to her illness. Her general health was much disordered ; her little eyes glissened most brilliantly ; the pupil was contracted, though expanding widely if she was suddenly excited ; the conjunctiva was reddened ; the head was hot ; the surface of the body of about the natural standard ; the extremities of a lower temperature, and the palm of the hand had as completely the peculiar feel of the nervous as a grown person ; her person had a disagreeable odour ; the bowels were much disordered, from the various strange things she had eaten.   Dr. B—— saw her in conjunction with me ; and we endeavoured to improve her general health, hoping that by so doing we should remove some exciting cause for her disturbed feelings: we were disappointed. As she grew worse, and her parents by mismanagement, sometimes humouring her, sometimes harshly correcting her, were likely to render her still more disordered, I took her into my own house, and placed her under the care of my wife. At this time she had taken to eat her own fæces and to drink her urine, and she would swear like a fish-woman, and destroy any thing within her reach ; yet she was fully conscious of every thing she did, and generally appeared to know well that she had done wrong. Having committed some mischief or destroyed something which was fragile, she would often run to my wife, and exclaim, " Well ! Mrs. H——, I have done it ! I have done it ! I know you will be angry, but I can't help it ; I felt I must break it, and I could not let it alone until I had !" Amongst her pleasures was that of dirtying herself as frequently as she had clean clothes ; indeed she would rarely pass her excretions at the proper place, but reserved them for the carpet of the sitting-room, or for her own clothes. When she had accomplished this end, she would jump about and exult ; but the little creature would often induce my wife to smile at her, when, with an expression of countenance, which was always intelligent, made up of cunning, feigned regret, and a subdued smile, she would say, " Well, Mrs. H——, 'tis too bad of me ; 'tis really very foolish, and I will try to be better ; but you must forgive me because I am mad." At other times she would be so far conscious of her situation as to cry bitterly, and express her fears that she should become like her aunt, who was a maniac. In addition to all these indications she lied, stole any thing which she thought would be cared for, and either hid or destroyed it ; and swore in language which it is difficult to imagine that the child could ever have heard.

"I could never detect in her any fixed idea, either of fear or belief, which influenced her conduct. She acted from the impulse of her feelings, and these were unnatural and unhealthy.

" She recovered in about two months.

" *Case* 3.—The following case has some interesting points, and I therefore transcribe it. A gentleman of good connexions, of good education, and of mental capabilities far above the general average, was brought up under the most advantageous circumstances that wealth can command, to the surgical branch of our profession. He was fond of literary pursuits, and had rendered himself an ornamental member of society by a careful and critical course of general reading. In his disposition he was mild, kind-hearted, obliging, and generous, and his attachments and affections were strong and ardent. Educated as a gentleman, he possessed what is essential to the character—the highest moral and religious principles without enthusiasm or fanaticism, and the strictest regard for that correct conduct which is due to those of his own rank in society. An unfortunate excess to which he was seduced when his duties in London were fulfilled, laid the foundation for a complete subversion of his character. He became irregular in his habits, negligent of his person, careless of the society he fell into, addicted to drinking, suspicious of his friends, wantonly extravagant, perverse in disposition, irritable and overbearing. Indulging himself in idleness for several years, and in dissipation when he had the means, he reduced himself to the condition in which he became known to me. My first acquaintance with him was under the effects of a long debauch, and the history of that will contain the recent history of the man. Being still fond of reading, he prosecutes his studies quietly but ardently for some weeks together, during which time indications of excitement show themselves. He becomes more inclined to talk and less disposed to read. In his conversation he assumes a loud and dictatorial tone, is impatient of interruption, intolerant of contradiction, and bears with ill grace the most modest expression of an opinion differing from his own. He becomes abrupt in his manners, speaks coarsely of mankind generally, and ill of all his friends and relations. Of those most nearly connected with him he speaks disrespectfully, and holds them up to ridicule upon all occasions, introducing their names when totally uncalled for, merely to gratify his perverted feeling. A greater degree of impatience is occasionally felt with some bodily sensation, which leads him to the use of ardent spirits for its relief or removal. Excepting at such times, this gentleman's habits are most abstemious ; he never drinks any thing stronger than beer, and frequently tastes water only for weeks together. When, however, this thirst for ardent spirits comes on, a fondness for low society accompanies it. On these occasions he repairs to a *pot-house*, takes his mixture amidst the lowest of mankind, treats all the brick-layers and hod-carriers who will drink with him, tells them tales, and recites to them for days and nights together, if they will listen to him, and ceases only when the reluctant integrity of mine host will draw no more for him, or, which is more commonly the case, when his cash is exhausted and his credit of no avail. During these lamentable debauches he seldom gets drunk, although drinking and smoking incessantly ; he falls into a state of abstraction for a time, and dozes and sleeps until the uneasy sensations within the stomach rouse him, and impel him to call for more drink. His condition, when no more drink is allowed him, is distressing ; he intreats and orders, implores and commands, grows violently enraged, experiences a hysterical or epileptic convulsion, sinks into a chair or on the ground, and falls into a sound sleep. This continues from twenty to thirty hours, when he awakes to the horrors of his situation, and to the mortification arising from his folly. No longer is to be found the high tone, the overbearing demeanour, or the authoritative language ; he is the humblest of the meek, and continues depressed for several weeks. Then he enjoys a period of tranquillity, to be succeeded by the overbearing conduct before-mentioned, and to be finished within the period of three months by another visit to the society of tinkers and labourers. In his state of depression I first saw him, free from any kind of delusion, and regarding the world as having in it no spot that was not too good for so mean a being as himself. He was desirous of redeeming his past follies by a life of usefulness and activity ; was regardless of the kind of occupation to which he might be subject, provided only he was made useful and industrious. To sweep the shop and open the shutters of a huckster or tallow-chandler, would have been regarded by him as a valuable appointment by way of a beginning. When, however, employment of the simplest kind was *proposed* to him, he found himself wanting in resolution to engage in it. He could busy himself about nothing, change from one trifling engagement to another, but would not steadily employ himself. In about three weeks the depression had left him, and for some time he was enabled to enjoy the rational amusement of reading, in which he greatly delighted, particularly works of history and philology, memoirs, &c. For about six weeks he spent his time usefully and rationally in this occupation, when he began to think himself entitled to his liberty ; he requested permission to take some exercise, which was permitted him without superintendence ; he grew louder and higher in his tone of conversation, began to hold himself above his fellow-patients, and ceased not to quarrel and disagree with them ; his manners, formerly agreeable, were now much changed, but not so far as to allow us to remark such alteration to him without encountering the chance of failing to produce conviction. At the expiration of three months from the time I received him, he was discharged, ‘ having no disordered ideas, and having conducted himself upon the whole like a sane man.’ In five days I was requested to take charge of him again, and I found him in a village pot-house, in the midst of company low, vulgar, and disgusting; without money, almost without clothes, which he had sold to purchase liquor, to share with his contemptible companions. I removed him to confinement, where three other months were spent, much as those already described, and within ten days from his second release he repeated the same indiscretions, and was replaced in an asylum.

" *Case* 4.—A form of moral insanity striking to the mere observer, but a most disagreeable one to those whose duty it is to take charge of such cases, is described in the following notes. It is the case of ———— ————, an account of whom is given in the ‘ *Sketches of Bedlam.*’ p. 135. Having been an inmate of numerous asylums both public and private, the directors of which I believe were glad to get rid of him, and some of whom, to my knowledge, rejected him, he became a patient of ours. Notwithstanding all that has been said of his delusions on the subject of property by the author of ‘ Sketches of Bedlam,’ I could never discover a permanently delusive notion in him during nearly two years spent with me. He enjoyed, for I may in truth use the term, the art of lying and the pleasure of boasting to an extreme degree. To a stranger he invariably represented himself as a man of great wealth—vast importance, in his neighbourhood—a magistrate, and all that was grand. His tale was never brief ; he had the art of making it so plausible that few were in haste to leave him, and none ever left him without feeling a regret that a man apparently so sane should be shut up from society. He usually laughed at the effect of his tale when the visitor was gone, and especially if he succeeded; which he always attempted, in obtaining money or snuff. He would then ridicule the *flats*, as he termed them, and chuckle over his success, considering the tax thus levied as a legitimate toll, taken, no matter how, from those whose ill-directed curiosity prompted them to look at the afflicted as they would at an exhibition of wild animals. His proneness to lying was not confined to the gratification of his own wants and wishes by false representations ; his most general application of this well educated propensity was in the production of mischief and disturbance. He had always a false report to me of the servants who superintended him—his food was withheld from him—his beer was drunk by the keeper or a fellow-patient—his clothes were worn by others, and he was robbed of his snuff and tobacco. Amongst his fellow-patients he ever delighted in creating a disturbance, and when this occurred, he invariably reported the offended party to be the aggressor. He would prepare himself, on every day when the visiting magistrates were expected to examine the house, with a budget of lies and misrepresentations, and with the most unfounded and malevolent calumnies against the officers and servants of the establishment. If he succeeded in exciting attention to his complaints, and to create a suspicion that there existed some ground for the serious charges he preferred, his next pleasure was to abuse the gentleman who had lent an ear to his calumnies, and to boast how easily he could deceive the wisest magistrate or the most careful examiner. He was equally an adept in stealing as in lying. Once in a week at least it was necessary to unpick the lining of his coat, waistcoat, and breeches ; to open the ticking of his bed ; to remove the head of his bedstead, and to examine holes in the wall of the airing-ground, which he was known to have made and to have partly filled with dirt or leaves. Here were found the knife-cloths, spoons, forks, and all small articles belonging to the gallery ; the night-caps, handkerchiefs, combs, and brushes of his fellow-patients ; half-picked bones which he had abstracted from the plates of his fellow-patients unobserved ; portions of bread and cheese taken in a similar manner, and articles of mere rubbish taken for the mere pleasure of stealing ; these were secreted, as observed, in holes or in his bed, or *sewn up in the linings of his dress*, and not unfrequently a pocket was made in the tail or back of his shirt. He was not often passionate ; sometimes he was violently so, but on ordinary occasions he had the power of controlling his anger. He was, in reality, one of the happiest fellows alive, but he was ever complaining and expressing dissatisfaction and discontent. He had no bodily ailment, but he would be always sick, if thereby he could improve or vary his diet. He was very fond of novelty, and would devise various plans in order to be moved to different parts of the establishment. Sometimes he would become noisy for this, purpose, at others dirty. He was extremely malevolent if offended, but the feeling did not last long, for as soon as the bodily inconvenience attending his offence had subsided, his disposition to injure ceased also. Though he was one of the most depraved men that I ever saw, he yet possessed many good qualities. He was extremely watchful and anxious for the sick ; was always ready to assist the servants when a patient was turbulent and likely to do mischief ; ever defended the keepers, if other patients charged them with unkindness ; would make himself extremely useful when any thing was to be done in his gallery ; corrected obscene or impious language in others, and seemed to tolerate no mischief or wickedness which was not entirely his own.

" In general his judgment was quick and correct ; he had quick perception, strong memory, great discretion in matters of business, was a good calculator, and would tell me what his quarterly expenditure had been, and from what sources the amount should be paid, with all the accuracy of a banker. Though he was occupied with calculations for the sake of boasting, and swelled a small property into an enormous wealth, he knew and spoke frequently of his exact income, and was always careful that his expenses should not exceed it.

" His madness appeared to me to consist in part in *a morbid love of being noticed*, perhaps admired and approved, though he had too much acuteness and too long an experience in the reverse of approbation to expect that any one could admire the extent to which he prosecuted his ingenious art of tormenting.

" He is now at large, and has been in the management of his affairs for *three* years, in which time he has sold an estate advantageously, and conducted his business with profit. He is still addicted to lying, but I believe is too wary to commit theft, excepting amongst his immediate friends.

" *Case* 5.—The following case displays a change of habits and feelings and a sacrifice of natural affections consequent upon causes which had previously generated ' a bad temper.' Mrs. ——, aged thirty, the wife of a man engaged as a cloth-worker, is employed, when equal to her work, in a department of the same business. She appears to be in good general health, and is reported to have always enjoyed it. She is the mother of eight children, is in comfortable circumstances, was always industrious and careful, took much pleasure in her domestic duties, and was fond of her husband and children. Her friends report her to have had naturally *a bad temper*, over which she never exerted any control ; and they add that its too frequent indulgence, to the great annoyance of her husband's peace, has on some occasions suggested remedies not the most mild. She appears to have given way to the most violent paroxysms of passion, followed by a morose and unyielding sullenness. About twelve months ago a change was observed in her habits ; she took less interest in her domestic concerns, neglected her children, abused her husband, and evinced the greatest hatred of him. Shortly after this change appeared, she quitted her husband's house and went to lodge with a neighbour ; here her habits were so disagreeble, and her disposition so dissatisfied, that she soon received a dismissal. She then resided with her sister, who parted with her on like terms, and many others received her and removed her from them for similar reasons. She at length obtained admission to the parish workhouse, where she found herself treated as people usually are in that hospital of idleness, and she made return for such attention and accommodation as she had received by breaking the windows and the crockery of the poor inmates. She escaped the punishment threatened her for this by seeking refuge in her husband's house, when she returned the kindness he had shown in receiving and protecting her by destroying all of his that was frangible. She had previously discovered a small sum of money, his occasional savings, which she spared him the trouble of expending, by giving away a part and throwing away the remainder. Her husband then consigned her to the Lunatic Asylum, and I have her under my care.

"Her leading desire is to lie in bed, where, if I would allow her to remain, she would stay the whole week. She frequently refuses her food. When up, if no notice is taken of her, and no inquiries made of her as to her health and feelings, she will conduct herself with propriety for some days. Sometimes, however, she will roll on the ground and indulge in the most violent screams and exclamations without apparent cause or object, and then return to whatever occupation she had been previously engaged in. If requested to do any kind of work, she declares her incapability, from weakness, pain, or some other cause, and in a few minutes sets about some other employment requiring greater exertion. When addressed by me in my *usual* visits to the wards, she throws herself into a violent rage, and without replying to my inquiries, falls suddenly to the ground as though she had fainted, or she rolls herself as before mentioned and screams, or she seats herself and cries and sighs as if in the greatest distress ; but if I enter into conversation with another patient on any subject with which she is familiar, as the localities of her neighbourhood, the clothing business, or such matters, and take an opportunity to address a question for reply, she joins in the conversation with the full command of her intellect. As a disagreeable and unmanageable patient, without actual violence, she exceeds most with whom I have met. Her mind appears totally unaffected as to its understanding portion, but in the moral part completely perverted.

"*Case 6.*—A man was discharged from this establishment about two years ago, reported cured, whose eccentricities and extravagant conduct had drawn upon him the anger and almost the dread of an extensive neighbourhood. He was about thirty-five years of age, a shoemaker by trade and married ; addicted to an irregular life, and fond of drinking. His natural disposition was lively ; he abounded in a peculiar kind of wit, and had an endless series of marvellous tales at his command, which, when excited, he told with great humour, and he rendered himself thereby a welcome guest at the village alehouse. Here he was also prone to those petty mischievous tricks which are vulgarly denominated ' fun,' and he was an amusing companion in his sphere. However, his love of sport did not rest in the gambols of the beer-house : he became restless and disinclined to his own business, made frequent excursions to different towns and villages under the pretence of seeking fresh work, was noisy and coarse in his play at the tavern, and eventually left the neighbourhood of his residence. He took with him the kit of a travelling tinker, and set up the business of a knife and scissors-grinder, of which he knew nothing. He exulted in the havoc he made in the cutting-instruments which were entrusted to him, but did not continue his new trade more than a day or two, when he disposed of his kit and began to sell old clothes. This pursuit he exchanged for another, and that for something new. In about a fortnight he returned home, and instead of entering his house by the door, he ascended the roof, removed the tiles, and entered through the ceiling. This he continued to do, making his entrance and exit from the top of the house. He would amuse himself at night by driving a pig fastened to a cord through the village, upon whose nose and tail something had been fastened to cause him to squeak, and thus disturb the neighbours. He would exchange the farmers' cattle and remove their gates during the night, and before morning was some miles out of the way. He would often run ten or twelve miles in a straight line without any motive, disregarding fences, corn-fields, brooks, or any thing. Whatever his fancy led him to want he made no scruple to take, regardless to whom it might belong, and when he had made the use of it which he thought proper, was not particular in returning it. For many of these acts be was taken before a magistrate; but his assumed simplicity or his sagacity, added to a plausible tale, saved him from punishment on all occasions but one, when he was sent to a house of correction for a month as a disorderly vagrant. He eventually was deemed to be mad, and sent to me. I found him one of the most mischievous of beings; his constant delight was in creating disorder to effect what he called ' fun ;' but he had no *motive*, no *impression* on his mind which induced him to this conduct, he was merely impelled by his immediate feelings. When he recovered his tranquillity, he had a perfect recollection of all that he had done, and wondered how he could have taken so much trouble to make himself appear ridiculous ! In this man's state of health I found nothing wrong, excepting that he did not sleep. His eye was not glistening, but his pulse was, as I so constantly observe it, *easily compressed.*

" *Case 7.*—A personal friend of mine was of sanguine temperament, possessed quick perceptions, warm feelings, strong attachments, the most delicate sense of what was due to others, and a high sentiment of honour. He was a member of the legal profession, in which he stood high; he worked hard, and had been amply rewarded for his talent and industry. He was hasty in disposition, and from defective management in early life had never been led to keep his warm feelings in check. He often grew hot in argument, and almost violent if offended, but he quickly became cooled, and was as friendly as ever. An affront was once offered him in public, which he instantly resented by violence ; this was followed by a repetition of annoyances and insults offered to him by parties who were under personal obligations to him, but who, as he felt, ought to have been beneath his resentment. His mind dwelt much upon the subject, and his life was embittered by it. Although his disposition was of that generous kind, that, excepting in the instant of danger, he would always have done a kind more readily than an unkind act, yet towards these parties he always felt malignantly : he watched opportunities to cross them in their purposes, helped them more deeply into their difficulties if he found them in a dilemma, and readily lent himself to oppose them in any and all ways. So completely were his good feelings perverted, that if in the midst of his pleasures, and he was a man who enjoyed the refined pleasures of polite society in the highest degree, the name of either of these parties was mentioned, or any circumstances caused him to think of them, a damp would be thrown upon his feelings, his face would flush, his brows lower, and those who knew him could but too well read the commotion that was within. For about two years he was the subject of this loss of self-control, and died of a paralytic seizure, upon which apoplexy supervened in a few hours, whilst preparing his mind to encounter a disagreeable duty in adjusting some family matters of a pecuniary kind which were in dispute.

"During the time when my friend was thus the subject of morbid irritability on one point, he was also a martyr to headache of a very severe kind, attacking him with the suddenness of an epileptic fit, and varying in intensity of pain to so great a degree as to produce convulsion, almost that of epilepsy. He, however, never lost his consciousness, even for a minute, during these paroxysms. On every other subject he could control his temper as much as usual, and had no disorder of ideas. He was well aware and admitted how contrary his malevolent feeling was to those religious principles to which he subscribed, and in his attachment to which he was sincere and fervent ; but his best efforts could never remove the demoniacal impulsion.

" *Case* 8.—A young lady, of no striking personal charms, but of good general appearance and of fashionable manners, had received the best possible education to fit her for ' *the world of fashion,*' and she had availed herself of the opportunities presented to her to render herself accomplished. Indeed, she was conspicuous for the share she had acquired of those merely external accomplishments which by many are deemed indispensable. In a word, she was a clever and a fashionable young woman. She had attained the age of twenty-three years, and had been ' introduced,' or, as I believe the term is, *she had come out*, and was distinguished in 'the beau monde.' She became greatly shocked on learning suddenly the embarrassed circumstances of her father, which must necessarily remove her in some degree from scenes of pleasure. She became dejected and melancholy ; soon afterwards sullen, obstinate, negligent of her person, idle, and disgusted with her accomplishments ; coarse and unpolished in her language, abusive, and passionate. She appeared to have no other delusive idea than that in which she was educated, viz. that 'the only world was the world of fashion;' and that as she was now out of that world 'she was dead,'—a delusion, which was not a change in her ideas. However, her friends associating these expressions with the lamentable change in her habits and feelings—for I should have added that she *hated* all her family but one sister—very properly placed her under treatment. In private lodgings she was unmanageable. Never subject to be opposed, she of course could not brook control; and the efforts ineffectually made to execute my directions only aggravated her case. As she was left solely to my management, I removed her to the Asylum. She was just as I have described her ; I soon became to her an object of dislike and derision: my necessarily firm conduct was to her the extreme of coarseness and cruelty ; and she represented me as fit only for the post I held, that of a jailor. Under these feelings I received her, and had the good fortune to restore her within three months to her friends, not *perfectly* recovered, but much relieved; for there had been originally an error in her education, which would have required that her mind should have been remodelled ere she could have been pronounced sane.

" To these cases I could add many others, varying in the manner in which the disease shows itself, and influenced by the habits, associations, education, &c. of the patients; but it does not appear to me that you will desire them; and I will, therefore, add one, and almost the only *clear* case I ever saw, of monomania.

" *Case* 9.—The son of a wealthy tradesman, residing in a country town, was one of several children, having the blessing of kind and discreet parents. He was educated carefully, and as a school-boy was particularly attentive to his duties; passed through his labours with credit ; was never considered wanting in capability ; but his diffidence, for I will use that word for the present, was so great, that he always dreaded the repetition of his lessons, fearing that he should be rejected, though this scarcely ever occurred. On leaving school his father gave him a choice of pursuits, and he selected his father's business. With the commencement of his duties his father assigned him a liberal allowance of pocket-money, and placed within his reach every convenience and comfort a young man of domestic habits could desire. For awhile everything proceeded satisfactorily; when suddenly he announced to his father that it was no longer of any use for him to be deceived,—he felt his mental capabilities unequal to the execution of what was assigned to him, and he should injure the trade. So far was this from being the case, that at the time alluded to, although young in the business, he was quite as competent to it as any one connected with it. The ground of incapacity was of course debated in the family, and all that the young man could advance was, that *he knew his talents were inferior to his brothers', and that he should never do his business correctly.* His father, a man of judgment, proposed to him a change of scenery and objects. He sent him to Manchester, where he entrusted him to make extensive purchases. These he effected very much to his father's satisfaction and advantage. The young man thought otherwise ; returned in low spirits ; bemoaned his want of talent, and returned to his former occupation. Here he still dwelt upon his want of ability ; and fearing he should injure his father's business, he preferred making a personal sacrifice; and with only a small sum of money and a few clothes he set off clandestinely for Liverpool, intending to embark for America. He did not find the Liverpool ship-owners so ready to make sacrifices as himself; and as his funds were inadequate to pay his passage-money, he was obliged to write to his brother for pecuniary assistance to effect his object. His brother very properly replaced him under his father's roof. He very soon repeated his attempt to escape with like effect ; and soon after his second return took poison with a view to destroy himself. Upon this he was placed under my care in the Asylum. I found him in every way a man calculated for business, excepting in the estimate he entertained of himself. He was quick in perception, active in body, persevering, fond of money, knew the value of articles, possessed very good general judgment, and was a very acute calculator ; but he distrusted his capabilities. His general health was much disordered, probably from the laudanum he had taken : this was restored. He was treated with great mildness and with an unbounded confidence, to which encouragement of every kind was added ; and having spent three months very usefully to me, he returned to his father's house and prosecuted his business most satisfactorily for upwards of a year, when his want of confidence returned, and he left home again. He now does so frequently, and after a short absence returns, takes no notice of what has occurred, and no remark is made by his family. They perceive, however, that his affections are changed ; he avoids his father, speaks harshly to him and angrily of him, and is suspicious of the rest of his family.

" An elder brother, without evincing any symptoms of madness, had destroyed himself ; and I fear the same event in this case.

" We have at the present moment a woman in the house, sent to us in consequence of her repeated attempts to destroy herself. She has been with us but a few days, and is at present suffering from having swallowed a quantity of diluted sulphuric acid prior to her admission.

" She is perfectly intelligent ; has not one disordered idea that I can detect, but the impulse of destroying herself. She states that she has been always subject to hysteria, which has at times occasioned her much suffering; that her desire to destroy herself is preceded by hysteric sensations—fulness of the bowels, flatulence and rising in the throat, and constriction of the fauces—but that these symptoms are followed by a rush of something, not of blood, into her head. Her head and face at these times feel hot, but the skin is not so reddened or flushed as her sensations would lead her to suppose. She says that a ringing or burring noise is heard in and about her head, and that these sensations last from a few minutes to a quarter of an hour; that during their continuance she feels prone to inflict injury upon those who are about her,—to do mischief to the surrounding furniture, &c.; but that on the sensation 'going down,'—that is her expression,—she becomes more and more wretched, and would then gladly destroy herself. Her health is much impaired.

" We had a similar case, a short time since, in a respectable farmer upwards of sixty years of age, whose mind was unaffected with disordered ideas, and who, by means of a nail, made a hole in the skin of his throat, into which he forced his finger, and actually tore a large rent. He had no motive likely to incite him to self-destruction."

Sect. IV.—*Of Mania, or Raving Madness.*

Characteristics of the disease.—In mania, or raving madness,[*] the derangement of the understanding is not limited, as it is in monomania, to one subject or to one train of thoughts, nor does it cease to be manifest, as in that disease, during intervals, when the attention is withdrawn from a particular subject. In the form of insanity now to be described, the mind is perpetually in a state of confusion and disturbance, which affects all the intellectual faculties, and interferes with their exercise even for the shortest period. Mania may be observed to differ from monomania in two respects : first, in the circumstance already noticed, that the derangement of the intellect is not partial, or involving but one series of ideas : secondly, that the mind being generally in a state of perturbation and excitement, the patient talks with vehemence, or raves on every subject which for the moment occupies his attention. This last characteristic is often the most striking, since maniacs, though their thoughts are not clear and collected on any subject, are often chiefly intent upon impressions of a peculiar description. Some rave incessantly about subjects connected with religion, and repeat texts of scripture with the greatest volubility. Some imprecate curses upon those who surround them and restrain their violent efforts. Others talk in the most obscene and indecent manner. Thoughts which associate themselves with some particular idea or feeling are often uppermost in the mind. This, however, is not invariably the case. In some instances the mind passes in rapid transition from one subject to another, and the current of ideas, always hurried and confused, is liable to be turned aside by any casual association or suggestion.

Description.—This form of madness generally makes its appearance and reaches its highest pitch more rapidly than others, and it

---

[*] The term *raving madness* may be used with propriety as an English synonym for mania. All maniacs display this symptom occasionally, if not constantly, and in greater or less degrees. The verb from which mania is derived means precisely what we express by the verb *to rave*.

is termed accordingly, when that is the case in a marked degree, *acute mania*. There are, however, in most instances premonitory symptoms, lasting for some days or even for some weeks, before the existence of mania becomes fully established. During this period the individual experiences occasional fits of excitement and confusion, by which his understanding is disturbed. He passes some days in a state of feverish agitation and general uneasiness : he is full of activity, and displays a morbid energy in the pursuits on which he is intent, in which, however, he performs nothing ; his projects are for the most part trifling and absurd. He neglects food, loses his appetite, passes sleepless nights, either lying awake and fatiguing his mind with anxious speculations, or rising often, walking to and fro in a state of uneasiness and perturbation. At length his reason is found to be disordered : he appears scarcely to know what he says, talks nonsense, repeats his words frequently, is unable to complete the sentences which he begins, and makes ineffectual efforts to recollect his thoughts, utters rapid and confused expressions in an impetuous manner ; cries, laughs, appears irritable and prone to anger, though, perhaps, naturally of mild and sedate temper ; is impatient of the most trifling opposition, and absurdly obstinate and capricious ; expresses his feelings with an unreasonable degree of warmth and enthusiasm. It is often remarked by their relatives and others, who have an opportunity of observing the conduct of individuals thus affected, that the state of their minds resembles that of persons intoxicated, and that their attempts to collect their thoughts and express themselves with correctness are like the efforts of men half drunk to continue conversation and prove themselves to be sober. The morbid state of a person under these circumstances is always apparent to those who surround him; but it is sometimes doubted whether he is completely mad and a proper subject for restraint, until some attempt being made to oppose him and interfere with his wild pursuits, he breaks out into a degree of violence which obviously requires coercion, and sometimes, though this is not a constant phenomenon in mania, shows that he has laboured under the influence of an unperceived delusion, an insane and absurd impression as to his own person, or his relation to others. Such an impression, if it exists, is not found to be a permanent delusion, like that of the monomaniac ; it is soon forgotten, or gives way to some other phantasm.

The disease generally increases in violence, and is several days, perhaps weeks, before it reaches its highest degree of intensity. During this period the phenomena of derangement vary according to the predominance of particular feelings. In some fear, in others anger, in all some violent emotion has the sway. Many individuals are seized occasionally with painful agitations, with fits of terror ; they are under apprehension of some undefined evils impending over them ; they pass sleepless nights, and cannot even lie in their beds ; and by day they are in a constant state of uneasiness and restless action. Others break out frequently into the most violent expres-

sions of rage and enmity against their relations, who are under the
necessity of exercising more or less of restraint and resistance to
their absurd proceedings, and have, perhaps, threatened to put them
into confinement, or have even carried the proposal into effect. They
utter imprecations against those persons who have deprived them
of their liberty, declare that they will obtain vengeance, and bring
them to condign punishment. The nearest relatives and the most
affectionate friends of the lunatic are now among the objects of his
most vehement displeasure. As the disorder approaches its highest
pitch, the current of ideas becomes more and more turbid ; the
thoughts and feelings are expressed with cries and ejaculations, with
agitation displayed in the manners and countenance, with violent
and irregular movements and jestures ; the internal sentiments or
feelings so absorb the attention that the patient becomes almost
unconscious of external impressions. Many individuals abandon in
their own persons all regard to cleanliness and decency, and become
filthy and disgusting in the extreme. All the functions of the body
are in these circumstances of the disease affected ; the bowels are
irregular, the tongue is furred, the skin cold and clammy. The
patient excreates saliva, mixed with mucus. His features become
haggard and maniacal ; his eyes watery and suffused. In some instances the countenance of the individual is so much altered in expression, that his nearest relatives would scarcely recognise him.

The state of highest excitement, which may be termed the acme
of acute mania, has been ably described by Pinel, though perhaps in
colours somewhat too vivid. He says, " the patient sometimes keeps
his head elevated and his looks fixed on high; he speaks in a low voice,
or utters cries and vociferations without any apparent motive ; he
walks to and fro, and sometimes arrests his steps as if excited by
the sentiment of admiration, or wrapt up in profound reverie. Some
insane persons display wild excesses of merriment, with immoderate
bursts of laughter. Sometimes, also, as if nature delighted in con-
trasts, gloom and taciturnity prevail, with involuntary showers of
tears, or the anguish of deep sorrow, with all the external signs of
acute mental suffering. In certain cases a sudden reddening of the
eyes and excessive loquacity give presage of a speedy explosion of
violent madness, and the urgent necessity of a strict seclusion. One
lunatic, after long intervals of calmness, spoke at first with volubility, he uttered frequent shouts of laughter, and then shed a torrent of tears ; experience had taught the necessity of shutting him
up immediately, for his paroxysms were at such times of the greatest
violence. It is often observed that extatic visions in the night are
the preludes to fits of maniacal devotion ; and by enchanting dreams,
or by the fancied apparition of a beloved object, it sometimes happens that erotic madness breaks out with violence, when it may
either assume the character of a calm reverie, or display nothing
but extreme confusion in the ideas, and the entire subversion of
reason."

When the disease has taken a firm hold on its unfortunate victim, it sometimes gives rise to all the internal effects, and displays all the external phenomena which the most intense feelings of human misery, resulting from the real calamities of life, may be imagined to produce. The maniac who becomes the subject of violent excitement " is seen in a state of extreme agitation, with his face flushed, his eyelids inflamed, and his eyes sparkling, his temples beating violently ; he talks, cries, sings, grieves, gets into fits of rage by night and by day, and is incapable of taking rest. The melancholic, also, in extreme agitation, but wrapt up in himself, goes to seek in some quiet and dark recess a refuge from his panic terrors, from his gloomy and despairing thoughts ; or the means of putting into execution his baneful designs. The insensible and stupid, incapable of any thing, remain unconscious of surrounding objects, and do not exert themselves to satisfy their most urgent wants. At this period of madness there is a constant want of sleep : the patient often experiences a feeling of tension and of heat in the head, without, however, complaining of it." Sensibility to external impressions, as well as to all bodily changes, is so much lessened, that blisters, cauteries, as well as exposure to intense cold, will sometimes produce but little expression of pain or distress.

A striking and graphical description of the phenomena of raving madness in cases which display the greatest intensity of the disease, has been drawn by Chiaruggi, and has been cited with high commendation by Professor Heinroth. The following is an abstract of it.

Among the phenomena of the first stage of this disease, we are at first struck by impetuous, audacious, shameless habits, a bold menacing aspect ; the natural evacuations are deficient ; the skin becomes of a slaty colour ; the forehead contracted ; the eye-brows drawn up ; the hair bristled ; the breathing hurried. The countenance begins to glow ; the eyes become fiery and sparkling ; the looks are wandering and scarcely ever fixed ; the eye-lids are by turns drawn widely open and closely shut ; the eye-balls are prominent, as if pushed forward out of the orbits. With this wild and menacing appearance is combined a patient endurance of hunger, and a remarkable insensibility of cold. If sleep visits the patient at all, it is short, unquiet, and easily disturbed. In the second stage, anger, violence, and the loss of reason manifest themselves in their greatest intensity ; shrieking, roaring, raging, abusive expressions and conduct towards the dearest friends and the nearest relations, who are now looked upon as the bitterest enemies. The patient tears his clothes to tatters, destroys, breaks in pieces whatever comes in his way. A striking and characteristic circumstance is the propensity to go quite naked. Whoever touches the patient is abused or struck by him. Strange confused ideas, absurd prejudices occupy the mind. Stillness soon follows, or a murmuring sound, as if the patient were alone : on the other hand, when he is alone, talking and gesticulating as if he were in company. If such individuals are confined and tied during the height of their paroxysms, for their own security or that of others, nothing can be compared to the truly satanical expression which their countenances display. In this state they throw hastily away with cries and shrieks all the food presented to them, except fluids, which thirst compels them to receive. When after some days hunger begins to be felt, they swallow every thing with brutal greediness ; they even devour, as it has often been observed, their own excrements, which, black and offensive, escape from them in great quantity, or smear with them clothes, beds, and walls. Notwithstanding his constant exertion of mind and body, the muscular strength of the patient seems daily to increase ; he is able to break the strongest bonds and even chains ; his limbs seem to acquire a remarkable nimbleness and pliability, and a singular aptitude of performing movements and actions which appear almost supernatural. Chiaruggi saw a woman who, clothed in a straight waistcoat and laced down in her bed like a child in a cradle, drew out her limbs from this double confinement with the greatest nimbleness and pliancy. Bold, however, and impudent as such patients are, yet they are, according to common observation, although not without exceptions, easily daunted by a strong threatening voice, by the sight of stocks, by close though harmless restraint. After their violence has expended itself, they become still, gloomy, appear to be reflecting or brooding over something ; but they break out again, before it can be anticipated, into a new storm of rage. At length comes on *the third stage.* A real cessation of violent paroxysms now ensues, exhaustion, sleep though unquiet, disturbed by fearful dreams. The pulse is small, the aspect of the whole body squalid, the countenance pallid and meagre. The patient is obdurately silent, or sings and laughs in a strange manner, or chatters with incessant volubility. These uncertain intervals, which often put on the appearance of fatuity, are frequently interrupted by new but short renewals of violence. Memory for the most part remains unimpaired through all the stages, and during the highest intensity of the disease the senses appear to acquire an unusual degree of acuteness and susceptibility. A patient who had recovered described to Chiaruggi all the scenes of his wild reverie and long-continued mental perturbation. It has often been observed that maniacal patients of this description are never attacked by any epidemic, and are seldom affected by any contagious malady.* According to Mead and many others, even consumptive disorders, dropsies, and other chronic maladies have disappeared on the accession of violent insanity. When patients are not freed from the disease after a succession of attacks, which come on like so many paroxysms of fever, one or the other of the following events ensues : either the powers of mind are exhausted to that degree that the disease subsides into a permanent fatuity ; or this appearance of fatuity is only a space of calmness interposed between relapses of violent madness, which now and then break out, like the eruptions

* This observation is not without exceptions.

of a volcano after a long period of repose ; or the patient falls into a state of melancholy or of complete mental confusion ; or, finally, his madness becomes chronical, and he scarcely recovers from this condition, in which sense and understanding appear to be lost in incoherence. Chiaruggi saw a woman who had sat during twenty-five years on a stone floor, in a fearfully demented state, beating the ground with her chains without ceasing by day or by night.*

It has often been observed that acute attacks of mania attain their utmost degree of intensity, and begin to decline or undergo a remission or a species of imperfect crisis, at a period of no long duration after the first appearance of severe symptoms. It is the opinion of M. Esquirol that such a change may generally, or at least frequently, be perceived to take place within the course of a month from the commencement of an acute attack. Certain it is that in the generality of cases the symptoms of extreme violence subside in a greater or less degree after a time, and that intervals at least of comparative quietness are perceived. From such a remission may be dated the commencement of the chronic or advanced stage of madness.

SECTION V.—*Of the Phenomena of Protracted Insanity, or of the advanced or Chronic Stage of that Disease.*

The ultimate tendency of insanity is to pass into a state of mental decay, or of obliteration of the intellectual faculties, which will be described hereafter under the designation of Incoherence or Dementia; but before the transition into this deplorable state has completely taken place, there is, in most cases of protracted mental derangement, a stage of uncertain duration, which may be termed the chronic period of madness. This is the state in which the majority among the inmates of lunatic asylums continue for years to exist. In some instances it lasts during life, the mental faculties never becoming entirely obliterated even after the lapse of twenty or thirty years. It is, however, itself a state of great intellectual weakness, in which none of the operations of the mind are performed with energy or effect. The memory, the judgment, the powers of attention and of combination are so much impaired, that the individual is wholly inadequate to the duties of society, and incapable of any continued conversation ; his actions and conduct are without steadiness and consistency : his thoughts are deficient in concentration and coherence. In fact this may be considered as a prelude or commencement of that state of incoherence or dementation which will be described in the sequel. It is a combination of the phenomena of mania or monomania with those of dementia.

On comparing the modes of action which are to be observed in an assemblage of lunatics in the advanced stage of insanity, we find

* Chiaruggi, della Pazzia in genere ed in spezie. Heinroth's Stoerungen des Seelenlebens, 2 abschn : Formenlehre.

the different forms of the disease in some measure blended and passing into each other; they are at least not so distinctly marked as in the early period. The symptoms belonging to one form of madness are often confounded with those of another, and from the combination there results, as it has been remarked by a writer of extensive observation and research, an assemblage of phenomena which bears little or no similitude to the description found in books and commonly entertained.

An opinion has been maintained that, in all cases of insanity, periods of monomania, of mania, and of dementia or incoherence, take place successively.* Nothing can be more erroneous than such a notion, although it is true that the two former of these morbid conditions sometimes pass into each other. Many individuals continue long to display the characteristics of mania, but except during particular periods of renewed violence or agitation, to which most are subject, they become more tranquil than at the commencement of their complaint. They display signs of incipient dementia, combined with morbid activity of body, in which the excitement characteristic of their disease exhausts itself into almost perpetual action. Lunatics of a different class fall into a state of calm reverie; their imagination, abandoned to itself without the control of judgment, gives itself up to wanderings without end: even in attempting to converse, or when their attention is excited by questions, these individuals exhibit a strange mixture of reason and of mistakes, both as to facts and inferences. Others, and these are a greater number, are chiefly governed by some particular passion or mental habit: many of the latter are under illusions as to their own persons and their relations to other individuals. M. Pinel says, " I was frequently followed at the Bicêtre by a general, who said that he had just ben fighting an important battle, and had left fifty thousand men dead on the field. At my side was a monarch who talked of nothing but his subjects and his provinces. In another place was the prophet Mahomet in person, denouncing in the name of the Almighty. A little further was a sovereign of the universe, who could with a breath annihilate the earth. Many of them seemed to be occupied by a multiplicity of objects, which were present to their imaginations. They gesticulated, declaimed, and vociferated incessantly, without appearing to see or hear any thing that passed. Others, under illusive influence, saw objects in forms and colours which they did not really possess. Under the influence of an illusion of that kind, was a maniac who mistook for a legion of devils every assemblage of people that he saw. Another maniac tore his clothes to tatters, and scattered the straw on which he lay, under the apprehension that they were heaps of twisted serpents."

These cases belong to monomania, the morbid impression having reference to one subject or favourite idea; but after the vigour of intellect has broken down under protracted disease, the mind is not

* M. Bayle, Nouvelle Doctrine des Maladies Mentales. Paris, 1825.

so tenacious of particular impressions as in the early stage of gradually approaching insanity. The illusions displayed at this period
are not, like those of the melancholic in distinctly marked cases of
partial insanity, silently cherished in the recesses of the mind,
brooded over in solitude or in gloomy reserve : they are less unconnected with the present objects of sense, and are for ever changing
with the casual alterations of feeling or temper. In a great number
of those lunatics who are threatened with general paralysis, or in
whom this affection has already displayed its symptoms, a very
remarkable form of monomania has been observed. The prevailing
state is most frequently one of exaltation and joyous delirium. The
imagination in patients of this class is puffed up with the belief of
great possessions; "they fancy themselves the owners of millions
of money, of towns, provinces, empires, worlds." Intoxicated with
their good fortune, they abandon themselves to the flattering ideas
which occupy their minds. Their joy diffuses itself over their
features, their gestures, and they beam with a sort of tumultuous
gladness, so much the more lively as they fancy it to be partaken
by all who surround them, and on whom they lavish promises of
bestowing fortunes, jewels, palaces, and gardens. " A man, says
M. Calmeil, " who had been employed in a gaming-house, said to
me one day with a mumbling articulation, and supporting himself
with difficulty by one hand against a table, ' Being the most puisant
of emperors, I shall build a new Paris in four hours : the streets
shall be paved with gold ; they shall meet in a great square which
shall occupy the midst; they shall have on each side two rows of galleries like a bazaar; every where there shall be a display of bronzes,
statues, and marble columns. The beds in the apartments shall be
made of rosewood ; in the place of curtains there shall be mirrors,
which shall be fixed at the four corners by hinges of diamonds.'"
This writer observes that the particular aspect of illusion now
described has often afforded a prognostic of general paralysis several
months before its actual appearance.* It continues during a great
part of the duration of paralysis, of which the course will hereafter be
described, but gives way gradually to the increase of dementia, and
the morbid ideas of exaltation are obliterated with the last traces of
intelligence. In other instances this joyous monomania undergoes
a transition into a variety of maniacal delirium, with excessive
agitation and violent anger ; and this state has continued, with short
intervals of quietude, until the death of the individual: in some
instances it terminates in dementia.† Monomania with melancholy
dejection is, according to the observations of M. Calmeil and others,
rarely the condition of the mind in these protracted complicated
cases.‡
   In a great number of protracted cases the disorder has a very
different aspect: the principal phenomena of disease refer themselves
to some particular habit or active propensity: in these examples no

---

* M. Calmeil, p. 325.   † Ibid. p. 330.   ‡ Ibid. p. 332.

distinct hallucination or illusion can be traced, and the condition of the individual come under the description of moral insanity. I have frequently seen one person in a group of lunatics who is perpetually and busily employed in numerical calculations. He has generally a slate and a pencil in his hands, and runs up to any stranger who presents himself to show some reckoning which he has just made, and ask if it is correct. The subject is perfectly unimportant, and generally turns upon dates taken from an almanack. Another lunatic, who was under my own care during a long period, was never so happy as when he was busily employed in making rhymes: he was a man of colour from St. Domingo, and wrote verses in French, which had occasionally some glimmerings of wit and point. He would immediately accost any person whom he saw, and demand a subject for an acrostic, which was very soon finished. An individual, who has been many years in confinement, is for ever carrying on law-suits, and wearing out the patience of all his visitors by a hurried but circumstantial detail of a case which, as he flatters himself, is to come on at the next quarter sessions. Almost every variety of human pursuit becomes occasionally the subject in relation to which madness is exhibited, and the disordered state is displayed in many instances rather in the mode of action and conduct, combined with a degree of general weakness or diminished vigour of mind, than in any of the hallucinations or illusions which are commonly regarded as characteristic of monomania.

SECT. VI.—*Of Incoherence or Dementia.*

Incoherence is a very peculiar and well-marked form of mental disorder. The mind in this state is occupied, without ceasing, by unconnected thoughts and evanescent emotions ; it is incapable of continued attention and reflection, and at length loses the faculty of distinct perception or apprehension. Numerous examples of this disease, or decay of the mental powers, are to be met with in every receptacle containing a considerable aassemblage of deranged persons. It was termed by Pinel *démence* or *dementia*, and that designation has been adopted by many late writers. Pinel complained of the poverty of the French language in words fit for denoting the different varieties of mental disease. We have no reason for bringing a similar imputation against our own, or for adopting, in this or in other instances, Latin terms. Such a practice is very inconvenient on many accounts,* and a more appropriate epithet cannot be

---

* There are many reasons which render it advisable to adopt English rather than Latin technical expressions, as far as the former are available. For example, if a physician informs a jury summoned in an inquiry "de lunatico," that the person who is the subject of examination is in a state of dementia, he will probably convey no information, and must be prepared with a definition of the term, which involves a discussion. By using the term incoherence he will convey a correct idea, if not a complete one, of his meaning.

7*

devised for the disordered state now to be described than that of incoherence, which expresses, in fact, its most striking and general feature. This consists in a want of coherence, or of the usual and natural connexion or association between ideas, thoughts, and emotions. Pinel has thus briefly defined it: " Idées incohérentes entre elles, et sans aucun rapport avec les objets extérieurs." He afterwards explains this definition or expands it, and I shall cite his own expressions, which I find it difficult to translate with perfect precision. " Une mobilité turbulente et incoercible, une succession rapide et comme instantanée d'idées qui semblent naître et pulluler dans l'entendement, sans aucun impression faite sur les sens; un flux et réflux continuel, et ridicule, d'objets chimériques qui se choquent, s'alternent, se détruisent les uns les autres sans aucun intermission et sans aucun rapport entre eux; le même concours incohérent, mais calme, d'affections morales, de sentimens de joie, de tristesse, de colère, qui naissent fortuitement et disparoissent de même sans laisser aucune trace, et sans avoir aucune correspondance avec les impressions des objets externes; tel est le caractère fondamental de la démence dont je parle."

Incoherence is either a primary disease, arising immediately from the agency of exciting causes on a constitution previously healthy, or it is a secondary affection, the result of other disorders of the brain and nervous system, which, by their long duration or severity, give rise to disease in the structure of those organs. The causes which produce the state of incoherence as an original disorder are nearly the same with those which in other cases excite madness in the first instance ; they are such agents as break down the powers of the mind by their overwhelming influence, or destroy them by vehement emotions.* Secondary incoherence or dementia follows long-protracted mania, attacks of apoplexy, epilepsy or paralysis, or fevers attended with severe delirium. This decay of the faculties has been termed fatuity or imbecility, and it has been confounded with idiotism, which in all its degrees and modifications is a very different state. The distinction, which is very important, has not always been kept in view by writers on disorders of the mind, and even in the works of Pinel we find it sometimes overlooked. M. Esquirol has the merit of having drawn more accurately the line of discrimination. He refers to dementia all the cases of effete or obliterated intellect which are the results of maniacal or other diseases, and are incident to persons originally possessed of sound

---

* M. Calmeil has described two cases of dementia, in which incoherence and the loss of the rational faculties commenced, and reached the last degree, without any symptoms of other insanity. Several strongly-marked cases are reported by Pinel. The individuals mentioned by M. Calmeil had paralysis complicated with dementia. In these instances weakness of memory and intellect came on gradually together with the first symptoms of general paralysis, and increased until all traces of understanding, moral feeling, and even of the instinctive impulses or merely animal powers were entirely obliterated, no degree whatever of maniacal agitation having been displayed through the whole course of the disease. (M. Calmeil, ouvrage cité, p. 324.)

faculsies, and includes those defects only under idiotism, which are original or congenital. "The imbecile," he observes, "have never possessed the faculties of the understanding in a state sufficiently developed for the display of reason. The victim of dementia was once endowed with them, but has lost this possession. The former lives neither in the past nor the future ; the latter has some thoughts of times past, reminiscences which excite in him occasional gleams of hope. Imbecile persons in their habits and manner of existence display the semblance of childhood ; the conduct, the acts of the demented preserve the characteristics of consistent age, and bear the impress derived from the anterior state of the individual. Idiots and cretins have never possessed memory, judgment, sentiments : scarcely do they present, in some instances, indications of the animal instincts, and their external conformation plainly indicates that they were not organized to be capable of thought.

A want of sequence, or connexion between the ideas, a failure of that aptitude in the mental constitution by which in the natural state one momentary condition of the mind follows in the train of its antecedent, seems to be the fundamental or essential circumstance in this state of disease; and it not only constitutes the most striking phenomenon of incoherence, but perhaps accounts for all the peculiar features which accompany it. Hence the defect of memory, which appears in the first and slightest degrees of this affection, and the incapability even of distinct apprehension which occurs in the advanced stage, when sensations are no longer the antecedents of perception or recognition ; and hence the moral indifference as to the present and the future for which demented persons are remarkable. The faculty or capability of receiving impressions is found in all demented persons to be impaired ; and this circumstance has been strongly pointed out by M. Esquirol, whose description of dementia is the best and most original that has been drawn.*
"Dementia," says this excellent writer, "deprives men of the faculty of adequately perceiving objects, of seeing their relations, of comparing them, of preserving a complete recollection of them; whence results the impossibility of reasoning correctly. Demented persons are incapable of reasoning, because external objects make too feeble an impression upon them ; because the organs of transmission have lost a part of their energy ; or, lastly, because the brain itself has no longer sufficient strength to receive and retain the impression which is transmitted to it; hence it necessarily results that the sensations are feeble, obscure, incomplete: being unable to form a true and just idea of objects, these persons cannot compare them, or exercise abstraction or association of ideas; they are not capable of a sufficiently strong attention ; the organ of thought has not energy enough : it has been deprived of that vigour which is necessary for the integrity of its functions. Hence the most incongruous ideas succeed each other; independent of each other,

* Dict. des Sc. Méd. t. viii. p. 13.

they follow without order and connexion ; patients repeat words
and entire sentences without attaching to them any precise meaning;
they talk, without being conscious of what they say. It seems as
if unreal expressions were heard by them in their heads, which they
repeat in obedience to some involuntary or automatic impulse, the
result of previous habits or of fortuitous association with objects
which strike their senses."

The following table, taken from M. Esquirol's treatise, will serve
to illustrate the forms of disease which are included by medical
writers under the common term of dementia. It is styled by M.
Esquirol a table of causes. The table exhibits the distribution of
235 cases of dementia ; the first column contains the number of patients admitted at the Salpêtrière during the years 1811 and 1812 ;
the second column is the report of the author's private establishment, and is limited to persons of the higher or more opulent classes
of society.

TABLE OF CAUSES.

	Number of individuals.	Total.
Physical Causes.		
Disorders connected with the catamenia .	11	4
Critical period	29	6
Consequences of childbirth . . .	5	3
Blows upon the head	3	0
Progress of age	46	3
Ataxic fever	1	2
Suppression of hemorrhoids . . .	0	2
Mania	14	4	195
Melancholia	13	2
Paralysis	3	2
Apoplexy	3	2
Syphilis and abuse of mercury . . .	6	8
Faults of regimen	0	6
Intemperance	9	6
Masturbation	4	7
Moral Causes.		
Disappointed love	1	4
Fright	4	3
Political excitement	0	8	40
Disappointed ambition	0	3
Poverty	5	0
Domestic griefs	8	4
	192	73	235

Of the several degrees of incoherence.—Incoherence, or dementia, exists in several stages or degrees, which present different phenomena ; and the description of one is, therefore, not applicable to
another. We find no difficulty in recognising four degrees in this
state, each of which is characterised by peculiar features. If the
disorder commences in the first degree, it goes on successively to
the more advanced ; but the more severe degrees, or the greatest

development of the morbid phenomena, may appear at once, as the immediate effect of causes which destroy the powers of mind, or produce disorganization of the brain.

The first stage or degree may be termed that of *forgetfulness*, or *loss of memory.* Its chief characteristic is a failure of memory, especially as to recent events.

The second degree brings with it a total abolition of the power of reasoning, depending on a loss of voluntary control over the thoughts. It may be termed the stage of *irrationality*, or *loss of reason.*

In the third degree the individual affected is incapable of comprehending the meaning of any thing that may be said to him. It may be styled the stage of *incomprehension.*

The fourth stage is characterised by loss of instinctive, voluntary action. The individual is found to be destitute even of the animal instincts ; he cannot obey the calls of nature. This is the stage of *inappetency*, or *loss of instinct or volition.*

First degree of incoherence or dementia. Impaired memory. —The first stage of this affection is distinguished by forgetfulness of recent impressions, while the memory retains a comparatively firm hold of ideas laid up in its recesses from times long past : the power of reasoning within the sphere of distinct recollection is not remarkably impaired, and the faculty of judgment is exercised in a sound manner when the attention can be sufficiently roused.

The disease of incoherence approaches most gradually and slowly when it comes on as the symptom and accompaniment of old age ; it is in such instances that its several degrees are most clearly recognised and distinguished. It is particularly in this modification of dementia, that we have an opportunity of tracing most distinctly the approach and observing the phenomena of the first stage; of noting its commencement and slow advances. It seems to begin with dulness of perception or apprehension. The organs of sense are not so perfect in advanced age as in the more healthy and vigorous periods of life : sensation is not so acute ; but it is rather in the subsequent recognition which the mind makes of the ideas presented to it, than in sensation itself, that the defect chiefly lies. Perception, indeed, takes place, but the impression is momentarily evanescent. The individual sees and hears ; he replies to questions, but his attention is so little excited that he speedily forgets what he has said, and repeats the same remarks or inquiries after a few minutes. At the same time ideas long ago impressed upon the mind remain nearly in their original freshness, and are capable of being called up whenever the attention is directed towards them. Sensations produced by present objects are so slight, and the notions connected with them so confused and indistinct, that the individual affected scarcely knows where he is ; yet he recognises without difficulty persons with whom he has long been acquainted, and if questioned respecting his former life, and the transactions and pursuits of his youth or manhood, he will often give pertinent and sensible replies.

The disorder of his mind consists not in defective memory of the past, but in the incapacity for attention and for receiving the influence of present external agencies, which, in a different state of the cerebral organization, would have produced a stronger effect upon the sensorium, or seat of sensation and perception.

I well remember conversing more than once with a gentleman advanced in age, who had passed the greater part of his life in active exertions, which he had relinquished when his memory had rather suddenly become defective. He remembered the events of his youth, talked of his father, who, as he said, had come from Scotland with a pack upon his back to settle in the town where he afterwards resided; he said that the latter had thriven in business and had become rich, mentioned a variety of particulars which proved that impressions made upon his mind up to a certain period of his life were still fresh, and made some remarks and general reflections indicating that his reason was yet sound. The same person could scarcely give any account of what had passed during the last fifteen or twenty years. He could not recollect the names of his grandchildren, though they had been frequently in his society, and he scarcely seemed to be aware of their existence. He appeared not to know where he was, but often fancied himself travelling and at an inn when he was at home, in the house which had been his abode for many years.

The following description of a case of senile dementia will serve perhaps still further to exemplify the state of the sensorium and of the mental faculties in this affection.

A. M., aged about seventy years, was in his youth a farmer, but changed that occupation for the business of a baker, which he followed until he had accumulated property sufficient for his maintenance. He has been living for several years in retirement, and without any regular employment. His memory is said to have undergone a gradual decay. When he is questioned respecting present objects and circumstances, he generally gives clear and distinct answers, but can seldom recollect what has occurred but a short time previously. In half an hour after he has been visited by his medical attendant, who is an intimate acquaintance, he will say, if asked, that he has not seen him for several days. His recollection of persons whom he knew in the former periods of his life, and of events which then happened him, is tolerably clear, but at times, and especially after sleep, he does not know where he is. He sometimes fancies, at night, on waking from a short sleep, that he is engaged in his former occupations. He then rises from bed, and sets himself busily to prepare for lighting a fire in his oven, beats the wall, calls his men up, and asks if the faggots are ready. He cannot be persuaded without great difficulty that he is in ———— street, and has nothing to do with the baking business. At other times he will get up in great haste to go down and see somebody who is waiting for him on business, or thinks that there is a horse standing for him at the door, calls for his clothes, and wonders that his friends are so tardy in assisting him. At these periods his state is not that of ordinary somnambulism. He sees and knows some at least of the persons who are about him, and will converse with them. He sometimes, during the daytime, wonders where he is, does not know the place though he has resided in the same house for some years. The hostess, who is an old acquaintance, at length convinces him that he his at her home. When his recollection is roused, and his thoughts are drawn into the right channel, he has a correct knowledge of persons, and shows not the slightest trace of maniacal illusions, or of any thing approaching to the character of ordinary madness. He is glad to see his old friends, shakes hands with them in his wonted cordial manner, is on the best terms with his relatives, and never displays the least deviation from the natural and habitual state of his feelings and affections.

Senile dementia, or the decay of the mental faculties, is not the lot of old persons universally, though it is a condition to which old age may be said to have tendency, and to which in the last stage of bodily decay some approximations are generally to be perceived. The change which time alone will perhaps sooner or later bring on, in those who long survive the allotted duration of man's days, may be accelerated by a variety of circumstances. Among these is a life of too much activity and excitement, of mental exertion beyond what the constitutional strength of the individual is capable of supporting without constant effort ; excessive anxiety and eagerness in the pursuit of business, or intense and unremitted application to studies of whatever kind. The minds and bodies of men are only fitted for exertion in certain degrees, which, however; differ in different individuals; but the powers of all are limited. All have need of occasional respite from labour, and the appointment of rest during one day in seven is, from physical considerations alone, calculated to promote the well-being of individuals and of society. We may observe that among those who have neglected this ordinance, there have been many who have suffered the penalty in this life. Some have terminated a rapid and perhaps brilliant career of unremitting and successful exertions by suicidal madness, of which too many and too well-known examples might be cited ; others, though in a longer measure of time, have accelerated the period of intellectual decay.

A second cause of senile dementia, next in the frequency of its operation to that which we have just mentioned, is the too liberal use of vinous or other alcoholic liquors. The same affection has been observed frequently to make its appearance in men long engaged in active pursuits, soon after they have relinquished their business or professions, and have laid themselves by to enjoy ease and leisure for the remainder of their days. The disease often appears in a more marked and sudden manner in elderly persons who have sustained a slight attack of apoplexy or paralysis, which has perhaps been speedily recovered, and might be expected to have left but slight traces of disease. That expectation is verified so far as the sensitive and motive powers are concerned, but the seat of intellect is found to have been shaken in its very centre.

Senile dementia is entirely distinct from that species of moral insanity which appears occasionally, as we have already observed, in aged persons. The former is merely a loss of energy in some of the intellectual operations. It brings with it nothing morbid or unusual in the state of the feelings or affections, no tendency to depraved or unaccustomed habits, nor, commonly, any change in the temper and general disposition of mind. Individuals to whose lot this complaint has fallen are seldom unhappy on account of it, and if they are in any degree aware of their condition, they bear it with patience and cheerfulness.

These remarks are only applicable in their full extent to dementia when limited within the first degree. This disease, as it advances, involves the feelings and moral affections : in the higher stages of dementia, whether occasioned by the progress of age or by other causes, the temper becomes changed and the disposition perverted.

It is in senile decay that the phenomena of incoherence in the first degree are most strongly marked. Traits of the same description may, however, be observed in other cases of dementia. The memory of those who labour under this disease in the early stage from whatever cause and in whatever period of life it may have arisen, is that of aged persons, more tenacious of long-past than of recent events : the latter make so feeble an impression that it is speedily obliterated. In such persons all the powers of the mind are greatly weakened : they have no aptitude to any train of thought or action, and they are quite unable to fulfil the duties of their business or profession : they cannot combine a variety of considerations in order to come to any practical conclusion; cannot enter with earnestness into any affairs of importance, or comprehend any continued conversation: all their discourse is marked by diffuseness and incoherence.[*]

The second degree takes place in every instance in which the disease continues. It is, perhaps, most conspicuous in cases which are the sequalæ of mania, or ensue after that disease has lasted for a considerable time : in some instances, as I have before remarked, it is the condition which disorder of the understanding assumes in the onset, and as the immediate effect of some powerful agencies which overwhelm the mind, as of sudden grief or joy, amazement, fright, which, in popular language, are said to render their victims idiots.

Second degree of incoherence—Loss of the reasoning power.—The second degree of incoherence brings with it a total abolition of the power of reason: the energy of the will in directing the course of the thoughts, which is essential to every process of reasoning, is impaired to such a degree as to preclude the exercise of this faculty.

Difficulties have engaged the attention of metaphysical writers

[*] M. Calmeil de la Paralysie chez les Aliénés.

with reference to the power of the will over the thoughts in the healthy and sound state. It has been said that the mind is so subjected to physical laws, that we cannot by an effort call up a single idea; that the thoughts follow each other by laws of succession independent of voluntary control, that the will has in some way a power of modifying the succession of ideas is, however, certain, otherwise we should be incapable of conducting any process of reasoning or argument. Professor Dugald Stewart has shown that this controlling influence is exercised by fixing the attention exclusively and by voluntary preference on certain trains of thoughts. It is, however, still through the associations which exist among the ideas, and by modifying the results to which the important principle of association gives rise, that this voluntary control can alone be exercised, and it is easy to conceive that when any morbid change has ensued in the connecting faculty by which the ideas, if we may so speak, cohere, when they become disjoined and incoherent, no longer following each other in their natural order of suggestion, the mind loses the power of reasoning through the shattered condition of its instrument. The loss of voluntary power over the succession of ideas is so great in a certain period of dementia, that the individual affected is incapable by any effort of mind of carrying on the series of his thoughts to the end of a sentence or proposition. He hears a question, apprehends sometimes its meaning, and attempts to answer; but before he has uttered the half of his reply, his mind becomes confused and bewildered, some accidental suggestion turns aside the current of his ideas, which are too loosely associated to remain, even in a short train, coherent: his expressions become consequently absurd and irrelevant. It is sometimes easy to observe the point at which the intention of the speaker ceases to direct his words, and at which the ideas are drawn aside into a different course. The individual begins to talk of one thing and before he has spoken half a minute he has wandered into subjects so remote from it that some care is required that the by-stander may be enabled to trace the links by which his thoughts have reached the point at which they are found. This degree of incoherence is generally to be observed as a prelude to a more severe and complete form, which will next be described. Until the mind has passed into the more advanced stage, glimmerings of sense and reason are displayed: the individual affixes some meaning to his words, though he soon forgets it. The memory is not entirely lost, though much impaired; its defects resembling in kind those of senile memory, but exceeding them in degree. Many individuals in this degree of dementia know and remember their friends or relatives, but scarcely display signs of emotion or sensibility on being visited by them. Not a few even in this state are capable of being employed in mechanical occupations. Females knit or sew, or perform any work with their hands to which they had been previously habituated; and men draw, or write letters or sentences, in which, however, their imbecility is generally conspicuous.

Some patients have occasional periods of greater excitement, in which the symptoms of a more active state of madness resume their prevalence. The physical health of patients thus affected is in general tolerably good ; they are often fat, have good appetites, digest their food, sleep well, and if in the previous stages of the disease they had been emaciated, they often recover their natural degree of plumpness on the approach of dementia. Hence the return of physical health without a corresponding improvement in the state of the mental faculties, is, as it has been remarked by M. Esquirol and others, an unfavourable prognostic in cases of maniacal disease. There are, however, some rare cases of recovery from this stage of dementia. Pinel informs us that many, especially young persons, who had remained in the Bicêtre several years or months in a state of absolute fatuity, have been attacked by a paroxysm of acute mania of twenty, or five-and-twenty, or thirty days' continuance. "Such paroxysms," he adds, "apparently from a re-action of the system, are in many instances succeeded by perfect rationality." The same result has been observed on the restoration of demented persons or of maniacs in the advanced stage of insanity after severe attacks of fever attended with delirium. Such attacks are often fatal to lunatics ; but of those who recover them, not a few are subsequently restored to the possession of their faculties.

Third degree of incoherence—Incomprehension.—The third degree of dementia is characterised by inability to comprehend the meaning of any question or proposition, however simple, that may be addressed to the person affected. If the attention can be ever so slightly roused, the reply attempted is always so remote from the subject as to indicate plainly that the question has not been understood.

This may be termed the confirmed stage of incoherence ; that epithet applying to it in a still more striking manner than to any other degree of the disease. It might also be termed the instinctive stage. Reason being entirely lost, and the instinctive or mechanical principles of action, as they are termed, still remaining in vigour, the latter display themselves more remarkably. The demented person is the creature of instinct and habit.

Physical activity is often remarkably displayed by persons reduced to this state, and it assumes the appearance of trick or habit. Some jump or run to and fro, or walk round perpetually in a circle. Some dance and sing, or vociferate frequently. Many talk incessantly in the most unmeaning jargon, attaching no ideas whatever to their words; others pass their time unceasingly in muttering half sentences and broken expressions, in which it is scarcely possible to discover any link of connection ; or if any association can be traced in their thoughts, it is of the most trivial kind, and depending on a word or on some sensible object which for a moment attracts a degree of attention. Many, on the other hand, sit in silence, with a sedate and tranquil look, sometimes with a vacant smile or with an unmeaning stare, and scarcely pronounce a syllable for weeks, or months, or even for years. A few remain crouched in a particular posture, which they always prefer, though to bystanders it seems the most uneasy and even painful ; if placed in a different manner by those who have the care of them, they soon resume their habitual position. Many demented persons crowd round a stranger who happens to visit a lunatic asylum and gaze at him, having just enough intelligence to perceive something new and to which they are not accustomed in his aspect. Some individuals in this state have a propensity to adorn themselves in a strange manner: they take any thing that happens to be in their way, and append it to their dress, which is singular and ridiculous.

M. Esquirol has described in a striking* and accurate manner the aspect of countenance peculiar to dementia, and especially belonging to this stage of the disease. " To the disordered state of the intellectual faculties," he says, " the following symptoms are added : the face is generally pale, the eyes moistened with tears, the pupils dilated, the look wandering, the countenance motionless and devoid of expression ; frequently the muscles of one side are relaxed and give the face a distorted appearance ; the body is sometimes lean and emaciated, at others it is loaded with fat ; in such instances the face is full, ruddy, the neck short; in a few persons no outward sign can be perceived indicative of the decay of intelligence."

Fourth and last degree of Incoherence. Loss of Instinctive Action : Inappetency.—In the last stage of this affection even the animal instincts are lost. The miserable victim of disease, when reduced to this state, has merely organic or physical existence; he appears scarcely conscious of life, has neither desires nor aversions, and is unable to obey the calls of nature.

Scarcely any exhibition of human suffering can be more deeply affecting than the aspect of a group of lunatics reduced to the last stages of fatuity, and those who have never witnessed such a spectacle can hardly imagine so abject a state of mental degradation. In a group of this description an individual may be seen always standing erect and immovable, with his head and neck bent almost at right angles to his trunk, his eyes fixed upon the ground, never turning them round, or appearing by any movement or gesture to be conscious of external impressions or even of his own existence. Another sits on a rocking chair, which she agitates to and fro, and throws her limbs into the most uncouth positions, at the same time chaunting or yelling a dissonant song, only capable of expressing a total inanity of ideas and feelings. Many sit constantly still, with their chins resting on their breasts, their eyes and mouth half open, unconscious of hunger or thirst, and almost destitute of the feelings which belong to merely physical life ; they would never lie down

* See the description of Démence, by M. Esquirol. Dict. des Sc. Méd. tom. viii. p. 13.

or rise were they not placed in bed and again raised by their attendants. A great proportion of the patients who are reduced to this
degree of fatuity are found to have lost the use of their limbs in a
greater or less degree by partial or general paralysis.

From such a state it is scarcely imaginable that recovery ever took
place, but patients in the last stage of fatuity often linger for many
years. Their state, however, is not always uniform : some of
them have comparatively lucid intervals, in which nature seems to
make an effort to light up the mind and recal lost impressions and
ideas. I have often observed a patient who sits all day in a wooden
elbowed-chair, with his chin hanging over his breast, appearing
hardly conscious of existence, and unable to assist himself in the
calls of nature, who would not eat if food were not actually put into
his mouth. He has been for several years in the same state, except
that he ocasionally appears to rouse himself, and for a short time to
recover an unusual degree of animation. At such periods he will
sometimes read a chapter in the Bible with a clear voice and a distinct and intelligible articulation. Such occasional variations in the
state of demented persons are not infrequent. They are capable
of being raised by favourable influences from a lower degree of
their disease into one which is above it in the scale.

The last stages of this mental disease are commonly styled idiotism
and fatuity; but these terms are liable to the objection that they tend
to confound dementia, which is an acquired state and the result of
disease, with a natural and congenital defect.

Dementia is often complicated with paralysis of a peculiar kind,
which will be described in the following section.

SECT. VII.—*Of General Paralysis complicated with Insanity.*

A variety of disorders are occasionally complicated with insanity.
The proper place for describing most of these will present itself in
a future section of this work. But there is one morbid affection
which, on account of its frequent occurrence in conjunction with
mental derangement, as well as for some other reasons, must be
looked upon as nearly related to that disease, and must therefore be
described in connection with its history. I allude to a peculiar
modification of paralysis, which is often observed in the advanced
stages of insanity, and especially in cases which are passing or have
already degenerated into dementia.

M. Esquirol was the first writer who directed the attention of
physicians to this morbid state, and pointed out the incurable nature
of insanity complicated with paralysis.* General paralysis, he says,
is often indicative of inflammation of the meninges, and must not be
confounded with those paralytic affections which are consequences
of cerebral hemorrhage, of cancers, or tubercles in the brain, or of

---

* Dict. des Sciences Médicales, tom. viii

ramollissement of that organ.* It sometimes appears with the first symptoms of insanity, during the acute period often so remarkable at the outset of the disease; in some instances it precedes, and in others supervenes on mental derangement. Its commencement, at whatever period of insanity, is often without any striking appearances. It has a course peculiar to itself, ever increasing while the mental powers diminish. Whatever character the disorder of the mind may have presented, it soon passes, when complicated with paralysis, into a state of chronic dementia ; and paralytic lunatics seldom survive, according to M. Esquirol, longer than from one to three years. Their last moments are ushered in by convulsions, cerebral congestions, diarrhœas, gangrenes affecting those parts of the body which sustain its weight after all muscular movement and support have been lost.

This form of paralysis is much more frequent in men than in women. Of one hundred and nine paralytics under the observation of M. Esquirol during three years at Charenton, ninety-five were males. "When I was charged," says that writer, "two years since, with the service of the department of the insane at Bicêtre, during the absence of M. Pariset, who had been sent to Cadiz, I was struck with the difference on comparing the number of paralytic men at Bicêtre with that of female paralytic lunatics at the Salpêtrière. The same observation has been made elsewhere. It has not escaped Dr. Foville, physician-in-chief to the asylum at St. Yon, near Rouen. Of three hundred and thirty-four lunatics at that hospital, an eleventh part, or thirty-one, were paralytics, of whom twenty-two were men and nine women."

At Charenton, according to M. Esquirol, the proportion of paralytics is more considerable : it forms one-sixth of the whole number of admissions ; of six hundred and nine lunatics admitted in three years, one hundred and nine were paralytics. The proportion among males is enormous, compared with that among females.

Thus, of 366 male lunatics . . . . 95 were paralytics.
     "   " 253 females . . . . . 14 "   "

Paralysis is complicated more especially with the mental disorder of those lunatics who have been previously addicted to excessive libertinism, or such as have suffered from the abuse of mercury or of spirituous liquors. Do these circumstances account for the different proportion between male and female paralytics? They appear at least, says M. Esquirol, to explain the fact of the greater number of paralytic males at Charenton compared with that at Bicêtre. The lunatics admitted at Bicêtre are poor men, whose laborious life has given them more energy of resistance against the causes above pointed out as exciting paralysis. These causes must have exercised less influence on men of active life, given to manual labour, exerci-

---

* Rapport Statistique sur la Maison Royale de Charenton, par M. Esquirol, Médecin-en-Chef. Annales d'Hygiène publique et de Médecine Legale. Paris, April 1829.

sing less intelligence, and fatiguing less their brains. The lunatics
of Charenton have been persons in easy circumstances, possessing
greater means of satisfying their passions, exercising professions
which excite the brain, and accustomed to less activity of body.
The pathology of this disease has been very much illustrated by
the excellent work of M. Calmeil, who has investigated its causes
and relations with great accuracy at the hospital of Charenton, both
during the superintendence of M. Royer-Collard, and subsequently
to the death of that distinguished physician, under the auspices and
availing himself of the information of M. Esquirol.*

In extensive hospitals devoted to the reception of lunatics, are to
be found, as M. Calmeil observes, a large number of individuals
deprived in a greater or less degree of the power of voluntary
motion. Some cannot speak without difficulty ; others totter in
walking, or are unable to keep themselves erect without some point
of support ; some are affected with hemiplegia or with paraplegia ;
others are crippled in all their four members; in a certain number
we observe contractions either of an arm or a leg. All these disorders of the locomotive power are included under the common term
of paralysis by authors who have written on mental derangement.
By the use of terms so comprehensive, many things are confounded
which are very different in their nature. The form of paralysis
now to be described is very distinguishable in its symptoms and
history from those affections which result from sanguineous congestion in the brain, from sanguineous effusion, and from acute ramollissement, though occasionally complicated, as we shall observe,
with these accessory changes of structure and their results. The
former affection constitutes a distinct species of disease, having its
peculiar causes, symptoms, course, and terminations.

M. Calmeil has observed three degrees in the general paralysis of
insane persons, of which the distinguishing characters are as follows:—

1. *Paralysis in the first degree.*—An impediment in the movements of the tongue is the first indication of this form of paralysis,
and it has often become already very apparent while no embarrassment is as yet discovered in the movements of the limbs. The
articulation is no longer perfect, the patient is obliged to use effort
in speaking, his words are uttered tardily and with a sort of mumbling and stammering like that of persons intoxicated. If the patient
is desired to put out his tongue, he does it without any discoverable
deviation ; the muscles of the mouth and face preserve their natural
position ; nothing unusual can be perceived except a kind of muffled
articulation, which might escape remark from a person not directing
attention to the circumstance.

2. *Paralysis in the second degree.*—The symptoms of the second

---

* De la Paralysie considérée chez les Aliénés. Recherches faites dans le
service de feu M. Royer-Collard et de M. Esquirol. Par L. F. Calmeil, M. D.,
&c. Paris, 1826.

degree are those of the first period with increased intensity. The power of the tongue in articulating is more imperfect ; scarcely a word is pronounced distinctly, and it is necessary to guess the meaning of every word. When the individual is sitting and attemps to walk, he raises himself slowly by fixing his hands upon the arms of his chair ; being once erect, he does not immediately go forward with security, but like a child who measures his first steps he seems to balance himself, and to totter from right and left ; he then ventures to walk, and goes a greater or less distance, but with a vacillating movement according to the degree of strength that remains to him. When reposing on his bed, he is able to move all his extremities in every direction. The upper extremities display less evidently the effects of paralysis ; yet in certain subjects there is a degree of stiffness in the arms, which are with difficulty raised to the summit of the head. The muscles of the neck participate in the general weakness ; the chin has a tendency to rest upon the chest ; the muscles of the trunk are impaired in strength, and the body rests ill at ease upon the pelvis.

These individuals feel, see, hear, and perceive odours ; but the energy of sense is singularly obtunded. Slight impressions upon the skin and the nostrils are disregarded ; it is evident that those points of the brain which are subservient to sensation are not less affected than those which belong to locomotion.

Persons in this stage of paralysis are generally in an advanced degree of dementia ; their want of cleanliness is extreme ; their clothes are continually imbued with their excretions, which escape without notice, either through want of attention, or, what is less probable, from a real paralysis of the sphincters.

During the second as well as the first stage of general paralysis, the functions of merely physical life are nearly in a healthy state ; the circulation is natural, sleep undisturbed ; digestion and other functions of the alimentary canal are performed in a healthy manner, and the flesh is firm and plump.

3. *Paralysis in the third degree.*—Nothing is more deplorable than the aspect of a lunatic affected with general paralysis in the third degree. Those injuries of the brain which affect the intellect and the powers of movement, now approach the very last point. These patients, motionless and insensible, are reduced to a state of mere vegetation ; there existence is a kind of slow death. Some individuals are not able to articulate a single word, and only utter vague and confused sounds. The lower extremities are so weak that standing is impossible. A period arrives when even, in sitting, the individual can no longer raise or extend his legs ; the hands and arms have not lost so entirely their power of action, but it is evident that they participate in the general weakness. Often there remains no trace of intelligence ; food must be put into the patient's mouth ; he is totally insensible to excretions, and pays no attention to surrounding objects, and is almost destitute of impressions. He hears

indeed, sees, tastes, and perceives strong odours ; but is scarcely affected by any sensation.

Digestion, which at first was strong, is at length lost with the other physical powers; the body becomes more and more emaciated; at length the skin sloughs. The lateral parts of the back, the lumbar regions, the cellular tissue which covers the coccyx, the sacrum, the sciatic tuberosities, become the seat of suppuration. Œdema takes place in the depending parts ; hectic fever accelerates the exhaustion of physical life.

M. Calmeil has well observed that death seldom follows, as the simple consequence of the cerebral disease ; the abdominal or thoracic viscera generally become affected ; the lungs are found to contain suppurating tubercles, and the intestinal canal to be inflamed or ulcerated.

The disease of general paralysis, simply considered, runs the course above described gradually and even slowly, the symptoms appearing and developing themselves in a regular succession. This is not the proper place for entering upon the statement of necroscopical observations, but it is necessary to remark that, according to the results obtained by M. Calmeil, the phenomena displayed by dissection are very uniform in the disease now described when uncomplicated with accidental disorders. Dissection has proved that this species of paralysis arises not from effusion of blood in the brain, from acute ramollissement, or sanguineous congestion ; it almost uniformly depends upon a chronic inflammation which takes place in the substance of the brain, especially at its surface or circumference. But this appearance is liable to deviations from accessory or supervening disorders ; the changes above enumerated are sometimes found in addition to that alteration which is proper to general paralysis, and in such instances additional symptoms have displayed themselves during life. The principal of these accessory diseases are the following :—

1. *Congestion in the brain.*—In general paralysis there is throughout a marked tendency to accumulation of blood in the brain, and this tendency is in some instances so strong that the individuals affected are liable to attacks of coma, which threaten and at length end in the sudden extinction of life. To these attacks lunatics are equally liable in each degree of the progress of general paralysis, and having once experienced them are exposed to relapses, to prevent which the utmost care is required on the part of the physician. In some instances the first onset of general paralysis is dated from an attack of this description.

Necroscopy displays in such cases injections and infiltrations of blood or of bloody serosity in the tissue of the membranes and on the surface of the brain.

2. *Hemorrhage in the cerebral substance.*—One example only of this complication occurred within the observation of M. Calmeil. The patient, after labouring under dementia with general paralysis

was suddenly attacked by hemiplegia of the left side. Besides other phenomena an apoplectic cyst was found in the corpus striatum on the right side of the brain.

3. *Simple hemorrhages between the two laminæ of the arach-noid.*—This is a much more rare event than effusion into the substance of the brain, and its diagnosis, as M. Rostin has observed, is very obscure. It takes place in the course of general paralysis, and is followed by sudden death with phenomena somewhat various.

4. *Ramollissement, properly so termed, seated in a point of the cerebro-spinal system.*—In cases in which this morbid change existed, additional symptoms had been complicated with those of general paralysis, such as occasional agitations or convulsions, and total abolition of locomotive power in the lower limbs.

5. *Erosions of the cerebral surface.*—M. Calmeil has remarked, with reference to the nature of convulsive phenomena, that he has never been able to detect any clearly marked differences in the morbid appearances found in the brains of paralytics who have expired in convulsions, and in those of paralytics who have never suffered any such attacks.

It results, from a great number of observations purposely made by MM. Calmeil, Esquirol, and others, that general paralysis commences sometimes long after mental derangement ; in other instances simultaneouly with it ; while in comparatively a few cases it precedes the manifestation of disorder in the mind. There are many lunatics who never become affected by this disease. Among those who are affected by it, some have experienced it after labouring under insanity during many years. According, however, to M. Calmeil, among the lunatics at Charenton its appearance has taken place almost always soon after the commencement of insanity. A few individuals have continued to display all the vigour of intellect for some time after they were attacked by this form of paralysis, and derangement has afterwards supervened. This observation might be subject to some doubt if it were not a fact clearly ascertained by M. Esquirol, in whose practice it was exemplified by a very remarkable instance.

The duration of general paralysis is various. M. Calmeil says that the mean duration in the cases which have been observed by him has appeared to be thirteen months. M. Calmeil confirms the observation of M. Esquirol that some live eight months, a year, or two, and that few survive more than three years under this complaint. The disorder is generally progressive, the symptoms becoming slowly more and more aggravated; but exceptions have occurred to this remark. A few individuals have recovered suddenly such a degree of strength as to be able to walk several miles in a day, and even to resume their occupations for a time. The ultimate prognosis, however, is most unfavourable. M. Royer-Collard, whose opinions were formed with great caution and reserve, had come to the conclusion that lunatics who displayed undoubted indications of general paralysis were incurable. During the experience of twenty years in a vast establishment for deranged persons, he had not seen one established recovery among the patients who had been attacked by this disease. M. Esquirol likewise regards it as generally incurable, though three instances to the contrary have occurred within his experience. At Charenton, as M. Calmeil assures us, it is so regular an observation that individuals who on their entry into the wards display any of the well-known signs of paralysis perish at the end of no long period of time, that the attendants who are ignorant of medicine, could scarcely be persuaded that there was for such patients any chance of cure. General statements are, however, seldom without exceptions, and two cases of recovery are reported by the writer last mentioned.

It appears that general paralysis is a much more frequent accompaniment of insanity in the hospitals of Paris than in some other places. Thus, in the south of France, Dr. Delaye found only five paralytics among one hundred and eleven lunatics at Toulouse ; and Dr. Rich has not recognised the disease among one hundred and thirty-two insane patients in the hospital at Montpellier. Vulpes, who was well acquainted with its phenomena, reported to M. Esquirol that there were scarcely three or four cases among five hundred lunatics at the asylum of Aversa, in the kingdom of Naples. Yet M. Esquirol seems inclined to doubt the correctness of this observation of Dr. Burrows, that general paralysis is a comparatively rare disease in England. He says that when English physicians shall have become able to distinguish the symptoms of this disease, they will find in England, and particularly in London, as many paralytics among the inmates of lunatic asylums as there are in Paris. I have made many inquiries with a view to determining this question, but have met with considerable difficulties in obtaining satisfactory information. This has arisen in part from the want of discriminate arrangement of cases in some of the public lunatic asylums, and in part from the circumstance that this particular form of disease is not well known in England, and distinguished from other modifications of paralysis. I have, however, in several instances obtained satisfactory results. The opinion which these inquiries have led me to adopt is that the disease in question is by no means an unusual phenomenon in this country, especially in the public hospitals for lunatics, or among the classes of persons who are principally found in such hospitals. It has been distinctly recognised by physicians and others who have the superintendence of English asylums. But it appears to be comparatively rare in private establishments ; at least this has been the fact in those particular ones to which my inquiries have been directed. The difference apparently depends on the classes of persons from which the inmates of these establishments are respectively drawn. Dr. Bompas has assured me that this paralysis has occurred in strongly marked cases in the private asylum under his care at Fishponds, near Bristol ; but it appears to have been there not more frequent than in the south of France. Out of two hundred and eighty-five patients received into this asylum during a given period of years, only five became the victims of general paralysis. Two of these were mariners, and one a dealer in spirits ; one was a military man, and the fifth a gentleman's groom : the two last were supposed to have been of temperate habits. Dr. Bompas adds that the speech of all was sooner or later affected, but that the first symptom generally observed by him has been a degree of unsteadiness in locomotion, and an inability to walk straight. In the Retreat belonging to the Society of Friends, near York, this disease is of still more rare occurrence. Mr. Tuke has sent me the following reply to my inquiries on this subject. " We have had one case, and but one, of the ' paralysie des aliénés.' It occurred a few years ago. The patient was one of our highest class, wholly unconnected with our religious society ; a man who had lived freely, to say the least, till nearly sixty years of age. The symptoms corresponded most accurately with the description of this disease. We have just now an old colonel who has been with us about two years, and who, as our surgeon* informs me, is likely to afford another example of this form of paralysis."

At Bethlem I was assured by the house-steward, who is a man of great sense and acute observation, that he has in many instances recognised the early symptoms of this disease. Patients are dismissed from Bethlem when they manifest any indication of paralysis, and the events of such cases cannot, on that account, be correctly noted ; it was, however, known that most individuals so affected have died within a year or two after leaving the hospital. The disease, as it has occurred in Bethlem, is characterised by the same symptoms as at Charenton, viz. by imperfect muffling articulation, by tottering in the gait, weakness and inaccuracy in the voluntary movements. Monomania, with pride and the illusive belief of great possessions, is the mental disease which has been noticed in the majority of these cases. This was a spontaneous remark of my informant, who, previously to my inquiries, had never heard of the disease described by M. Esquirol ; and it confirmed in the belief that the same affection has been recognised by him. Among the lunatics in St. Peter's Hospital in Bristol, general paralysis has frequently occurred. Some cases have been strongly marked, but I am not able to state with confidence of accuracy their proportional number. Dr. Whally, physician to the Lancaster Asylum, assures me that there are always cases in that hospital exactly coinciding with M. Calmeil's description of the " paralysie des aliénés." He has not mentioned in what proportion they occur. The asylum contains three hundred and fifty patients, of whose diseases one principal cause is the prevalent habit of dram-drinking. I have been informed by Mr. Hitch, the resident medical officer at the Gloucester Lunatic Asylum, that many instances of the same disease have occurred in that hospital. He says, " I find in the records

* Mr. Caleb Williams.

of the establishment, that sixteen well-marked cases of this disease have passed under our view since May, 1828. Of the sixteen cases which I have had under my charge, fifteen were males and one female." This proportional excess in the number of male paralytics is in accordance with the observations of M. Esquirol. With respect to the event of these cases, it is reported that they were all ultimately fatal. The female died after an attack of menorrhagia, and her death was thought to be its consequence. Of the males, five died in the house, six were discharged as incurable and harmless, and three were removed by their friends. Mr. Hitch adds,—" Of the individuals *discharged* and *removed* by their friends, *all are since dead,* at least so I am informed."*

There is a modification of paralysis, of much more frequent occurrence in conjunction with protracted insanity and dementia, in English hospitals for lunatics, which differs in duration and in some of its features from the paralysie générale of Esquirol. It resembles the debility of old age. Patients labouring under it are crouched, with their heads hanging forwards ; if they attempt to raise themselves into the erect posture, their limbs tremble, they stoop and totter, like men in the extremity of old age ; some stand leaning against a wall for whole days, with their bodies curved forward, and their heads and necks at an angle with the perpendicular line ; their upper extremities shake and hang useless ; such individuals are always in an advanced stage of dementia ; but in this state they remain for many years : others become bed-ridden, and remain long incapable of any voluntary movement, till at length the powers of physical life become impaired and gradually extinguished.

SECT. VIII.—*Observations on the State of the Sensorial and Intellectual Functions in Cases of Insanity.*

The inquiry in what precise changes from the healthy state, whether in structure or functions in the brain or in any other part of the organized fabric, the proximate cause of madness consists,

---

* Mr. Hitch has added to the above remarks the following details :—" Of the patients who died in the Asylum, three were examined *post m rtem* The scalp was found preternaturally thickened and fully injected ; the periosteum of the skull was also more than usually turgid ; the skull firmer than natural, the diploe wanting, and its place filled with solid osseous matter, resembling ivory more than bone ; the vessels of the dura and pia mater highly turgid ; the arachnoid raised in patches by fluid between it and the pia mater ; fluid in the ventricles ; the substance of the brain generally firmer than in other subjects, and its vessels dilated and full of dark-coloured blood."

" With reference," he adds, " to your short sketch of the progress of this peculiar palsy, I cannot omit a remark which I find in my notes on several of these cases, viz. that the tongue appeared flabby or relaxed, and larger than natural, and tremulous. I have at the same time noted a suspicion that such an indication was unfavourable. Some of the cases, however, in which this appearance was observed, have terminated in recovery, although I have also noted that a slight difficulty of utterance accompanied the tremulous state of the tongue."

belongs to the *theory* of the disease. The present is not a suitable opportunity for entering into this subject. But a correct statement of the phenomena, and, as far as these are accessible to research, of the relations of the phenomena to each other, is requisite in order to complete the *history* of insanity.

The state of the faculties is very different in the several forms of mental derangement.

The conditions of the mind and of the nervous system connected with *moral insanity*, is a subject involved in deep obscurity. The phenomena observed in this form of mental disorder are so difficult to explain, that we might be tempted to doubt its existence as a primary affection, and to refer the appearances ultimately to the unperceived influence of delusive notions impressed upon the understanding. In spite, however, of all the considerations which might incline us to this view of the subject, it must be acknowledged that the disordered feelings of insane persons, and the perverted state of their affections, are not to be explained by attributing them to erroneous impressions on the belief, which might seem sufficient to account for them. The morbid phenomena which this disease displays in the moral constitution or feelings are independent of any corresponding affection of the understanding. This is an assertion which may be proved as matter of fact ; and the appeal for proof must be made to experience and observations. The sudden anger of a person labouring under moral insanity, and subject to paroxyms of rage, is not the result of fancied provocation which the individual has sustained from him who is the victim or object of his malice. It is not the revenge of supposed injury, but an immediate impulse arising spontaneously in the mind, which is diseased only in its moral constitution.

M. Broussais, adopting M. Pinel's opinion, has admitted this fact, and offers an explanation according to his peculiar theory. He says, " There results from a perversion of the natural desire of society, cruelty, a delight in destroying, an impulse unreasonable, and even condemned by the individual by whom it is experienced, to inflict suffering upon the friends whom he tenderly loves, and to put them to death. This perversion and that of suicide are often found in conjunction. *The causes of this morbid state,"* continues M. Broussais, *" consist always in irritation of the trisplanchnic apparatus, and especially in that of the stomach, acting on the brain.* This last viscus," continues M. Broussais, " may be such, by its normal constitution, as to give a propensity to cruelty ; but in the morbid state it is a sense of uneasiness perceived through the whole splanchnic apparatus, comprehending the brain itself, which renders ideas of murder predominant in spite of reason. This horrible perversion may be considered, as well as that of suicide, as a species of chronic anger or hatred, which impels the individual sometimes against himself, sometimes against other men or against inanimate objects. We have already considered it under a subacute form in furious mania ; but in the modification in which we now describe it, it is entirely chronic and apyretic. In fact it may be extremely obstinate, and conceal itself under the appearances of calm, of joy, of benevolence, until the lunatic finds the opportunity of executing his horrible project."

" In the mediate degree of irritation, monomaniacs who are aware of such growing aversions for their friends or associates condemn these feelings, and are afflicted by the consciousness of entertaining them. There are lunatics, females especially, who grieve at the thought of no longer loving their husbands, their children, their neighbours, and for that reason alone think themselves unworthy to live."

"In its slightest degree this perversion produces moroseness, impatience, and dislike to certain individuals ; a state which we so often observe in children of different ages, and in many adult persons whose imperious, ungrateful, and selfish dispositions, skilfully dissimulated under ordinary circumstances, are sure to discover themselves on the slightest uneasiness, and especially under the existence of irritation in the digestive apparatus."*

Such is M. Broussais' theory of these phenomena. It must be allowed that various irritations, and especially those in the digestive organs, often give rise to irritability of temper; but that any such state as that which M. Broussais has described is a cause, and even the principal cause, of moral insanity, and in particular of that intense excitement of malevolent propensity which leads to murder and suicide, is a position which, before it can be admitted, requires proof ; and no such proof has been afforded by the ingenious writer who has advanced this hypothesis. It must be confessed that this subject is as yet enveloped in obscurity.

I shall now offer a few remarks on the state of the mental and sensorial faculties in other varieties of insanity.

Consciousness is generally unimpaired in persons labouring under this disease. There have been some instances in which lunatics have appeared to make singular mistakes in relation to the objects of consciousness. They have been known to talk and reason about their own feelings as if the latter belonged to or were experienced by another person. These are not frequent cases ; and in general the insane have distinct apprehension of their personal identity, and refer their sensations correctly to themselves.

Sensation likewise generally remains unimpaired in lunatics : nothing proves, at least, that the organs of sense are the seats of disease, or that those processes in the nervous and cerebral structures on which sensation depends are in a disordered state. The sensations produced by light and sound are sometimes morbidly acute ; but this arises from temporary and accidental affections of the organs of sight and hearing, or of the brain, independent of the principal disease, and is by no means characteristic of insanity. The insensibility to painful impressions which lunatics occasionally

* M. Broussais, sur l'Irritation et la Folie.

display is more nearly related to their state of derangement ; it results from the intense excitement of internal feelings, and from the attention of the mind being powerfully directed to other objects and sensations. Such instances are perhaps not so frequent as they are supposed to be ; and in general lunatics are not remarkably insensible of external impressions.

Perception of external objects is generally unimpaired, in cases of insanity, when unmodified by other contingent disorders. In some instances, however, this faculty is singularly affected by morbid impressions on the mind, or by the influence of some prevailing hallucination. Such impressions pervert the convictions to which sensation gives rise, even when that faculty itself is uninjured. I have seen an insane female confined in an asylum, who had a firm persuasion that her husband was dead. When he came to visit her, she asserted that it was the devil, who had assumed his form. Perception and memory here gave a true evidence, but the mind was preoccupied by a false opinion, and disregarded their testimony. These are instances of what Dr. Cullen terms "false judgments," or "errors as to the relations of things." Cullen very correctly divides maniacal illusions into two kinds. "There is sometimes," he says, " a false perception or imagination of things present that are not : but this is not a constant nor even a frequent attendant on the disease. The false judgment is of relations long before laid up in the memory."* This means that the illusion seldom refers to the scene actually present, but to the impressions of memory. When, however, morbid reverie becomes very intense, it produces hallucinations or false impressions which represent unreal objects as actually present. Even in this case it does not appear that perception is impaired. Some particular phantasms, the creations of reverie, are presented to the mind, otherwise diseased, in colours so vivid as to produce an effect similar to that of actual perception ; the patient in the mean while makes no mistakes with regard to place or time ; his perceptions of external objects are correct and uniform whenever his attention is directed to perceptible things ; but he is so intent upon his reverie, that for the most part he totally neglects them ; his fancy becomes so intense in its operation as to carry him away from the influence of his external perceptions, and to environ him with unreal scenes.

That insanity does not consist in disease of the sensitive or perceptive powers appears the more clearly when we compare the state of a lunatic with that of individuals who have really laboured under affections of the organs of sense, giving rise to false impressions on the sensorium. The celebrated histories of Nicolai, the father of Bonnet, and Pascal, have been cited in connection with this remark by Jacobi ;† and nothing can be more complete than the proof

---

* First Lines, ¶ 1558.
† Beobachtungen über die Pathologie und Therapie der mit Irreseyn verbundenen krankheiten, bd. i. § 99.

which they afford, that however erroneous may be the impressions
which take place under circumstances of disease in the organs of
sense themselves, the evidence of such impressions is corrected by
a sound judgment, and fails of producing erroneous belief. Such
cases are entirely distinct from those of insanity. The hallucinations of the insane, as M. Esquirol has well observed, are intellectual
phenomena totally independent of the organs of sense, and may take
place even though these organs may have been destroyed or so affected as to be no longer capable of any function. Thus there are
deaf persons who fancy that they hear words and speeches; and
blind men who think they see a variety of objects. These phenomena depend on processes carried on entirely in the brain, without any
participation on the part of the sensorial organs.*

There are cases of a morbid state coming under the denomination
of insanity which form an exception to the preceding remark, for
in them sensation itself appears to be disordered, or if not so, sensation modified by bodily disease becomes the occasional cause of
mental aberration. In these instances there is some local disorder
which gives rise to painful or unusual feelings or preternatural sensations, and the mind mistakes the cause. Reil mentions the case
of a female who became insane after suffering under a disease which
affected the nerves. She believed, in mid-day and with her eyes
open, that she was pursued by spectres of different forms and sizes.
When her eyes were covered, and light intercepted, the illusion
ceased. In a case cited by Dufour, a cataract gave rise to disorder
of the understanding, but this was only at first; when the patient
became habituated to the disease, he recovered his reason. Caspar
mentions the case of a youth who perceived the smell of fuel and
smoke, and afterwards refused sustenance under an impression that
all his food was impregnated with this offensive odour. M. Guislain, who has referred to these examples of sensorial disease, remarks that the faculties of smell and taste being more especially
connected with the functions of physical life, afford fewer instances
of morbid alteration than the other senses.†

To all those instances in which there is disorder of sensation, or
at least a diseased state of parts without the brain, affecting the organs of sense in such a way as to occasion, the mind itself being in
an unsound state, erroneous impressions and false belief, M. Esquirol proposes to affix the term *illusion*, which he distinguishes from
hallucinations, before described. As instances of illusion, M. Esquirol mentions the case of a female who fancied that she had a
living animal in her stomach, and was found on examination to have
laboured under a cancer of that viscus; and another instance of a
woman who believed that the pope was holding a council in her
belly, and who was discovered to have laboured under chronic in-

---

* Observations on the Illusions of the Insane, by M. Esquirol. Translated by
Mr. Liddell. Lond. 1833. P. 2, 3.
† Guislain, Traité d'Aliénation, tom. i.

flammation of the peritoneum. A general officer, who had become insane when labouring under rheumatism in his knee, used to seize the affected part, and striking it with the other hand exclaim, Wretch, thou shalt not escape ! supposing that he had seized a malefactor. All these are probably cases originally of the nature of hypochondriasis, in which, after that disease has long continued, the judgment gives way, and illusive notions are admitted, nearly as in the ordinary examples of monomania, the mind receives and cherishes hallucinations which coincide with the prevailing state of the sentiments and disposition. Perhaps the term *hypochondriacal illusions* would sufficiently characterise this form of mental error or disorder, without making so great a change in the ordinary acceptation of terms as that proposed by M. Esquirol.

With the exception of these cases, in which there is some previous disorder distinct from insanity and affecting the organs of sense themselves with morbid and generally painful impressions, it would appear that sensation and perception are nearly in their usual state in persons deranged as to their understanding, and that it is in the latter that the disease, or manifestation of disease, is principally seated.

But in what disturbance of the understanding itself does insanity consist ? What particular intellectual process is that which undergoes the peculiar modification characteristic of madness ? and what precisely is this modification ? It must be confessed that to these inquiries nobody has yet given a satisfactory reply. No modern writer, however, with whose works I am acquainted, has examined the subject with more attention and with greater acuteness of analysis than M. Guislain ; and if he has not succeeded in illustrating it, his failure is perhaps owing to the inscrutable nature of the research. This writer has compared the opinions of Aristotle, Descartes, Locke, Condillac, Leibnitz, Kant, and others, on the nature of the intellectual processes termed comparison, judgment, and ratiocination. He cites with peculiar approbation La Romiguière, who, in his Leçons de Philosophie, has drawn an ingenious and correct distinction between the mental operations of comparison and judgment. It is erroneous, according to La Romiguière, to term, with Condillac, this last faculty a mode of sensation. " In judging," he says, " the mind does not act. We have already acted when occupied in performing comparison ; but the perception of the relation between ideas compared comes subsequently to the act of comparing itself, and is its immediate result ; the exertion of the mind is finished in the instant when it perceives the relation." The perception of relation is, then, *judgment* in the sense which La Romiguière attaches to the expression ; comparing is the antecedent process. The relation being once recognised by the centre of perception, a new idea is acquired. "Judgment," says M. Guislain, "has for its elements our sensations ; but the *ideal object* which the mind by it perceives is totally distinct from every sensation previously obtained through the sensual organs.

"Reasoning or ratiocination is the recognition by the mind of a certain connexion between a number of such ideal objects. In this process we pass from one proposition to another: it enables us to recognise the order and disorder which exists in our thoughts, their resemblances and differences, the connection by which they approach to identity.

"If in ratiocination we recognise the act of judging as a part of the process, we yet do not confound these two operations of the understanding. Ratiocination is conversant with superior orders of ideas, which have no longer the external world for their foundation. This is the peculiar faculty of man. Some brutes appear to be endowed with a species of intelligence, but they never distinguish cause from effect, or form comparisons and judgments on the internal objects which the mind furnishes to the centre of perception."
—"We reserve the term judgment for the perception of relations which the mind receives from the external senses, while we adopt that of reasoning for the comparison which the centre of intellect makes between ideas furnished spontaneously by the understanding without the immedate aid of external sense. The act of ratiocination comprehends in it as subordinate processes—first, imagination, which furnishes the store of ideas ; secondly, attention, directed towards the ideas furnished by the mind ; thirdly, judgment exercised on its appropriate objects.

I have endeavoured to abbreviate the observations of M. Guislain on the processes of the mind in some morbid changes of which insanity may be thought to consist. He has defined them with accuracy, but has not succeeded in the discovery, what precise deviation from the healthy and usual state of these processes constitutes mental derangement. He cites the example of a man confined at Ghent, who reasons with perfect correctness on every subject, and even, his premises being allowed, on a false conviction that his wife has destroyed her children, which is the particular illusion under which he labours. To which of the intellectual operations whose united exertion constitutes the power of reasoning, are we to look, in this instance, for the deviation from health ? The individual can reason soundly on all subjects, only he can never be brought to doubt or to exercise his faculty of judging and reasoning on the subject of this false impression. The will seems in default or defective as much as or more than the power.

Perhaps we may observe in general, that the power of judging and of reasoning does not appear to be so much impaired in madness as the disposition to exercise it on certain subjects. There is often a manifest unwillingness to admit any evidence which appears contradictory to the false notion impressed upon the belief, while great ingenuity is even displayed in the attempt to find arguments which may seem to render it more reasonable.

I have endeavoured to prove in the preceding sections of this chapter, that monomaniacs begin by having disordered feelings and inclinations, and that their intellectual disease appears to follow. It is often said that judgment is independent of the will, that men are therefore irresponsible for belief or disbelief, which depends upon the evidence submitted to their judgments. Yet nothing is more certain than the great influence which the will and inclinations exercise over the understanding in the processes of ratiocination and judgment. The exercise of the mind in attention, in the performance of comparison, reflection, abstraction, judgment, reasoning, is so far a voluntary exercise that the will and inclination perpetually interfere without our consciousness, and modify the result. Most men think, believe, opine on particular subjects in harmony with the general temper of their characters, or of their sentiments and inclinations. If we could discover the particular rationale of this influence, by which the previous habitude of the mind modifies the operations which are termed, by eminence, *intellectual,* we should perhaps approach the clue which may explain the deviations from the natural state of the human mind constituting insanity.

By some writers it has been supposed that a great part of the derangement of lunatics depends on a disordered state of the faculty of attention. Professor Hoffbauer, who translated the work of Crichton, and who has been best known out of his own country as the author of a celebrated treatise on medical jurisprudence, has maintained in his "Untersuchungen über die krankheiten der seele," that many disorders of the intellect orginate from certain defects in the power of attention.* Attention has been observed to be too concentrated in monomania, and in mania altogether distracted, or in fact totally impeded in its exercise. Hence the melancholic broods particularly over one train of thoughts, and the maniac continually wanders: his attention passes in rapid transition, or rambles from one object to another. There is truth in these observations, but they do not furnish a solution of the principal difficulties which environ the subject of our investigation.

It has been well observed by M. Georget, that insane persons uniformly entertain a full conviction of their perfect sanity. "They are convinced that all that they feel and think is true, just, and reasonable ;" in a word they believe themselves in perfect health, and they often treat as fools those who do not think like them ; nothing can shake them in this conviction ; no arguments, not even the most positive proofs, can cause them to change their impressions and opinions. When they are confined, they exclaim against the injustice of the proceeding, and imperiously reclaim their liberty ; inculpate one person after another ; and accuse men and demons, actuated by envy, jealousy, revenge, as having caused their sufferings, and as persecuting them by hidden means even in their most secret thoughts." Yet, as the same author observes, there are some patients who are well aware of the disorder of their thoughts or of their affections, and who are deeply afflicted at not having sufficient strength of will to repress it.

* Hauptsitz der verstandeskrankheiten, vol. i. p. 82. in Hoffbauer's Untersuchungen.

SECTION IX.—*Disorders in the State of the Physical Functions attendant upon Madness.*

The phenomena of insanity, properly so termed as characterising the disease, are those which refer to the state of the mental faculties; but other processes of the living body, besides the functions of the brain, are likewise disordered in many, perhaps in most instances of madness. There is, in these cases, besides the morbid condition of the brain and nervous system, more or less of disturbance in the physical functions; the secretions, excretions, appetite, and digestive processes are frequently disordered. Medical writers have differed in opinion as to the relation which these affections bear to the cause of insanity. Pinel has stated it to be the result of his inquiries, that the primary seat of mental alienation is generally in the region of the stomach and intestines, and that from that centre the disease propagates itself, as it were, by irradiation, and deranges the understanding. Others have looked upon the disorders in the functions of the viscera as merely contingent results of a primary disease, seated in or immediately affecting the brain. Whichever of these opinions may be correct, the general, or at least the frequent co-existence of disorder in the physical functions with that affection of the brain from which the deranged state of the mind immediately results is an indisputable fact.

The physical functions are differently affected in different forms of madness. In disorders of slow and gradual accession, and especially in those cases in which the mind is melancholy and depressed, a torpid state of the vital and natural functions for the most part prevails; the circulation is languid; the pulse weak and generally slow; the skin cold and clammy; most of the secretions are defective; the bowels are torpid, and sometimes obstinately constipated and flatulent, requiring strong doses of aperient medicine. The appetite is defective; digestion is impaired. Emaciation and loss of strength inevitably result from these causes, but they are sometimes not so striking as any person would anticipate.

Attacks of maniacal disease, which break out suddenly with great excitement of the passions, with general disturbance of the intellectual faculties, or with incoherence, are almost always accompanied by symptoms of fever or of pyrexia more or less acute. The pulse is rapid, often full, and beating with disproportioned strength in the carotid and temporal arteries; the skin is hot and the tongue white; there is thirst, with loss of appetite, headache, sleeplessness, and great irritability; the secretions are deficient, the urine is highly coloured and scanty, and the bowels are constipated. The face is often flushed; the eyes are glossy and suffused; the conjunctiva is injected with blood, and the pupils are contracted. The patient sometimes complains of pain in the forehead and temples, with a sense of weight upon the head, or of constriction, as if the scalp were tightly drawn. Want of rest is often a troublesome and distressing symptom. Many patients pass whole nights without closing their eyes, or when they obtain sleep, it is short and agitated. In other instances a few hours of sound sleep are the prelude to a paroxysm of renewed excitement, the maniacal symptoms breaking out, on waking, with increased violence.

All the symptoms which refer themselves in a perceptible manner to the head are liable to undergo occasional exacerbations during the continuance of madness. Increased heat of the scalp, redness of the eyes, fulness and strong pulsation of the carotid and temporal arteries, want of sleep and consequent irritation of the temper and feelings, indicate and precede or accompany renewed periods of violence in the symptoms of mental derangement.

In many instances of maniacal disease there is much disturbance in the functions of the intestinal canal. This observation has been made more particularly in persons whose general health has been previously much neglected ; in the inmates of some lunatic asylums ; in individuals of the lower class, who have been subjected to hardships and unwholesome diet, as well as to cold and a damp unwholesome atmosphere ; in cases in which the disease has followed excesses of various kinds, or confinement on ship-board, with the use of salt provisions. In many instances of this description it has been found that the bowels had been long in a confined and torpid state. In those instances in which it is stated that the bowels are open and even more loose than natural, it often appears on further examination that a long-continued torpor and constipation have given way to diarrhœa ; the abdomen, which had previously been swelled with indurated matter, has become more distended than before, flatulence being added to the load of solid contents but partially discharged. The evacuations are thin and watery, or contain mucus mixed with vitiated bile and recent aliment in an undigested state. Sharp and transient pains are experienced in various parts of the abdomen, which is often tender on pressure ; at length, in very neglected cases, dysentery supervenes and brings on extreme emaciation. The tongue is often red or covered with a brown fur, and the mouth and fauces with a viscid mucus, which, together with saliva, the patient spits out in all directions. There is great thirst and a peculiar fetor of the breath, which extends to the whole person. The appetite is depraved ; in many cases the patient has an aversion to all food ; in other instances he has a keen and voracious desire for it, and greedily devours without selection every thing eatable that falls in his way. The skin is cold ; there is a remarkable coldness of the extremities, resulting from the damp state of the skin and the want of energy in the circulation through the extreme vessels. In some cases of long duration papular or scaly eruptions are observed ; and in exhausted and debilitated subjects, furunculi appear in various parts of the body, which are much disposed to slough.

Cases of madness, coming on with some degree of rapidity are often preceded and sometimes accompanied or followed by suppres-

sions of natural or customary discharges, by the disappearance of
external diseases, or the cure or suspension of internal complaints.
The relation which these changes bear to madness as causes or
results may be different in different cases ; they are connected circumstances of that disease. The catamenia, if not suppressed
previously to the manifestation of maniacal symptoms, soon become
scanty, or cease entirely after its actual appearance. Lochiæ and
other analogous effluxes are suppressed ; ulcers, which had become
habitual and had long discharged, are dried up; chronic eruptions
generally disappear, or are materially lessened ; symptoms of pulmonary phthisis in various stages cease or become mitigated in a
remarkable degree. On the decline of mental disorders, it is often
found that the return of such discharges, or the revival of suspended
trains of morbid phenomena, is the harbinger of restoration to a sound
state of mind, though not to complete bodily health.

CHAPTER III.

OF THE TERMINATIONS OF INSANITY.

SECTION I.—*General Remarks on the Duration and Terminations of Insanity.*

THE duration of insanity is various, and admits of no general
estimate. In some instances this disease has subsided within a few
days after its commencement ; in others it has continued many
years. It was observed by Dr. Greding, and the remark has been
repeated by M. Esquirol, that it is by no means uncommon to meet
with inmates of lunatic asylums who have been twenty, thirty, or
even forty years in confinement. The same observation must have
occurred to every person who has been in the habit of visiting such
establishments.

Recoveries as well as deaths take place at various intervals from
the commencement of the disease. If neither of these events occurs
at an early period, the confirmed stage of mental derangement succeeds, in which the disease begins sooner or later to assume the
character of dementia or incoherence. In this case the ultimate event
is death. For the sake of distinctness in completing the history of
insanity, it is usual to consider this disease as having three terminations ; first, in *recovery ;* secondly, in *dementia ;* and thirdly, in
death. I have already described the second of these events, and I
shall now proceed to state the facts and circumstances which are
connected with the terminations in recovery and in death.

SECTION II.—*Of Recoveries from Insanity, and, first, of the various Circumstances which have an influence on their proportional Number.*

It is important, in relation to the history of this disease, to determine, as far as this can be done, the proportion of cures or of recoveries, which take place in a given number of cases. This is also of practical importance in respect to the arrangements to be adopted for the care or restoration of lunatics. Information connected with the same inquiry is likewise of advantage for prognosis, or for estimating the prospect of recovery in particular instances of the disease.

Recovery is the event of insanity in a large proportion of cases, especially of such as occur under particular circumstances. The circumstances which have the greatest influence on the event of the disease are, its existence in a simple form, or as complicated with other disorders ; the particular character of the mental affection, some modifications of insanity being, according to universal experience, more susceptible of cure than others; the duration of the complaint, or the interval of time which has elapsed from its commencement ; the age, sex, and constitution of the patient ; and the nature of the causes which may have given rise to the disease.

I shall now consider the influence of these several circumstances and conditions before I proceed to the estimates which have been formed of the proportion of recoveries in any given number of cases.

ARTICLE I.

Of the Complication of Insanity with other Cerebral Disorders.

There are several disorders occasionally complicated with insanity. Those which have their seat in the brain may be supposed, for obvious reasons, to render, by their complication with mental derangement, recovery from that state much more difficult and improbable than it otherwise is found to be.

The complication of insanity or dementia with general paralysis is, perhaps, without exception, the most unfavourable. In the attempt to form a prognosis in any particular case, or in separating curable from incurable patients, those who are acquainted with the history of insanity examine with care whether *progression* is performed with perfect freedom and security, whether the *articulation* is free from embarrassment, or is affected by lisping or mumbling. If any of these phenomena of general paralysis are discoverable, however slight in degree, the case is usually considered as hopeless.*

Epilepsy is likewise a disease the combination of which with

* M. Calmeil, de la Paralysie des Aliénés, p. 8.

insanity is most unfavourable. But we must distinguish those instances in which fits of convulsion, more or less displaying the epileptic character, occur in maniacal cases during the periods of high excitement, from the violent mania which appears as the sequel or occasional interlude of severe and inveterate epilepsy. It is the latter combination which is so deplorable: fits, more or less resembling epileptic paroxysms, sometimes occur under the circumstances above described, without rendering the case desperate, or even appearing to exercise much influence on its tenor; yet they are to be regarded, under all circumstances, as unfavourable indications.

ARTICLE II.

The form of the disease.

The form of the disease is of great consequence in respect to the probable event. "At Charenton, as every where," says M. Esquirol, " a greater proportion in the cases of mania are cured than of any other variety of madness. He adds that dementia is scarcely ever cured.† Out of 209 recoveries at Charenton, the numbers were as follows:

Mania	115 cases out of	226
Monomania ·	91 ,,	289
Dementia	3 ,,	99
	209	614

It must be observed that in the aggregate of cases were included 109 paralytics, 19 epileptics, and 4 idiots ; so that the number of curable cases of insanity from which an estimate is to be formed of the success of medical treatment is reduced to 487 ; and of this number upwards of two-fifths were cured. It is remarkable that the greater sanability of maniacs, in comparison with monomaniacs, had place only in males. From this it would appear that monomania is comparatively a more curable disease in females than in men.

ARTICLE III.

The period of the disease.

The previous duration of the disease is a circumstance of great importance in estimating, at any given time, its probable termination. The probability of recovery is very much greater in the early than in the advanced periods. Dr. Willis declared that 9 lunatics out of 10 recovered, if they were placed under his care within three months from the attack. Dr. Burrows has reported 221 cures out

* Statistique, p. 136, in the " Annales d'Hygiène ; item, art. *Folie* in Dict. des Sciences Méd.

of 242 recent cases. Dr. Finch has stated that 61 out of 69 patients recovered who were received into his asylum within three months after the first attack of their disorder. From the experience obtained at the Retreat near York, to which I shall have occasion again in the sequel to advert, it appears that 7 out of 8, or perhaps a larger proportion of recent cases have terminated in recovery.

The inquiry during what time recovery is still probable, and what degrees of probability there are at different periods, has been frequently pursued, especially by French writers. Some facts, tending to illustrate this question, were contained in a memoir presented by M. Pinel to the National Institute in 1800. It appeared from this memoir that the greatest number of recoveries from madness take place in the first month of its duration ; the recoveries during the first being compared with those of succeeding months. The mean time for the duration of the disease, in cases terminating favourably, was fixed in the same document at from five to six months. This result was deduced from a selection of cases from which the author excluded all those which had been under previous treatment, as well as cases of long duration. A longer term is assigned to this disease, in cases terminating in recovery, by Mr. Tuke in his account of the Retreat at York ; and M. Esquirol, whose accuracy of research in subjects of this nature gives to his authority the highest value, confirms the opinion of Mr. Tuke. He has drawn this conclusion from a statement of the cases admitted into the Salpêtrière during ten years, as shown by the following table:—

Table of recoveries at the Salpêtrière during ten years.

Admissions.	1804.	1805.	1806.	1807.	1808.	1809.	1810.	1811.	1812.	1813.	1814.	Totals of Cures.
209	64	47	7	4	3	2	..	1	1	..	..	129
212		73	54	4	2	2	1	..	..	..	1	137
206			78	49	10	3	1	1	1	..	..	143
204				60	55	11	1	..	2	..	..	129
188					64	57	4	2	1	..	2	130
209						48	64	9	4	1	3	129
190							48	51	7	1	3	110
163								44	30	8	3	85
208									75	41	11	127
216										50	49	99
2005												1218

It seems that the report on which this table was founded extended from the year 1804 to 1813; 2804 female lunatics were admitted during this interval, of whom 795 were considered as incurable, on account of their advanced age, or because they were idiotic, epileptic, or paralytic subjects. The remaining 2005 were put under treatment without regard to the duration or peculiar character of their disease. Out of this number, 604 were cured during the first

year, 497 in the second, 86 in the third, and 41 in the seven succeeding years. From these data M. Esquirol draws the following
conclusions : first, that the greatest number of recoveries are obtained
in the two first years ; secondly, that the mean duration of cases
that are cured is somewhat short of one year ; thirdly, that after
the third year the probability of cure is scarcely more than one in
thirty.

From another table published by M. Esquirol, it appears that, out
of 269 maniacal patients, 27 were cured in the first month of their
illness, 34 in the second, 18 in the third, 30 in the fourth, 24 in the
fifth, 20 in the sixth, 20 in the seventh, 19 in the eighth, 12 in the
ninth, 13 in the tenth, 23 after the first year, and 18 after two years.
The same writer has made a remark in illustration of the greater
proportion of recoveries observed in the early period of madness,
which is worthy of attention. He says, " I have constantly observed that in the course of the first month from the commencement of
the disease a very marked remission takes place. About that period
the maniacal excitement, which had previously run its course as an
acute disorder, seems to have reached its termination as such, and it
is then that it passes into a chronic state,. the crisis having been
incomplete. This remission, which I have watched with the greatest accuracy, must be attributed to the complaints which are complicated with madness at its commencement." The author implies,
though he does not clearly express himself, that the natural termination of the disease, when not interrupted by the coexistence of
other maladies, or by organic lesion in the brain, is in the very
early stage.

The following table of recoveries at the Gloucester Lunatic
Asylum,* drawn up by Mr. Hitch, affords similar results. It
includes cases of very long duration, and will be found so much the
more interesting.

* The Gloucester Lunatic Asylum is under the superintendence of Dr. Shute.
Mr. Hitch is the resident medical officer.

MALES.—TABLE I. *Showing the time that each case required for its treatment to effect recovery; arranged in a line with the length of time it had existed prior to admission.*

Time occupied in the treatment to effect recovery.

Duration of the disease prior to admission.	No. of Cases
1 week ...	91
2 "	11
3 "	11
4 "	17
5 "	5
6 "	3
7 "	3
8 "	8
12 "	14
4 months..	5
5 "	1
6 "	6
7 "	1
8 "	1
9 "	0
10 "	1
1 year ...	6
2 "	11
3 "	7
4 "	1
8 "	1
10 "	3
11 "	0
15 "	1
40 "	1

* These three cures occurred in the same individual, whose recovery from the time respectively stated. The relapses occurred at intervals of four months: he is now well. I usually denominate such cases "relieved."

FEMALES.—TABLE 1. *Showing the time that each case required for its treatment to effect recovery; arranged in a .ine with the length of time it had existed prior to admission.*

Time occupied in the treatment to effect recovery.

Duration of the disease prior to admission.	No. of Cases.	Y.	M.	Y.	M.	Y.	M.	Y.	M.	Y.	M.	Y.	M.	Y.	M.	Y.	M.	Y.	M.	Y.	M.	Y.	M.	Y.	M.	Y.	M.	Y.	M.	Y.	M.	Y.	M.	Y.	M.	Y.	M.	Y.	M.	Y.	M.	Y.	M.	Y.	M.
1 week ...	11	3			10		20		60		20		10		30		50		10		40		70		90		20		30		30		20		41		00		30		80		4
2 "	11	1			30		30		40		30		50		30		20		50		2		30																				
3 "	4				30		30	3																																		
4 "	22				60		40		20	3			20				11		100		40		30		3																
5 "	3				40		60		6		1		6																													
6 "	6	1			50		60	1			10		7	1																												
8 "	9	3		1			70		40		30		40		80																												
12 "	13	1		6	2		20		100		40		10		21		9						30		3																
4 months	3				20		70		7																																
5 "	9				100		100																																		
6 "	8				30		30	100			30		20		5						70																				
7 "	0																																								
8 "	2	1		3	0		40				90		30		3																										
9 "	1	1			0		50				90		50	40		9																									
10 "	6				0		40		40		20		40																												
1 year ...	5				02		50																																		
2 "	2				4																																				
3 "	1				0																																				
4 "	0				91																																				
8 "	2			9																																					
10 "	1	4		3																																					
11 "	1	3		3																																					
17 "	1	3		6																																					
20 "																																										

Although the probability of cure after the third year is so small, there are, notwithstanding, as we find from these tables, examples which prove that we ought never to despair of the recovery of lunatics ; and M. Pinel, from Baumes, cites the case of a lady who passed twenty-five years in a state of lunacy, within the knowledge of the whole country where she lived, and who suddenly recovered her reason. "I have seen," says the same writer, "a girl who from the age of ten years was in a state of incoherence, with suppression of the catamenia. One day, on rising from bed, she ran and embraced her mother, exclaiming, 'Mamma, I am well!' The catamenia had just flowed spontaneously, and her reason was immediately restored. M. Esquirol has repeated this relation, adding his own evidence. He has reported other facts of a similar kind. "Tout le midi a retenti, il y a quelques années, de la guérison d'une dame qui après vingt-trois ans fut guérie spontanément d'un accès de manie compliqué de fureur." M. Chambeyron observed, at the Salpêtrière, a young woman who fell into a state of dementia after a maniacal fit. She cut open her abdomen with a scissors. A portion of intestine and nearly the whole of the epiploon came out through the wound. As soon as suppuration was established, the intellects of the patient appeared sound. After the cicatrization a large blister was applied, and the improvement was for a time maintained. At the time when the report was given, the state of the individual still gave much greater promise of her restoration than could be entertained before the accident which changed the character of the disorder. M. Esquirol adds, "Que de faits je pourrais citer de guérisons inattendues ou tardives, qui ont trompé l'expérience la plus étendue, et les calculs les plus sévères."* These facts are sufficient to prove that in the duration of the disease alone there is no reason to despair altogether of recovery. A few instances of the same kind have occurred in several lunatic houses or public hospitals, from the superintendents of which I have obtained information. Some striking and, indeed, surprising examples may be seen in the above table of the Gloucester Asylum.

ARTICLE IV.

Age.

The age of patients is a consideration of great importance as to the prospect of recovery. M. Esquirol observes that the most favourable age for recovery is between the twentieth and thirtieth year, and that few are cured after the fiftieth year. The same writer has given a table of ages in reference to the 209 recoveries at Charenton, to which I have before alluded. In this it seems that the greatest number of cures were from the twenty-fifth to the thirtieth, and from the thirtieth to the thirty-fifth year. This is the period of life during which the greatest physical energy subsists, and in which

* M. Esquirol's notes to Hoffbauer.

acute madness breaks out most frequently, while intermittent or recurrent cases have not yet had time to pass into the continued form.   Recoveries diminish progressively from the forty-fifth year to the end of life.   The diminution is more abrupt in females, and more uniform in men.   We must observe that cases occurring before the twentieth year are the most numerous in males, and that the greatest number of attacks manifest themselves in men from twenty to twenty-five, and from twenty-five to thirty.   In females the greatest frequency begins between twenty-five and thirty, and it is not diminished until after forty-five.   The table before cited shows that advanced age does not preclude hope : twenty men are marked as having recovered after the fiftieth year, in which number were four out of twelve lunatics who had exceeded their seventieth years.*

ARTICLE V.

Sex.

It has been observed by many writers that insanity is, generally speaking, more curable in women than in men.

ARTICLE VI.

Season.

The summer produces a greater number of recoveries than other seasons. If we divide the aggregate of recoveries by trimestres, it appears that they are most numerous in that of the summer and autumn.   Summer being the season at which violent mania most frequently breaks out, and this form of the disease being more rapid in its course than others, it may be supposed the greatest number of males will probably be cured in the summer : females recover in greater numbers during the autumnal months.   These observations, made by M. Esquirol on the report of Charenton, coincide with those formerly obtained by him from the hospitals of Bicêtre and the Salpêtrière.†

ARTICLE VII.

Circumstances of the constitution.

When insanity is manifestly connected with some condition of the natural functions which is susceptible of change by the progress of life or by medical art, there is on this ground hope of a favourable termination.   Recoveries take place in females at critical periods. M. Esquirol has related that he observed two instances of dementia in females which had continued from early youth and terminated at the appearance of the catamenia.   Another female at the Salpêtrière,

---

* Statistique de la Maison Royale de Charenton, p. 135.
† Statistique, et artic. Folie in Dict. des Sc. Méd.

whose derangement began at that period, recovered at the time of life when the catamenia cease.*

SECTION III.—*Of the proportional Number of Recoveries in general.*

· The proportional number of cures effected, or to speak more accurately, of recoveries which take place in any given number of cases of insanity, is very differently estimated by different writers.

Dr. Burrows has reported from his own experience 240 cures in an aggregate of 296 cases of various descriptions ; 221 cures from 242 recent cases ; 19 cures from 64 old cases ; affording a proportion of 81 in 100 of all cases, and of 91 in 100 of recent cases.

So great a proportion of recoveries, which, however, coincides nearly with the statements of Dr. Willis, has surprised many persons. Dr. Maximilian Jacobi says that it can only be explained by referring to the practice which he believes to prevail in England, of discharging patients from lunatic asylums at a very early period after apparent recovery, or as soon as the phenomena of insanity have ceased for a time to be displayed, and before a real and permanent cure has been obtained. Dr. Jacobi has given a report of cases admitted into a new public asylum under his management at Siegburg in Westphalia, where he says that patients are always retained until their recovery is confirmed, and this he considers as affording a more just example of the ordinary proportion of recoveries, though still, as he supposes, more favourable than the general average in hospitals which admit patients of all descriptions. In this, out of 100 cases, 40 are marked as dismissed in a state of complete recovery, and 6 as improved and displaying alleviation of the disease.†

Dr. Jacobi is certainly under an error as to the practice which he imputes to the superintendents of lunatic asylums in England, of dismissing patients before their recovery is established. It is plainly not the interest of those who conduct private establishments to err on this side, and in most of the public hospitals in this country the proportion of recoveries is by no means so great as to require such an explanation. The subject to which these inquiries refer is one of so much importance that my readers will probably be interested with a more extensive collection of the facts which bear upon it.

M. Esquirol has for many years carried on very extensive and accurate researches into the statistics of lunatic establishments, in which he has been followed by physicians in different countries, particularly by Dr. Burrows and Sir A. Halliday in England, by M. Guislain in Belgium, and by Dr. Jacobi in the Prussian territories

---

* Esquirol. See Jacobi's Sammlungen für die Heilkunde der Gemüthskrankheiten, B. i. s. 339.

† Beobachtungen über die Pathologie und Therapie der mit Irreseyn verbundenen Krankheiten von Dr. Max. Jacobi. Elberfeld, 1830, p. 173.

on the Rhine. In these inquiries the proportion of recoveries forms
the most interesting topic.

In a table given by M. Esquirol in the Dictionnaire des Sciences
Médicales, we find the following calculation of recoveries taken
from the reports of French asylums.

French Lunatic Asylums.	Dates.	Admissions.	Recoveries.
Charenton . . . . . . from Nov. 22,	1798 to 1800, 22 July	97 ..	33.
	1803	499 ..	161
Salpêtrière . . . . from	1801 to 1805 ..	1002 ..	407
„ . . . . from	1804 to 1813 ..	2005 ..	1218
„ . . . . from	1806 to 1807 ..	531 ..	286
„ . . . . from	1812 to 1814 ..	891 ..	413
In M. Esquirol's private establishment . . . . from	1801 to 1813 ..	335 ..	173
	Totals ..	5360 ..	2691

In a more extended calculation given in the first volume of the
Memoirs of the Royal Academy of Medicine, we are informed that
out of 12,592 cases of insanity which were treated in the Salpêtrière
and the Bicêtre, 4968 cures were registered.

M. Esquirol has lately reported that at the Royal Hospital of
Charenton, on a totality of cases occurring in 1826–1828, including
incurable cases of all descriptions, one-third of recoveries was obtained,—a proportion which he says may be honourably compared
to that of any other hospital equally indiscriminate in admissions.*
Nearly the same results was declared in a report made officially in
Paris in 1825, of the state of hospitals for lunatics during the three
preceding years. Dr. Burrows has copied this report, in which it
appears that in an aggregate of 2506 cases, including those deemed
curable and incurable, the recoveries were 34 in 100 or 1 in 2.90.†

The following statements were collected by M. Esquirol from
English lunatic hospitals.

English Lunatic Asylums.	Dates.	Admissions.	Recoveries.
In Bethlem Hospital .. from 1748 to 1794	..	8874 ..	2557
„ „ . in . . . . , . . 1813	..	422 ..	204
In St. Luke's . . . . from 1751 to 1801	..	6458 ..	2811
In York Asylum		599 ..	286
In the Retreat near York from 1801 to 1814	..	163 ..	60
	Totals	16516 ..	5918

From this calculation it appears that the proportion of cures
formerly obtained in English lunatic asylums was in some instances
less than that which is reported from the celebrated hospitals in
France. This is the more remarkable when we take into our account the peculiar regulations of the great lunatic establishments
of London. The hospitals of Bethlem and St. Luke impose certain
exclusions elsewhere unknown. They reject all patients who have

* Statistique de la Maison Royale de Charenton.
† Dr. Burrows' Commentaries on Insanity, p. 251.

been more than twelve months insane ; those affected by paralysis, however slight, and by epilepsy or convulsive fits ; idiots, the aged and infirm ; those discharged uncured from other hospitals : there are likewise other exclusions besides those above mentioned, and all persons who have not recovered at the expiration of one year are dismissed. Yet, on comparing the reports of these hospitals with those of other institutions, the regulations of which are less favourable to a high proportion of cures, and where no selection or exclusion exists, we do not find, as Dr. Burrows remarks, the relative number of recoveries to be so great as might be expected. It is indeed surprising to observe that the reports of Bethlem Hospital, of a century and a half ago, give a greater proportion of cures than those of many years preceding 1817, when an improvement took place in the arrangements of that establishment. Dr. Burrows remarks on the authority of Stow, who derived his information from Dr. Tyson, physician to Bethlem Hospital, that "from 1684 to 1703, 1294 patients were admitted, of whom 890 were cured, which is a proportion of two in three. But from 1784 to 1794, 1664 patients were admitted, of whom 574, or rather more than one in three, recovered.

We cannot explain the difference which is displayed by this statement. It is impossible to imagine that any want of attention or of skill in the superintendence of the hospital or in the treatment of the disease would adequately account for so great a difference in the results, and there is, I presume, no ground for entertaining the suspicion that any such defect really existed.

A much more favourable average of recoveries has taken place in the recent admissions at Bethlem Hospital, since the removal of the institution to its new site, and the alterations that have been made in its arrangement. The following report, which I have obtained through the kindness of Mr. Lawrence, sufficiently proves this fact.

| Remaining from | Admissions. | Discharged. | | | | Died. | Remaining. |
		Cured.	Uncured.	By request of friends.	Improper objects.		
1819	81						
1820	124	60	33	11	22	4	
1821	135	43	36	7	28	6	
1822	165	66	43	5	27	11	
1823	145	72	49	4	19	5	
1824	155	59	55	5	31	6	
1825	170	70	48	7	29	12	
1826	162	70	63	6	24	6	
1827	149	64	41	2	15	9	
1828	204	111	48	6	34	6	
1829	195	126	42	2	29	10	
1830	201	110	45	4	30	6	
1831	212	98	55	5	41	6	
1832	163	92	41	2	35	5	
1833	184	83	44	4	21	7	124
	2445	1124	643	70	385	99	124

In order to estimate the result of the plan on which the hospital of Bethlem is instituted, we must subtract from the entire aggregate of admissions the number of patients who were subsequently excluded as improper objects. Thus 2445—385=2060 will be the total number from which 1124 cures were obtained, amounting to considerably more than one-half of the aggregate. It is probable, from the result of the facts before stated in reference to the periods of the disease at which recoveries are obtained, that a great proportion of patients discharged uncured were still curable. We have seen that among the patients of the Salpêtrière, the number cured during the second year are nearly as five in six to those who recovered during the first. If we might presume that among the patients dismissed from Bethlem at the end of the first year, which is understood to be the case with those who are still uncured, a proportion of curable cases still remains, approaching nearly to that which exists in the Salpêtrière among the patients who remain still uncured in the hospital at the expiration of their first year, this would raise the recoveries at Bethlem to a very high proportion indeed. We are not authorized to draw any positive conclusion on this subject, but we can hardly fail to entertain a strong doubt as to the propriety of the regulation still subsisting at Bethlem, and a suspicion that it is a relic of the ignorance of our predecessors which calls loudly for such a revision and adaptation to the improved state of knowledge, as would ere now have been obtained under our continental neighbours.

The following reports from English provincial lunatic asylums are taken from Dr. Burrows. They display a greater proportion of recoveries than the returns given by M. Esquirol, and very nearly agree with the report from Siegburg. I believe that in the hospitals to which they refer, no principle of selection is adopted.

In Stafford Asylum, from 1818 to 1828, admissions 1000 ; cured 429 ; or about 43 in 100.

In Wakefield County Asylum for the West Riding of Yorkshire, from 1819 to 1826, admissions 917; cured 384; or about 42 in 100.

I have obtained a later and more ample report of the Lancaster County Asylum, through the kindness of Dr. Whally.

Report of the Lancaster County Asylum.

Dates.	Admissions.		Recoveries.		Deaths.		Remain or dismissed uncured.	
Admitted before June 24.	Male.	Female.	Male.	Female.	Male.	Female.	Male.	Female.
1817	35	25	7	1	3	0	25	24
1818	75	48	12	4	10	10	70	59
1819	35	17	15	10	9	2	79	64
1820	44	36	24	14	26	6	71	77
1821	38	22	12	9	9	6	88	82
1822	62	42	16	16	12	5	117	102
1823	63	52	20	15	21	12	135	120
1824	44	43	21	25	14	18	137	117
1825	76	55	35	20	18	18	158	132
1826	60	48	39	26	38	27	137	123
1827	83	52	27	26	37	20	144	128
1828	57	57	31	18	24	20	143	146
1829	76	58	22	22	33	15	160	164
1830	76	63	35	30	30	16	166	178
1831	83	62	37	37	39	21	166	180
1832	90	72	34	35	42	37	177	186
Totals ..	997	753	389	308	344	233		
Gen. Totals	1750		697		577			

Here the recoveries are to the admissions within a small fraction of 2.5, or about 40 in 100.

The following is a similar report of the Gloucester Asylum drawn up by Mr. Hitch.

Report containing the annual statements of admissions into the Lunatic Asylum at Gloucester from the period of its opening.

	Before July, 1823.	1824.	1825.	1826.	1827.	1828.	1829.	1830.	1831.	1832.
Patients already in the house	0	57	75	78	79	90	91	101	103	92
Admitted in the year	68	43	47	37	67	54	55	63	35	45
	68	100	122	115	140	144	146	164	138	137
Recovered	7	11	23	16	31	29	25	40	23	26
Relieved*	1	4	8	5	4	2	0	6	1	1
Removed†	1	5	6	7	14	12	7	10	17	12
Died	2	5	7	8	7	10	4	5	5	4
	11	25	44	36	56	53	45	61	46	43
Total number admitted from the opening	68	111	158	105	262	316	373	436	471	516
Total of recoveries	7	18	41	57	88	117	142	182	205	231

* Many of these are stated to have been discharged on trial, and to have recovered in a short time after their dismissal.

† Removed either by request of friends or as harmless and incurable, some of them demented, or subject to epilepsy of long duration.

The proportion of recoveries, without taking into the account a considerable number which afterwards took place among those dismissed as relieved and on trial, is here very great, viz. 234 in 516, which approaches nearly to one-half of the total number admitted ; a circumstance the more striking, as no selection is used in the admission, lunatics of all descriptions being reckoned fit objects to receive the benefits resulting from this excellent establishment.

A highly favourable result has been afforded by the experience of the Retreat near York. I have obtained, through the kindness of Mr. Tuke, a table exhibiting the numbers of admissions into this asylum from 1812 to 1833 inclusive, with the results of all the cases. The admissions of each year are divided into three classes, one for cases of less than three months in duration, a second for cases of more than three but less than twelve months, and a third for cases of more than twelve months ; to these three a fourth class is added for cases of relapse re-admitted. The summary of this table will convey the general results : it is as follows :—

Cases classed as above.	Recovered.	Died.	Removed.	Removed improved.	Remain.
First class . . 63	51	8	1	2	1
Second class . 65	28	10	6	3	18
Third class . 101	31	15	17	4	34
Fourth class . 105	58	17	13	1	16
Total . 334	168	50	37	10	69

From this table it appears that out of three hundred and thirty-four admitted between the years 1812 and 1833 inclusive, one hundred and sixty eight have recovered, fifty have died, thirty-seven have been removed by the friends unimproved, and ten in an improved state, and sixty-nine remain.*

Of the eight deaths reported in the first class of cases, four took place very soon after admission ; one by phthisis, under which the patient laboured in an advanced stage at the period of admission ; one by apoplexy, of which the patient had had fits prior to admission ; one from self-injury ; one from fever, the case having been one, not of insanity, but of febrile delirium. It is obvious that these cases ought in all fairness to be subtracted from the number of admissions, when we attempt to estimate the probability of recovery ; and this, joined to another consideration, will raise the proportion in recent cases, as Mr. Tuke has pointed out, from somewhat below 7 in 8, the rate at which he has estimated it, to somewhat above 9 in 10. The consideration referred to is the following. Several cases entered in the most recent class were those of persons who had been long eccentric, and whose aberration had only advanced a short step beyond that state by which they had been always or long

---

* Previously to 1811 there had been twenty-nine cases admitted of the most recent class, of which twenty-six are reported to have been dismissed *recovered*.

characterised, but of which the partiality or the familiarity of friends and relations had hardly allowed them to suspect the real nature. " These," says Mr. Tuke, " are properly old cases ; and if we were to exclude these from our list together with those connected with disorders speedily terminating life as consumption and apoplexy, I should say that, according to the result of our experience, the probability of recovery from insanity in recent cases is greater than as nine to one."

Section IV.—Of the Termination of Insanity in Death.

Insanity is not to be reckoned among the diseases which are very dangerous to life. The state of the brain on which it depends, though incompatible with the continuance in a sound state of those functions with which the mental operations are associated, is yet such as to carry on other processes, dependent on the brain, which are subservient to physical existence.

This conclusion is established in a most convincing manner by the duration of insanity, and the cases even of longevity which occur among lunatics. We are informed by M. Desportes that among the lunatics at Bicêtre in the beginning of the year 1822, one had been lodged there fifty-six years, three upwards of forty years, twenty-one more than thirty years, fifty upwards of twenty years, one hundred and fifty-seven more than ten years. At the Salpêtrière the entry of patients was dated, seven cases from fifty to fifty-seven years, eleven from fifty to sixty, seventeen from forty to fifty.

I. The morbid state of the brain is, however, liable to increase beyond the limit above adverted to, and then the usual phenomena dependent on severe cerebral disease are manifested. It is well known that lunatics are subject in a much greater proportion than other persons to apoplexy, paralysis, convulsions, and all the trains of symptoms depending on different degrees or modifications of cerebral congestion.*

II. Another mode by which madness brings on a fatal termination is by the exhaustion arising from continued excitement. There are many cases of maniacal disease in which the ceaseless excitement of the feelings, the constant hurry of mind and agitation of body, the total want of rest and sleep, and the febrile disturbance of the system which frequently ushers in the attack of madness, and is a prominent feature in cases of this description, bring on a very marked reduction of strength as well as of flesh : the degree of emaciation is sometimes extreme. In general this state of excitement gradually abates, or the means adopted to lessen it and tranquilize the system are attended with success : but this is not uniformly the case, and some maniacs die completely worn out and exhausted. It is in part owing to this cause that the mortality among lunatics is more considerable during the two first years from the period of their attack than in the succeeding years, a fact which appears to be established by the calculations of M. Esquirol. In the Salpêtrière the number of deaths is even much greater in the first year than in the second. Of seven hundred and ninety lunatics who perished in that hospital between the years 1804 and 1814, it appears that three hundred and eighty-two died in the first year from their admission, two hundred and twenty-seven in the second year, and one hundred and eighty-one during the seven succeeding years.

Many lunatics are carried off by diseases of the abdominal and thoracic viscera, which are complicated with madness. Pathology does not enable us to explain the connection between organic diseases of the lungs or bowels and disorders in the condition of the brain, and hence many have been inclined to regard the combinations of morbid states to which we now advert as accidental. They are perhaps too numerous to be attributed to chance. The combination of madness, as well as of some other affections of the brain and nervous system, with morbid states of the liver and the intestinal canal, was pointed out some years since in my work On Diseases of the Nervous System. The conjunction of insanity with pulmonary phthisis is a fact established beyond doubt by the observations of M. Esquirol, who remarks that phthisis often precedes the appearance of melancholia, or accompanies it. The disease of the lungs is in such instances latent ; the patients lose their strength, become emaciated and suffer under slow fever, sometimes attended with cough and diarrhœa; the phenomena of madness rather increase than abate under these circumstances, and continue until death. On the examination of the body, the lungs are found tuberculated or affected by melanosis.*

Diseases of the heart are not unfrequently complicated with madness. We are assured by M. Foville, that, of the bodies of lunatics which he examined after death during three years, five out of six displayed some organic disease of either the heart or the great vessels. This was very frequently hypertrophy of the heart. These morbid changes, however, are probably, as M. Foville has observed, more frequently results of the continued agitation, the violent efforts and cries, which in such patients bring on diseases in the thoracic organs, than predisposing causes of cerebral disorder. That this, in some instances at least, is the true explanation of such facts I am convinced from my own observation.

Diseases of the intestinal canal, whether they exist or not at the

---

* Dr. Greding, of Waldheim, found that forty out of one hundred maniacs, and twenty of twenty-four melancholics, laboured under pulmonary phthisis. The same writer says that seventy-six among one hundred maniacs, and twenty among twenty-four melancholics, were found to have effusion either in one or in both of the cavities of the thorax.—See *Crichton's Extracts from Greding on Insanity.*

onset of the maniacal attack, are among the frequent causes
of death. A state of obstinate constipation often continues for
a long time, attended by its usual accompaniments. It gives way,
and is followed by or alternates with diarrhœa, which wastes the
strength of the patient and terminates in a fatal dysentery. When
the body is examined, the intestines are found sometimes distended
and loaded with indurated matter, at others empty and pale, with
disease of the mucous coat, discoloured and abraded patches or
ulceration, and gangrenous spots.

In protracted cases death either results from increase in the
disease of the brain, which disease up to a certain degree had only
interfered with the operations subservient to the mental faculties,
but at length becomes incompatible with the merely physical functions of the same organ ; or it is the result of accidental disorders,
which, owing to the peculiar state of the brain and other organs in
lunatics, are more than usually fatal to them.

Many lunatics in the advanced stage labour under a degree of
cachexia bordering on scurvy. The skin is beset with scaly or
papular eruptions, or discoloured in patches; furunculi appear in
different parts of the body, which are much disposed to become
sloughy; the gums become red and sore, and bleed; the surface of
the body is cold, with a clammy perspiration ; diarrhœa and abdominal pains accompany these symptoms; the patient apparently
suffers under defective nutrition and a gradual decay of physical life,
and dies in a state of extreme emaciation or marasmus.

The preceding are perhaps the natural results of the diseases
under which lunatics suffer in connection with their original complaint. A great number, however, are carried off by disorders
which may be considered as accidental, but to which the condition
of body in patients of this description renders them more than other
individuals liable. Fevers which assume more or less of the typhoid
character, severe catarrhs, and pulmonary affections, are the most
frequent of these. It will be supposed that fevers which affect the
brain are fatal to lunatics, and such is the fact in a very marked
degree.

The diagnosis of accidental diseases in lunatics presents, as M.
Georget has well observed, remarkable difficulties. Some patients
of this description are continually making unfounded complaints,
deceived by their erroneous or fancied sensations. " On the other
hand, many lunatics labour under very severe affections without
revealing them by any expression, either because these affections
are latent and do not occasion suffering, or because the disturbed
state of their minds does not allow their sensations to reach the
centre of perception. In this last relation the medical treatment of
lunatics is much more obscure and difficult than that of young children, because the latter are conscious of their ailments, and express
them by their cries. When we observe a lunatic, who had previously been agitated and furious, become morose and taciturn, and
at the same time lose appetite, seek repose, and display a suffe-

ring and dejected expression, we ought to examine him carefully: he is threatened with some acute disease. The development of symptoms will soon point out the seat and nature of the complaint, and consequently by what remedies it is to be opposed. But chronic affections are so slow in their approach and concealed in respect to their symptoms, that they often reach to a very advanced stage before their existence is suspected, unless the organs affected are examined before their diseased condition has manifested itself. We find the lungs full of tubercles, with cavernous excavations and abscesses, or in a state of atrophy, in the bodies of individuals who had neither coughed nor expectorated, nor experienced pain or dyspnœa during life ; they had become gradually debilitated, had taken to their beds, and after a continually increasing emaciation, had at length sunk. The disorganization of the lungs had only been discovered by the aid of auscultation and percussion. We must not then wait for the expression of complaints on the part of lunatics, in order to have due watchfulness excited to the means which are necessary for preserving their existence."

The following table given by M. Esquirol, in his statistical report of the Royal House of Charenton, serves to illustrate the comparative mortality resulting from different forms of madness.

Table of mortality in relation to different varieties of derangement.

	Men.	Women.	Totals.
Mania	39	21	60
Monomania	25	18	43
Dementia	89	26	115
Idiotism	0	1	1
Died after recovering from insanity	2	0	2
Totals	155	66	221

"The mortality fell chiefly on persons in a state of dementia. This," as M. Esquirol observes, "is to be expected, since dementia is almost always the ultimate condition to which continued insanity leads, of whatever form, and because dementia is the form of disease with which paralysis is chiefly complicated. There is likewise to be remarked a great difference between the numbers of men who sink under dementia and those of women : thus we have in the former eighty-nine, and twenty-six in the latter. Next to dementia mania is the most fatal, and it is more destructive to men than to women : this, however, is explained by the circumstances that we admit more men than women, and that men are more subject to mania than women."[*]

* Statistique, ubi supra, p. 108.

It appears generally that the mortality at Charenton was much greater among the male than among the female patients. This is attributed in part to the comparatively greater prevalence of general paralysis among the former. The fact is equally striking in the reports of some English hospitals, as in that of the Lancaster Lunatic Asylum, given in a previous section, in which the deaths of males are 344 in 997, or about 1 in 3, and those of females are 233 in 753, or about 1 in 3½. Among the lunatics in St. Peter's Hospital in Bristol, the difference is still greater in the relative numbers of deaths of males and females ; and Mr. Brady, the intelligent medical officer under whose immediate care the patients are placed, has assigned this difference to the cause suggested by M. Esquirol. With respect to the mortality at different seasons, it is observed by M. Esquirol that in general the months of December, January, and February, are the most fatal to deranged persons.

SECTION V.—*Of Relapses, and of recurrent Insanity.*

Recoveries from madness are in many instances complete. There are numerous persons who have been insane for six or twelve months, or during a longer period, and have afterwards entirely recovered the vigour of their intellectual faculties, so as to be capable of as great and effective mental exertions as previously to the attack. Others, and perhaps these are the majority, are curable only to a certain point. These persons remain, as M. Esquirol has observed, in such a state of susceptibility that the slightest causes give rise to relapses, and they only preserve their sanity by continuing to live in a house where no mental agitation or inquietude, no unfortunate contingency is likely to fall to their lot, and throw them back into their former state. There are other individuals whose faculties have sustained such a shock that they are never capable of returning to the sphere which they had held in society. They are perfectly rational, but have not sufficient mental capacity to become again military officers, to conduct commercial affairs, or to fulfil the duties belonging to their appointments. Such cases may be about one-tenth in the number of recoveries.

Convalescents are subject to relapse as are those who are advancing towards recovery from other diseases. But lunatics are in many instances likewise prone to a recurrence of the disease after it has been entirely removed, or at least after its manifestations have long ceased to be observed. The same observation may be applied to other disorders of the nervous system. It would seem that one attack of disease has in these cases left the patient with a stronger predisposition than he formerly had to the complaint, whatever it may have been, and that the morbid tendency is strengthened after every renewed incursion. The most trifling circumstances have in these instances sufficient influence to produce the morbid condition of the brain and of the mind. At length the patient is scarcely ever in a lucid state ; the intervals lessen in duration, and become more and more imperfect in degree, until finally the disease is in a great measure permanent.

The proportion of cases in which madness is recurrent has been overrated. According to M. Pinel, in 71 cases out of 444 recoveries relapse took place, or, rather, the disease was in those instances recurrent. This gives somewhat less than one-sixth of the whole number as recurrent ; but the same writer allowed that out of the 71 cases 20 patients had previously relapsed, or had undergone several attacks, 16 had left the hospital at too early a period, 10 came afterwards under treatment and recovered without relapse, 14 had given themselves up to grief and intemperance, and several others were under circumstances unfavourable to continuance in health. M. Esquirol published a report of 2804 recoveries, in which number only 292 recurrences of disease took place, that is, a little more than one-tenth. M. Desportes, however, has stated that, in 1821, 52 recurrent cases were recognized at Bicêtre, out of 311 admissions, that is, about 17 in a hundred ; at the Salpêtrière in 454 admissions there were 66 relapses, about 15 in a hundred, or one-seventh. But in the proportion of recurrent cases indicated by this last report, it is probable that there were, as M. Georget has well observed, many cases which had been discharged in a state of incomplete recovery, as well as a considerable number of drunkards, who come habitually every year to spend a few weeks in Bicêtre or the Salpêtrière, having been picked up in the streets in a state of intoxication. The following table, furnished by Mr. Hitch, illustrates this subject.

Table showing the number of cases in which relapses have occasioned re-admission ; distinguishing the paupers from the others, and the males from females.

The total number of cases admitted before June 30, 1834, is 546

Number of those whose names appear in the entry-book more than once 68

Of these 68, 49 are males.
             19 " females.

Of the 49 males, 1 has been admitted 14 times = 14
                   3   "   3 " = 9
              13   "   2 " = 26
              ——   ——
              17   49

Of the 19 females, 3 have been admitted 3 times = 9
                5   "   2 " = 10
              ——   ——
               8   19

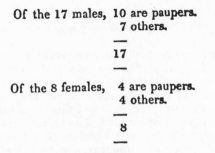

Of the 17 males, 10 are paupers.
                  7 others.
                  ——
                  17
                  ——

Of the 8 females, 4 are paupers.
                   4 others.
                   ——
                   8
                   ——

" It is to be observed that many persons re-admitted are such as had been removed uncured by the wishes or caprices of the friends. Others are cases of periodical excitement ; as, for instance, the gentleman admitted fourteen times, who spent his life in five weeks of excitement and five weeks of depression, with the variation scarcely of a day.   He died at Dr. ————'s, whither he had removed on account of our fire.   Some have been discharged 'relieved on trial,' whose friends have found it necessary to replace them, and some have relapsed after an apparently perfect cure."

In all instances we may consider it as certain that the improbability of recurrence increases with the length of the interval during which the patient has existed without manifesting signs of renewed disease, and that it is also greater in proportion to the completeness of the recovery.   When the energy of mind is fully restored, relapse is much less to be feared than when it remains weak and excitable.

CHAPTER IV.

OF THE CAUSES OF INSANITY.

Section I.—*Nature of the Causes of Insanity : Distribution under different Heads.*

There are many questions connected with the theory of mental disorders, which are yet and will perhaps always remain involved in obscurity ; but two departments of inquiry are accessible to us from which we may expect to obtain resources for elucidating that subject.   One of these comprehends the antecedents of insanity, or all that is or can be known as to the previous conditions of which mental derangement is the consequence or result.   The other includes necroscopical phenomena, or the appearances discovered by dissection in the bodies of the insane, and likewise a comparison of these appearances with the symptoms or manifestations of disease which had been observed during life. I shall devote the two following chapters to a consideration of these subjects.

The causes of insanity have been differently distributed. Some divide them into remote or predisposing, and immediate or exciting causes ; others into moral and physical causes. I shall adopt this latter division, but shall first, for the sake of clear and distinct arrangement, consider the facts which refer to predisposition, or the susceptibility of mental disorders, and the circumstances which modify it and tend to augment its influence. These may be comprehended under the term predisposing causes.

Under this head, of predisposing causes of insanity, may be considered, first, constitutional predisposition, whether hereditary or originating with the individual ; secondly, among the circumstances which modify this predisposition, the influence of sex and age; thirdly, the marks which denote or render it manifest, viz. external peculiarities of organization, form, and complexion; fourthly, circumstances which augment it, as previous attacks of insanity and other diseases of the brain ; lastly, the influence of education, moral and physical, in modifying the organization of the body and the predispositions of the mind.

SECTION II.—*Predisposing Causes of Insanity.*

ARTICLE I.

Of constitutional predisposition, whether hereditary or original.

A certain peculiarity of natural temperament or habit of body is a necessary condition for the development of insanity : without the previous existence of this condition the causes which give rise to the disease will either act upon the individual without any noxious effect, or they will call forth some other train of morbid phenomena. A natural predisposition may be inferred to have existed in every instance in which the disease has appeared.

The constitutional peculiarity whence arises the predisposition to insanity, is not generally distinguished, or to be certainly recognised by any remarkable external characters. The fact that it exists and is a necessary condition to the development of mental disease, is to be inferred from the consideration that the causes which induce madness in one person are precisely similar to those which in other individuals are observed to call forth disorders of a different kind. For example, we may observe that, among the physical agents which give rise to madness, there is none more influential than intemperance and the habitual use of ardent spirits. A very considerable proportion of lunatics in the lowest classes of society in some countries owe their disease to this habit. But it is only in a certain proportion of persons addicted to intemperance that the phenomena of insanity make their appearance. Others, under the influence of the same noxious cause, are affected with apoplexy or paralysis ; in many the brain escapes and the liver becomes disordered, or dropsy takes place, with or without disease of the liver ; in some the lungs become the seat of morbid changes. It is evident that there must be an original difference in the habit of body whence arises the diversity of results brought about by the same or very similar external agencies. This original difference is apparently a peculiarity in the congenital constitution of each individual. It may be transmitted from parents, or it may arise *de novo*, as other varieties in the congenital structure are known to do. Hence it is comparatively of little moment, as far as an individual is concerned, to inquire whether his morbid predisposition has been derived by hereditary descent, or has sprung up with himself. It may, indeed, be observed that peculiarities which arise in a race are often common to several individuals even in the first generation. Albinos, for instance, though the offspring of parents of ordinary complexions, very frequently have brothers or sisters resembling themselves. In like manner, diseases which appear for the first time in a family often affect several members of it. They partake of the same peculiarity of structure, which is congenital and constitutional, though not inherited.

If these remarks are well founded, it must be apparent that hereditary madness is not less curable than a disease having symptoms of the same description, which has not been previously observed in the family of the person affected by it.

That the predisposition to insanity, when it has once arisen, is frequently transmitted, is a fact too well established to admit of doubt ; it constitutes a feature in the history of the disease.

In a following section of this chapter I shall give some statements which are intended to indicate the proportional number of cases in which insanity has been known to arise from hereditary predisposition.

M. Esquirol affirms that persons born before their parents had become insane are less subject to mental disease than those who are born after the malady has displayed itself. He makes a similar remark as to individuals who inherit the disease only on one side, in comparison with persons whose ancestors on both sides had been affected by it. According to Burton the offspring of parents advanced in years are more subject than others to melancholy madness.

Another observation relating to the hereditary transmission of this morbid tendency is, that the disease is apt to show itself in different individuals of a family at a particular period of life. M. Esquirol has made this remark, and he has mentioned several facts in illustration of it. " Two sons of a merchant of Switzerland died insane at the age of nineteen years. A lady, aged twenty-five years, was attacked by puerperal madness ; her daughter suffered in like manner at the same age. In one family the father, the son, and the grandson, all committed suicide about their fiftieth year. There was at the Salpêtrière a prostitute who had thrown herself into the river seven times ; her sister drowned herself in a fit of intoxication. There exists near Nantes a family in which seven brothers and sisters are in a state of dementia. A gentleman, affected by the first events of the revolution, remained during ten years shut up in his chamber. His daughter, about the same age, fell into a similar state, and refused to quit her apartment." Dr. Burrows says that one of the youngest lunatics under his care was a boy of Jewish family, whose father and mother were insane : his six brothers and sisters became, like himself, deranged on arriving at the age of puberty : the individual who was under the care of Dr. Burrows recovered in three months. M. Falret has observed that melancholy occasioning suicide is perhaps the most frequently hereditary among all the forms of insanity. He mentions a case in which females of three successive generations either committed or attempted suicide.* Dr. Rush has also mentioned examples of hereditary suicide.

This predisposition to insanity, says M. Esquirol, is not more surprising than are the predispositions to gout, to phthisis pulmonalis, and other diseases, in a different point of view. "It may be traced from the age of infancy : it furnishes the explanation of a multitude of caprices, irregularities, and anomalies, which at a very early period ought to put parents on their guard against the approach of insanity. It may furnish useful admonitions to those who preside over the education of children. It is advisable in such cases to give them an education tending to render the habit robust, and to harden it against the ordinary causes of madness, and particularly to place them under different circumstances from those with which their parents were environed. It is thus that we ought to put in practice the aphorism of Hippocrates, who advises to change the constitution of individuals in order to prevent the diseases with which they are threatened by the hereditary predisposition of their family."

It is an inquiry highly interesting in many respects, what causes or previous circumstances lay the original foundation for the existence of that congenital or inborn peculiarity of constitution which renders certain individuals predisposed to become, when acted upon by exciting causes, the victims of this disease. In order to throw any light on this subject we must go back an entire generation, and inquire how and by what means the parents can be so affected as to render their offspring physically weak and predisposed to become, under circumstances which have no such effect on others, deranged in their understandings. It seems probable that any causes which tend to produce enervation and debility in parents will have an effect on their offspring.

It is a general opinion that marriages between persons near of kin have such an effect, and that the mental faculties, display it even more than the physical. The apparent results of frequent marriages within a confined circle have been noted in some royal familes, both

---

* Falret de l'Hypochondrie et du Suicide, p. 6.

in ancient and in modern times. The offspring of marriages between cousin-germans are very often observed to be weak and defective both in mind and body. The children of such families often die during infancy, or if they grow up, are frail and imbecile. M. Esquirol affirms that many facts have occurred within the sphere of his information, proving that a strong predisposition to madness has arisen from some accidental fright sustained by the mother during pregnancy. Marked cases of this description are said to have occurred during the period of the revolution.

In many instances one particular form of mental disorder seems to be transmitted in families. This has been observed already in respect to the derangement which occasions suicide. M. Pinel has mentioned an affecting instance in which dementia occurred in several individuals of a family, nor is this fact of very rare occurrence. As the particular form of insanity is determined in a great measure by the natural temperament, and as peculiarities of temperament are hereditary, the predisposition to mental disease, where it exists in a family, is likely to be determined in its type or character. This, however, is not uniformly the fact. There are many instances in which one individual is affected with melancholy dejection and a tendency to monomania, while another of the same kindred is subject to attacks of raving madness. Insanity displays in a similar way its alliance to other diseases of the brain. The relatives of insane persons labour frequently under diseases of the same class, such as paralysis, chorea, epilepsy, congenital idiotism. In many instances it has been observed that, while some members of a family are manifest lunatics, others are only eccentric in character, displaying peculiarities of habit, conduct, and disposition, which, though constituting in reality a degree of moral insanity, may not render such individuals altogether unfit to be at large, and to enter, as much as they are disposed to do, into the intercourse of society.

There is reason for believing that this one circumstance of constitutional tendency to mental derangement is by itself more important, in respect to the origination and the frequent occurrence of the disease, than all the other causes, both predisponent and occasional, taken together. It cannot be said with propriety to give rise to insanity alone and without any exciting contingency ; but if it be very strong, the disease will take place under the agency of ordinary and very slight causes.

ARTICLE II.

Of sex.

Cœlius Aurelianus, who lived in the age of Trajan and Hadrian, and who wrote with more accuracy of discrimination than any of his predecessors on disorders affecting the mind, stated that both mania and melancholia occurred more frequently in the male than in the female sex.* It is doubtful whether this writer made the assertion after adequate research, for which there were probably no data to be obtained in his age. His conclusion is at least contrary to the general fact observed in modern times.

The relative proportion in which the two sexes are affected with insanity has been a matter of discussion among those who have occu pied themselves with the statistics of this disease. The subject has, not long since, been investigated by M. Esquirol in the most elaborate and satisfactory manner, in his valuable report on the Royal House of Charenton. As this is not the place for the statistical history of insanity, it would be contrary to my present design to enter into an extended consideration of the evidence from which the conclusions are deduced, and I shall confine myself to a statement of the general results.

In the hospital of Charenton, during the years to which M. Esquirol's report has reference, the proportion of male patients admitted to that of female was three to two. This proportion is the result of peculiar circumstances, and is very different from that which obtains elsewhere, as well in France as in other countries. From a variety of public documents it appears that in the great hospitals of the Salpêtrière and Bicêtre an inverse proportion to that above stated holds in the numbers of the two sexes, male patients at Bicêtre being to females in the Salpêtrière only as two to three. This, however, does not hold throughout France. It appears from a great number of published and private documents which M. Esquirol has collected, that in the cities in the south of France the number of male is somewhat more considerable than that of female lunatics ; while in the northern departments the number of females predominates in a greater degree ; but that in all France the number of insane women is to that of insane men very nearly in the proportion of 14 to 11. From Spain, the returns which M. Esquirol has been able to obtain are very defective: the result, which can only be looked upon as a presumptive one, since it rests on few data, and may hereafter be modified by more copious information, gives an excess of one-fifth in the number of female lunatics compared with that of males. In Italy, it appears from the documents obtained that the proportion is different, there being more insane men than women, particularly in the kingdom of Naples. In all Italy, 5718 male lunatics were reckoned, and 5067 females. In Holland and Belgium, according to the information given to the world by M. Guislain, it appears that the number of females in the lunatic asylums is much more considerable than that of males, being as 34 to 29 ; and this excess on the side of females is rather greater in the southern, or Belgian provinces, than in those of the north, or in the present Dutch kingdom. In Great Britain and Ireland the proportion of male to female lunatics is as 13 to 12. In England the num-

---

* Cœlius Aurelianus, Morb. Chron. lib. i.—Esquirol, art. *Folie*, in Dict. des Sc. Méd.—Heinroth, Stoerungen des Seelenlebens, b. i. s. 85-87.

ber of men insane compared to that of women is more considerable than in Scotland and in Ireland. This excess in the proportional number of male above that of female lunatics in England is greater, according to Dr. Burrows, in the higher than in the lower classes of society. M. Esquirol who has cited this observation, adds a parallel remark in respect to the comparison of different orders of society in France, insanity being apparently more prevalent among men compared with women in the higher than in the lower classes.

In the same memoir M. Esquirol computed that in the north of Europe the proportion of male to female lunatics is greater than as above stated: he says that it is as three to two. In this are included the results obtained from reports of lunatic asylums in various parts of Germany, in Denmark, Norway, and Russia. Subsequently to the publication of this report by M. Esquirol, Dr. Max. Jacobi has given us extensive information on the state of lunatic asylums in the Prussian provinces on the Rhine. In the different establishments of that country the total number of male lunatics in the year 1824 was 1180, and that of females 835. The result nearly coincides with that deduced by M. Esquirol from other documents for the general proportion of Germany.

In a later memoir which appeared in 1830, M. Esquirol has given some new results from the statistical reports on lunatics in Norway, published by Dr. Holst. He reduces the proportion of male to female lunatics in that country to an excess of one-sixth instead of one-third part.

In the United States of America it appears from information given by Dr. Rush, by Portman of Massachusetts, and a report of the asylum in Connecticut printed in 1827, that the number of insane men is greater than that of female lunatics. Later researches have rendered this observation more precise. In the states of New York, Pennsylvania, and Connecticut the proportion of males to females is very nearly as two to one.

On summing up the results of his inquiries, M. Esquirol has shown that in a sum total of 76,526 lunatics, confined, though not all at the same period, in asylums or hospitals in various parts of the civilized world, there were 37,825 males and 38,701 females. Thus the proportion of males to that of females is, a fraction being neglected, 37 to 38. This difference is so much the less considerable, as in the general population the number of males somewhat exceeds that of females. Yet, small as it is, it is sufficient, as M. Esquirol observes, to refute the assertion of Cœlius Aurelianus, who supposed that women are less subject to insanity than men.

ARTICLE III.

Age.

Idiotism and imbecility are observed in childhood, but insanity, properly so termed, is rare before the age of puberty. Cases, however, have sometimes occurred which have exemplified almost every form of insanity at an earlier period, and almost as soon as the mental faculties begin to display themselves. One case of madness was observed by Dr. Joseph Frank in St. Luke's Hospital, when he visited that asylum in 1802, occurring in a child two years of age. Dr. Haslam has recorded three instances of insanity in children. In one of these the disease appeared after small-pox, attended by convulsions and delirium. In the two other cases insanity was combined with more or less of imbecility: in one of them there was inaptitude to mental application, combined with symptoms of moral insanity, a perversion of natural feelings, and an ungovernable disposition to give way to violent passion. In a preceding section of this work I have inserted the history of a strongly marked case of moral insanity occurring in a child. Another example, in which the symptoms were of a different kind, but still falling strictly within the definition of moral insanity, was reported in the Annales d'Hygiène et de Médecine Légale for 1832. On this case M. Fodéré has made some observations in his late work on the varieties of madness.*

M. Esquirol has described two cases of mania commencing at the eighth and ninth years, one occasioned by fright during the siege of Paris, the other following an attack of fever: he has likewise mentioned an instance of melancholia combined with marasmus in a child eleven years old, who had a remarkably large head, and for his age great application to learning.

After the age of fifteen mental derangement is no longer a rare phenomenon, but it assumes, generally speaking, various aspects at different ages of life. Soon after puberty, while in females the constitution is making efforts to establish the catamenia, or in young persons who grow rapidly, symptoms of mania or melancholia occasionally appear. In the three or four years which succeed this period, hysteria in females, and the excitement occasioned by the sexual passion in males, or the vices which are often consequent, give rise to the same diseases in more numerous examples.† "In the vigour of youth," says M. Esquirol, "mania breaks out with all its varieties of excitement : melancholia is more frequently the lot of the middle period of life, and dementia chiefly threatens advanced age. In youth," he continues, "derangement of the mind has a more acute and violent course, and more often terminates by a remarkable crisis ; in middle age it is a more chronical disorder, is more often complicated with diseases of the abdominal viscera, and is resolved by hemorrhages from the hemorrhoidal veins or by diarrhœas ; at a later period it is combined with paralytic affections or with apoplexy, and recovery is less to be expected. Yet these remarks are liable to exceptions. Dementia sometimes occurs to young persons. We have," says M. Esquirol, "in the Salpêtrière

* Traité Médico-Légale sur les differentes espèces de Folie, par M. Fodéré. Strasburg, 1832.
† Esquirol sur la Folie. Jacobi's Sammlungen, i. 294.

two women, one eighty and the other eighty-one years old, who
were attacked with raving madness, and who recovered." He
mentions another maniac who had been under his care at the age of
seventy-eight, but adds, that " these individuals still possessed the
vigour of constitution which is generally peculiar to a much earlier
period of life."

The years of life in which insanity is most frequent are, according to the calculation of M. Georget, those between thirty and
forty ; next .to these are the years between twenty and thirty ;
thirdly, come those between forty and sixty. M. Esquirol adds
that the proportional number of females attacked before their twentieth and after their fiftieth year is greater than that of men, whence
he concludes that females are more in danger of insanity at the
early and late periods, and men in the intermediate years of life.
The susceptibility of madness takes place rather more early in the
female than in the male sex, and in persons belonging to the opulent
than in those of the laborious classes of society.

According to a calculation given by M. Georget, the aamissions
of lunatics into different hospitals in England and France took place
in the following ages :—

From 10 to 20 years of age	. . . .	356
„ 20 to 30 „ „	. . . .	1106
„ 30 to 40 „ „	. . . .	1416
„ 40 to 50 „ „	. . . .	861
„ 50 to 60 „ „	. . . .	461
„ 60 to 70 „ „	. . . .	174
„ 70 and upwards	. . . .	35

4409

This table affords sufficient evidence to establish the fact that the
frequency of insanity as occurring at the different periods of life, or
the proportional number of individuals attacked by mental disease
at the several ages, is just what MM. Esquirol and Georget have
stated.   But though this is true absolutely and without reference to
the proportional numbers of individuals existing in society who have
respectively attained the several ages or periods of life, it is by no
means apparent that the same relative frequency holds when these
proportions are taken into the account.   For example, 174 individuals becoming insane between sixty and seventy is, absolutely, a
smaller number than 1416 who are seized with insanity between
thirty and forty years of age, but we have no evidence that the
former is a smaller number in proportion to the numbers of persons
existing between sixty and seventy, than the latter is to the number
of individuals existing between thirty and forty.

M. Esquirol is well aware that this relative computation puts the
matter in a different point of view, and he has expressed to me his
conviction that when due attention is given to it, the result wil l

indicate a proportionally increased frequency of mental disease with the advancement of age, or, in other words, that the longer men live after attaining maturity, the more obnoxious they continually become to the causes which give rise to derangement or lesions of the understanding. He has given a brief survey of the data from which this result is deduced, in an excellent memoir on the Statistics of Insanity, published in the "Annales d' Hygiène et de Médecine Légale for 1830." The general conclusion is, that the predisposition to mental derangement increases with advancing age, though in an irregular scale. The increased number of insane persons compared with the population of that age is very striking between fifty and fifty-five years. From seventy to seventy-five and from seventy-five to eighty it becomes enormous, owing to the frequency of senile dementia.

ARTICLE IV.

Of temperament: peculiarities of complexion and of form which are supposed to denote predisposition to insanity in general, or to particular forms of the disease.

No observation relating to madness is more common than the connection of particular complexions with its different varieties. Persons of the melancholic temperament, or those who have certain external peculiarities which are well known as characteristic of the constitution of body so termed, are certainly more often affected with melancholy madness than others, and they are more prone to this than to other forms of insanity. Individuals of the sanguine temperament are more frequently raving under accessions of violent mania. It has been observed by M. Esquirol, that when persons of the lymphatic or phlegmatic temperament, or those who have a pale exanguious constitution, fall into mania or monomania, their disorder is more liable than that which occurs in other constitutions to pass into dementia or incoherence. An apoplectic form, a thick head and short neck, mark a predisposition to dementia. Imbecile persons and idiots are not remarkably of one temperament more than of others.

According to M. Esquirol, insanity has a somewhat different course, as occurring in persons of different temperaments. Persons of choleric temperament, or those who have black hair and eyes, with warm vigorous constitution, become violently maniacal, but have a shorter and more acute distemper, and more frequently terminating in marked crisis than others : the sanguineo-phlegmatic, or persons of fair, pale complexion, with flaxen hair, fall more readily into a chronic disease : the dark-haired are gloomy monomaniacs : red-haired lunatics are disposed to anger and violence ; they are treacherous and dangerous.*

A table, indicating the varieties of temperament or of complexion

* Dict. des Sc. Méd. Jacobi's Sammlungen, b. i. p. 298.

which displayed themselves in the lunatic hospital of the Salpêtrière, proves that the numbers of individuals of each complexion in that establishment were nearly in the proportion of their respective numbers in the population of Paris. It hence results that no particular temperament indicates a greater tendency to madness than others, if we speak of that disease generally and including under the term all its varieties. The numbers are as follows :—

" Hair chesnut brown in one hundred and eighteen cases ; blond in thirty-nine ; grey or white in thirty-six ; black in thirty-one ; yellow or red in two. Eyes of a chesnut or brown hue in one hundred and two ; blue or light in ninety-eight ; black in seventeen."

The varieties of temperament and the peculiarities of organization belonging to individuals are so related to predisposition to mental disease, that I cannot omit the consideration of these subjects ; and it is impossible to enter upon the inquiries which are connected with them, without interrupting by a long digression a series of facts of which I am anxious to give a brief and distinct statement. I shall, therefore, refer to a supplementary note some further remarks on peculiarities of structure and constitution as connected with insanity.

ARTICLE V.

Previous attacks of insanity and other diseases of the brain.

Among the most powerful of the influences which tend to augment the susceptibility of mental disease in persons naturally predisposed to it, we must reckon previous attacks of insanity and the previous existence of some other disorders affecting the brain, which though totally unlike their madness in their phenomena, are shown by experience to be its frequent harbingers and antecedents.

There have been instances in which individuals have sustained repeated attacks of insanity during a certain period of their lives, and have seemed afterwards to have lost all predisposition to the disease. They have recovered their entire sanity and vigour of mind, without any relic or trace whatever of the calamity through which they have passed. The late admirable and truly excellent Robert Hall was a remarkable instance of this kind. Other morbid predispositions are sometimes of temporary duration. Some persons, for example, and even whole families, have a predisposition to phthisis or other constitutional disorders at a particular period of life ; and it has been noted, in the latter instance, by relatives or medical attendants, that if the particular period has passed for some years, the threatening malady ceases to give cause of apprehension, and the susceptibility of a disorder which has long been dreaded and with great difficulty warded off, entirely disappears for the remainder of life.

But there are likewise numerous instances in which an attack of madness leaves the individual affected more prone to the disorder than he originally appeared to be. His recovery is partial : he is more susceptible of impressions, more irritable, irascible, excitable than he previously was. This susceptibility augments with every renewed attack, and at length the individual has but short and imperfect intervals of comparative health and tranquillity.

Insanity is often consequent on, and intimately connected with various diseases of the brain. Maniacal symptoms sometimes display themselves in persons recovering partially from severe paralysis in the form of hemiplegia, or after fits of apoplexy. These instances are quite distinct from the combination of madness or dementia with general paralysis, of which an account has been given in the preceding chapter. In the cases now adverted to, the injury which the brain has sustained from the hemiplegic or apoplectic attack must be considered as laying the foundation of insanity. Epilepsy still more frequently gives rise to a similar affection. I am not at present alluding to the decay of intellect or the modification of dementia which ensues on long-continued or severe epilepsy. It occasionally happens that the paroxysms of this disease appear to usher in at every return an attack of violent mania, which generally continues for a few days and then subsides. In other instances signs of mental derangement become permanent, and either take place of the original affection and supersede it, or continue to be complicated with it.

It has often been observed, and the remark might be supported by many facts, that the form of insanity to which epileptics are subject is of the most dangerous and violent description. Individuals labouring under it are sullen and irascible, and commit occasionally atrocious acts. Moral insanity with a propensity to homicide has often been observed to take its rise under such circumstances. In other cases the moral derangement induced by epilepsy has been violent satyriasis, or these morbid dispositions have been combined in the same individual. There are instances of epileptic insanity, however, in which fits of boisterous mania, resembling attacks of drunkenness, have been the only symptoms of derangement.

ARTICLE VI.

Of Education.

The influence of erroneous education in increasing the susceptibility of mental derangement must be reckoned among predisposing causes, though of a different class from the circumstances already enumerated.

There are two different points of view under which the injurious effects of wrong education may be considered. By too great indulgence and a want of moral discipline, the passions acquire greater power, and a character is formed subject to caprice and to violent emotions : a predisposition to insanity is thus laid in the temper and moral affections of the individual. The exciting causes of madness have greater influence on persons of such habits than on those whose feelings are regulated. An overstrained and premature exercise of the intellectual powers is likewise a fault of education which predisposes to insanity, as it does also to other diseases of the brain. These are two considerations which are of the greatest importance with respect to the welfare of families to which an hereditary constitution may belong, rendering them more liable than others to cerebral diseases. They are distinct in themselves, and each might furnish a theme for an extensive treatise, most valuable in a practical point of view. Under the first head it would be necessary to consider the efficacy of those plans of education of which the professed object is to form a character remarkable for sedateness, for the strict discipline of the feelings, and, as far as this is attainable, for the abolition of strong passions and emotions. Such, undoubtedly, would be the kind of moral education best adapted for those who are constitutionally liable to insanity. The second remark, on the regulation of mental exercise in young persons whose nervous systems are feebly constituted, has a more extensive bearing than on the subject of insanity. It brings forward a suggestion which is of very general interest in these times, in which mental exertion is stimulated to the utmost ; and too great sacrifices are often made to the cultivation of intellect, or even to the mere acquisition of knowledge, while the education of the moral affections is considered as a matter of secondary importance.

SECTION III.—*Of the Productive Causes of Insanity: Moral and Physical Causes.*

I now proceed to consider the productive causes of insanity, or the conditions in which individuals predisposed or originally susceptible are found to promote the development of mental disease. Moral causes of insanity, as it is well understood, are all the circumstances which exert an influence immediately on the mind or they are states of the mind itself giving rise to disorder in the exercise of its faculties. Physical causes are those agents which affect the body, and exert their influence on the mind through the medium of organic structure.

Modern writers on insanity are by no means unanimous in the opinions they have formed, as to the comparative influence of moral and physical causes in the production of mental derangement. Some have ascribed the greatest importance to the first class of agents, and others to the latter. It must be observed that those who maintain the greater power of physical causes appear to have included among them many very important circumstances which are rather to be considered as influences predisposing to insanity, or as constituting a kind of preliminary condition, without the actual presence of which neither physical nor moral agents will produce their effect. Congenital predisposition must exist as the groundwork in all instances: this is reckoned a physical cause, and such it is in one sense, but for obvious reasons it is not to be taken in the amount in the comparative estimate to which I am now about to advert. If this article is abstracted from the comparison, a more decided preponderance will appear on the side of moral causes as the principal agents concerned in the development of mental disorders.

Several authors of various countries, who have differed widely among themselves in other respects as to the nature of insanity, have been of one sentiment in ascribing great importance in this respect to moral causes. Professor Heinroth, who is among this number, has maintained his opinion, as usual, in a speculative and theoretical manner: others, as M. Guislain and Georget, have deduced a similar conclusion from facts. A great part of the evidence on this question has been furnished by MM. Pinel and Esquirol, who incline, on the whole, to this view of the subject.

Some have argued in favour of this opinion from general considerations connected with the history of insanity, its alleged increase with the advancement of civil society. Among nations existing in a savage state, in which the human mind is uncultivated and its higher faculties remain undeveloped, it appears that mental diseases are comparatively rare phenomena. Travellers among barbarous nations, and naturalists and physicians who have resided among them and have described their physical characters and diseases, have generally reported madness to be unknown among such tribes of men. It comes forward with the dawning of civilization, and perhaps keeps pace, though its increase is modified by other circumstances, with the advancement of mental culture. The proofs of this general observation can only be collected from a survey of facts which refer to the frequency of mental derangement in different places and times. Such a survey belongs to the statistical history of insanity, a subject to which I must devote a separate consideration in a later part of this work ; and I must refer my readers to the facts which I shall there accumulate. For the present I have only anticipated the inference.

From the rare occurrence of insanity in rude nations, and its comparative frequency in those which are civilized, it has been argued that the most influential causes of the disease are circumstances connected with the improved state of human society. The restraints imposed by social order, the diversity of interests which are excited in civilized communities, the mixed and diversified feelings which are called forth by a variety of sometimes arduous pursuits, long-continued griefs and anxieties, disappointment of hopes long cherished, causes which act powerfully on the moral affections rather than on the animal passions, particularly great and long-continued exertion of the intellectual powers;—these are some of the most obvious traits which distinguish human life in the civilized state from the manner of existence peculiar to savage men. It is among these circumstances, as some celebrated writers have thought, that we are to look for the causes which are most influential in the development of mental diseases.

These considerations are entitled to some regard. We cannot deny or easily call in question the facts on which they are founded; yet the general assertion that insanity belongs exclusively to the civilized condition of our species goes beyond all probable expectation, and might be disputed on theoretical grounds, if we were at liberty to proceed upon such a foundation. In a barbarous state of society the passions are under no restraint; the emotions are impetuous; hatred and malignity are in perpetual exercise; the fierce and sensual desires which are common to mankind and the inferior tribes are indulged without limit. Nor are the intellectual faculties without their exercise in carrying on the stratagems of barbarous warfare. We should conjecture that such a state of society in which the passions are in perpetual and violent agitation would produce not unfrequently the moral causes of madness. The fact, however, appears to be otherwise.

I am not without a suspicion that there is something in the state of civilization which tends to promote the existence of that congenital state of bodily structure on which predisposition to mental diseases depends. This, however, is a subject on which I cannot enter further at present. I must now advert to the more strict results of observation.

Experience itself has led many to the conclusion that moral causes are mainly influential in the development of diseases of the mind. No writer has maintained this opinion to a greater extent than M. Georget. "The observations," says M. Georget, "which I have had in my power to make, the more numerous ones which I have compared in authors, have convinced me, that, among one hundred lunatics, ninety-five at least have become such from the influence of affections and of moral commotions: it is an observation become almost proverbial in the hospital—the Salpêtrière,—'qu'on perd la tête par les révolutions d'esprit.' The first question that M. Pinel puts to a new patient who still preserves some remains of intelligence, is, Have you undergone any vexation or disappointment? Seldom is the reply in the negative. It is," continues the same writer, "in the age in which the mind is most susceptible of strong feelings, in which the passions are excited by the strongest interests, that madness is principally displayed. Children, calm and without anxiety, incapable of long and extensive combinations of thought, not yet initiated into the troubles of life, and old men, whom the now vanishing illusions of their preceding age, and their increasing physical and moral weakness render indifferent as to events, are but rarely affected. The same remark applies to persons who in their constitution approach to the character of children or of old men."[*] M. Georget evidently supposed persons far advanced in life to be less subject to mental derangement than they are, according to the later researches of M. Esquirol. The derangement, however, so frequent in old age is senile dementia and not insanity in the or-

* De la Folie, par M. Georget, &c. Paris, 1820.

dinary forms, and to these the present question and the remarks of
M. Georget chiefly refer.

In a computation made by M. Pinel from the observations of five
years, cases of insanity produced by moral causes were, to those
occasioned by physical causes, in the proportion of 464 to 219.
The following are the particular numbers from which this result is
deduced.

Cases of mania . . . . { 285 arising from moral causes.
{ 165 arising from physical causes.

Cases of melancholia { 148 arising from moral causes.
{ 46 arising from physical causes.

Cases of suicide . . . { 31 arising from moral causes.
{ 8 arising from physical causes.

Cases of dementia . . { 26 arising from moral causes.
{ 31 arising from physical causes.

Cases of idiotism . . { 26 arising from moral causes.
{ 31 arising from physical causes.*

M. Esquirol's tables are more instructive as to the particular
causes of insanity and their respective influence. According to various calculations deduced by this writer, it appears that moral
causes are on the whole far more numerous and influential than
physical ones in inducing insanity. This is especially observed with
relation to the higher classes of society, physical causes having proportionally a greater influence on the lower orders. It appears also
that females are subjected to the operation of physical causes in
many respects more than males. In a memoir presented by M. Esquirol to the Society of Medicine in 1818, it was concluded that
cases of madness occasioned by moral causes are, to those arising
from physical causes, in the proportion of 4 to 1.

The following tables, by the same writer, include cases belonging
indiscriminately to the different forms of insanity, and display the
particular nature of the causes which are most powerful, as well as
their comparative influence. The tables exhibit cases of females
belonging to the lower classes in which the influence of physical
causes in the production of insanity is the greatest ; they likewise
exhibit corresponding aggregates from a higher grade of society.

* Journal de Physique; mois de Septembre, 1808. Guislain de l'Aliénation,
tom. i. p. 149.

Table of cases produced by moral causes.*

	In the Salpêtrière during the years 1811 and 1812.	In M. Esquirol's private establishment.
Domestic grief	105	31
Disappointment in love	46	25
Political events	14	31
Fanaticism.................	8	1
Fright....................	38	8
Jealousy ...·..............	18	14
Anger..................	16	—
Poverty, reverses of fortune	77	Reverses 14
Offended self-love	1	16
Disappointed ambition	—	12
Excess in study	—	13
Misanthropy	—	2
	Sum .. 323	Sum .. 167

Table of physical causes.

	In the Salpêtrière.	In M. Esquirol's private establishment.
Hereditary predisposition†	105	150
Convulsions suffered by the mother during pregnancy	11	4
Epilepsy	11	2
Irregularities in menstruation ...	55	19
Consequence of parturition	52	21
Critical period	27	11
Advanced age..............	60	4
Coup de soleil..............	12	4
Blows or falls on the head	14	4
Fever	13	12
Syphilis	8	1
Mercury	14	13
Intestinal worms	24	4
Apoplexy	60	16
	361	120

* Art. *Folie*, Dict. des Sc. Med. Jacobi's Sammlungen, band i. p. 309.
† This article is separated, and does not in propriety belong to the table of physical causes.

The causes of mania, separately considered, are given as follows:*

1. *Moral causes.*

	In the Salpêtrière.	In M. Esquirol's Establishment.	
		Males.	Females.
Domestic griefs	62	9	20
Reverses of fortune	6	13	6
Poverty (misère)	19	0	0
Disappointment in love	58	4	4
Jealousy	4	1	8
Injured self-love	1	15	7
Fright	36	1	6
Anger	2	1	1
Excess in study	0	10	0
	183	56	62

2. *Physical causes.*

Hereditary predisposition	88	38	37
Masturbation	8	6	2
Menstruation	27	0	11
Consequences of parturition	38	0	19
Critical period	12	0	8
Abuse of wine	14	0	0
Coup de soliel	2	3	0
Exposure to fire	12	2	0
Falls or blows	8	1	2
Mercury	2	2	1
Suppression of scabies	3	1	0
Suppression of tinea capitis	2	2	6
Ulcer healed	1	0	0
Fever	3	4	1
Apoplexy	0	1	1
	132	26	51

The causes of melancholia, meaning monomania with melancholy dejection, are thus stated by the same writer :—†

Moral causes.		Physical causes.	
Domestic cares	60	Suppressed catamenia	26
Reverses, misery	48	Critical age	50
Disappointed love	42	Puerperal state	35

* Art. *Manie*, Dict. des Sc. Méd. Tobsucht, p. 372, in Jacobi's Sammlungen. Guislan, Aliénation, i. p. 151.

† Art. *Melancholie*, Dict. des Sc. Méd. Jacobi's Sammlungen, i. 418.

Jealousy	8	Falls on the head	10
Frights	19	Masturbation	6
Injured self-love	12	Dissipation	30
Anger	18	Abuse of wine	19
	219		**165**

Hereditary predisposition is marked 110.

M. Guislain has cited, from Nasse's "Zeitschrift für psychischen aertze," a statement drawn up by Hayner from the Lunatic Institution at Waldheim, of which the result differs considerably from that of the French hospitals ; the report is, however, drawn up in so different a manner that it is scarcely possible to make a satisfactory comparison. It is as follows :—

Moral causes.		Physical causes.	
Immorality	25	Hereditary predisposition	23
Violent illusions	10	Malconformation	54
Obstinate passions	18	Mechanical injury	9
	53	Previous disease	41
		Metastases	12
			139

We have, from M. Esquirol, a later statement of the cases in the Maison Royale de Charenton, which is appropriated to persons of a higher rank in society than those who are remitted to the other hospitals near Paris. The following table contains the results of three years' observation.[*]

Physical causes.

Hereditary predisposition	93 cases.
Masturbation	23
Libertinism	24
Use of mercury	16
Abuse of wine	64
Insolation	7
Effect of carbonic acid gas	2
Suppressions of habitual evacuations	13
Consequence of parturition	10
Blows on the head	4
Total	256

[*] Annales d'Hygiène Publ. et de Médicine Légale. Avril, 182 .

Moral causes.

Domestic griefs	89
Excessive study and watching	8
Reverses of fortune	20
Passion for gaming	2
Jealousy	13
Disappointments in love	21
Injured self-love	6
Fright	7
" Dévotion exaltée"	18
Excess of joy	1
Reading romances	8

Total . . 192

M. Esquirol observes that it is from a variety of circumstances very difficult to obtain adequate information as to the previous condition of persons who are brought for treatment to Charenton, and that there is strong reason for believing that some of the causes marked down have been productive of madness in much more numerous instances than as displayed by the tables. He has found proof that hereditary predisposition has existed much more frequently than the accounts received indicate. He says that immoral habits and the use of mercury, of which the injurious results can be recorded only in a comparatively small number of cases, are yet very frequently productive of that deplorable species of paralysis which becomes complicated with dementia and monomania. Excess in the use of intoxicating fluids, which gives rise exclusively to delirium tremens, is also a frequent cause of mental derangement. Love, jealousy, *excessive devotion*, are principally causes of madness in females. In treating of the causes of insanity in general, we have only to estimate the different effects resulting from the circumstances of age, sex, education, and fortune, in order to ascertain the principal diversities which are to be found in the appearance and development of the disease in various departments of society.

I shall now offer some further remarks on the effects produced by the most important of the agents above enumerated.

SECTION IV.—*Of particular moral Causes.*

ARTICLE I.

Care and anxiety.

Care and anxiety, distress, grief, and mental disturbances, are by far the most productive causes of insanity. A sufficient proof of this remark may be found at once by inspecting the preceding tables drawn up by M. Esquirol. In the first table, domestic griefs, poverty, and reverses of fortune, taken together, comprise considerably more than one-half of the whole number of cases attributed to the influence of moral causes.

These causes are at all times influential in civilized countries, and hence one principal reason why insanity prevails in proportion to the cultivation of society. Poverty and reverses of fortune are sustained in very different degrees in different places and times; and this accounts for the fact that insanity appears under particular circumstances to be more frequent than under others.

Anxiety and agitation of mind caused by political events, have occasionally produced a very decided effect on the numbers of persons becoming deranged. M. Esquirol declares that the law of conscription increased the number of lunatics in France, and that at every period of this levy many individuals were received into the hospitals who had become insane through the excitement and anxiety occasioned by it: they were partly from the number of those on whom the lot fell, and partly from their friends and relatives. " The influence of our political misfortunes has been so great," says the same writer, " that I could illustrate the history of our revolution from the taking of the Bastille to the last appearance of Bonaparte, by describing in a series the cases of lunatics, whose mental derangement was in connexion with the succession of events." Political disturbances, like the mental impressions which give rise to insanity, are among the exciting causes. They set the predisposing influences in operation, and bring out some particular character of madness; but this impress, even if general, is still only temporary. At the destruction of the old monarchy many persons became mad through fright and the loss of their property. "When the Pope came to France, religious maniacs were very numerous. When Bonaparte made kings, there were many kings and queens in the madhouses. At the time of the invasion of France by foreign troops, terror threw many into derangement. The Germans had experienced the same effects at the era of our irruptions into their country."

Under the same head must be considered the influence which different professions or occupations exercise in the production of mental derangement. M. Fodéré, in his Treatise on Insanity, has entered into this inquiry : he has endeavoured to estimate the moral and physical influence of different habits and modes of employment. He concludes that the classes of society which furnish the greatest number of inmates to the lunatic asylums in France are those of traders, merchants, and military men.

ARTICLE II.

Passions and emotions.

Next to the examples of insanity produced by care and anxiety, the greatest number of cases in the preceding tables, and in the evidence afforded by general observation, are those arising from the influence of strong passions and emotions. The former class of influences produce their effect by slow and constant operation ; the latter, sometimes at least, by a sudden action, so vehement as to disturb those functions of the brain and nervous system which are subservient to the exercise of the mental faculties, and give rise to manifest derangement. The emotions of terror and of violent anger are the most powerful and sudden to which the mental constitution of man is subject, and by them the nervous system is most severely agitate I : this is apparent from other effects which sometimes ensue from the sudden efficacy of these emotions, and which take the place of mental derangement in persons who are not predisposed by nature to the latter disease : such are fits of convulsion, tremors, palpitations, and syncope. In M. Esquirol's table there are thirty-eight cases of madness produced by fright ; thirty-six of them were instances of mania or raving madness. There are sixteen cases produced by anger or rage. Mania is the form of insanity which generally results from the operation of the causes above mentioned. There are, however, instances in which dementia has displayed itself at once from the same causes, in an advanced degree. Some instances of this description are mentioned by Pinel.*

The passion which nature has appointed for the continuation of our race, and of which the influence and effects, though universal, are so greatly modified and varied by education and external circumstances, gives rise to numerous forms and varieties of mental derangement. One of the most palpable facts connected with this subject is displayed by comparing the numbers of married and unmarried persons in great public hospitals.

In a report on the numbers and condition of lunatics in the different hospitals devoted to their cure near Paris, from the beginning of 1801 to 1822, which was presented to the general council of civil hospitals near Paris, by M. Desportes, it appeared that married and unmarried persons were victims of insanity in the following proportions :—†

Total number of male lunatics, imbeciles, and epileptics in Bicêtre, Jan. 1, 1822. 764
Total number of females in the Salpêtrière at the same date . 1726
They are distributed as follows :—

	Females.	Males.
Unmarried	980	492
Married	397	201
Widowers and widows	291	59
Divorced	5	3
Not noted	53	9
Total . . .	1726	764

* Traité Philosophico-Médicale de la Folie, par M. Pinel.
† Rapport fait au Consul Général des Hospices Civils de Paris sur le service des aliénés, &c.. Paris, 1823..

In Germany the proportion of unmarried to married persons is much greater, as may be judged from the following enumeration, which I take from Dr. Jacobi's *Statistik*. The total numbers of 1180 male lunatics and 835 females are thus distributed :—

	Females.	Males.
Unmarried	599	974
Married	156	176
Widowed	80	30

The disproportion which here displays itself is a very striking and remarkable circumstance, and if a similar result were generally obtained, this would constitute a most leading feature in the history of mental derangement, and one which has not yet been adverted to in its due importance. The reports of most hospitals are not kept with sufficient accuracy to authorise a determination whether this is the fact or not, but it should become a matter of careful inquiry.

As it appears probable that celibacy tends to augment the numbers of lunatics, an inquiry will obviously be suggested in what manner this result ensues. Is it through the restraints which the condition of celibacy imposes, or through the vices to which unmarried persons are more frequently abandoned ? M. Esquirol is of opinion that where one case of insanity arises from the former cause, a hundred result from the latter.

We must take into our calculation that married persons lead in general more regular lives, in all respects, than the unmarried ; that they are for the most part more fixed in their pursuits, and their condition as to maintenance and employment ; and that they are in a less degree subjected to causes which agitate the mind and excite strong emotions. These remarks, however, apply principally to men, and the difference observed in respect to numbers is almost equally great among females.

After making allowance for all deductions, it still appears probable that the condition of married persons is, *cæteris paribus*, much less favourable to the excitement of madness than that of celibacy.

ARTICLE III.

Apprehensions relating to a future state.—Of insanity connected with religious impressions.

There is no subject connected with the history of insanity on which more crude and ignorant notions are expressed than on what is often termed *religious madness*.

It cannot be doubted that in persons predisposed to insanity by natural constitution, education, and other circumstances, anxieties connected with a future state of existence have been the exciting causes of mental derangement. This, indeed, would seem, *à priori*, more likely than that care respecting success in business, and in matters of comparatively trifling moment, should produce the same result. We should be inclined to suppose that the former cause would have the greatest influence, inasmuch as the interests concerning which fears and hopes are raised are in the one case incomparably more important than in the other, were it not for the observation daily repeated by moralists and divines, that men are far more concerned about the most trifling affairs of the present life than about the most momentous which regard the unseen and unchangeable state, and that this remark holds good to a vast extent, even to the exclusion of those who profess disbelief in a future existence.

As a matter of fact, there is reason to believe that the number of persons who become insane through the influence of religious hopes and fears, is much less considerable than it is generally supposed to be. The circumstance that the mind of a lunatic is occupied during the period of his disease with ideas and feelings connected with an invisible world, is no proof whatever that the derangement of his understanding was produced in the first instance by impressions related to the same subject. To a mind already prepared by disease to indulge fearful thoughts and gloomy forebodings, the unknown future opens a wide field which the imagination is likely to select, and it often dwells upon the evils which it anticipates in another stage of existence, when the original cause of derangement has been some misfortune of the present life, or perhaps some merely physical influence. It is the opinion of a writer, whose judgment on subjects of this nature deserves the highest regard, on account of the extensive research and the deep reflection with which he has investigated the history of mental disorders, that instances of the last-mentioned kind are in fact incomparably more numerous than those in which religious terrors have been the originating cause.[*]

There is, however, no room for doubt that distress occasioned by such anxieties has really given rise to disorders of the mind. Several instances of this kind have, indeed, fallen within my own sphere of observation. Some of these have occurred among persons who had frequented churches or chapels where the ministers were remarkable for a severe, impassioned, and almost imprecatory style of preaching, and for enforcing the terrors rather than setting forth the hopes and consolations which belong to the Christian religion. Foreign writers have supposed this to be the practice of the methodists in particular; and M. Falret, persuaded by the assertions of Darwin and Perfect, mentions the prevalence of methodism in England as a presumptive proof of the frequency of suicide among our countrymen.[†] That none of the preachers of this sect have been deserving of such a censure, I shall not venture to affirm; but in the present time at least, it cannot justly be laid either generally or exclusively to their charge. A vehement and impassioned mode of preaching has often been the practice in other sects, both among protestants and catholics, and in no instance more remarkably than among the itinerant missionaries of the latter church.[‡]

* Dr. Maximilian Jacobi's Sammlungen für die Heilkunde des Gemüthskrankheiten. Th. i.
† De l'Hypochondrie et du Suicide. Par J. P. Falret, M.D., Paris, 1822.
‡ "In the kingdom of Naples," says M. Berthollet, "a custom exists of

Such accidental excitements are sometimes the occasional causes
of insanity, or rather they are the immediate antecedents of its actual
appearance or out-breaking ; but the conditions on which the existence of this disease, under the modifications now described, seems
mainly to depend are of more extensive influence. It may be said
in one sense that a preparation is made for this species of derangement in the constitution of the human mind. Hope and fear,
anxiety respecting the future, are the principles in human nature by
which the care of self-preservation is insured. In the lower orders
of the creation this object is attained by blind mechanical impulses
termed instincts, counterfeits of that care and caution of the future
which are peculiar to man. This anticipation of wants, which
answers the end of foresight, varies in its reach according to the
necessities which are to be provided for ; in most of the irrational
tribes it extends forward only a few months, till the return of seasons brings with it new resources for sustenance.* The anticipations
of the human mind are alone bounded by no limit of time or physical
circumstances ; the hopes and fears of good and of evil which are
allotted to humanity reach forward into eternity. Hence the intensity which these anxieties are capable of acquiring when the mind is
fully excited to entertain them, and to yield itself to their influence.
Various as are the anticipations which human anxieties create or
embody in remote futurity, there is one feature common to them all.
Their prevailing character is gloomy : they are generally forebodings of evils and calamities. Horrible forms hang over the path
which the human imagination marks out to itself through the
unknown regions of futurity. Death is the king of terrors, not by
the dread of extinction, but by ushering us into an endless world of
anxieties. It has often been observed that in all the mythological
fables of antiquity, the representations that prevailed respecting the
state of the dead were full of gloom ; the abodes of the manes or of
souls were " loca pallidula, frigida." The explanation of this fact

preaching in favour of missions by a particular set of priests. In order to
animate the faith of believers, they accompany their orations with particular acts,
which are often of such a nature as to produce too powerful an effect on weak
minds. They hold their hands over flaming torches, and whip themselves with
scourges garnished with iron points. Their sermons are prolonged till the close
of day, and the feeble glare of a few flambeams heightens the effect of the scene."
" One of these sermons gave occasion to the case I am about to describe. The
subject was *hell:* to heighten the colouring of the frightful picture which the
preacher had traced, he took a skull in his hand, and having raised a question as
to the abode of the soul to which it belonged, he exclaimed, invoking it, ' If
thou art in heaven, intercede for us ; if thou art in hell, utter curses.' He then
cast it from him with violence." The lady, whose case is subsequently described
in M. Berthollet's Memoir, was instantly affected by a morbid change in the
nervous system.
Strong emotions excited by vehement preaching produce continually in females
and very sensitive persons fits of hysteria, and in those who are predisposed to
mania there can be no doubt that similar causes give rise to attacks of madness.
* See Dr. Hancock's excellent and truly philosophical work "On the Relations of Instinct to the Higher Principles of Human Action."

is, that such mythological fictions were the creations of fancy, but of
the fancy under a strong and predominating influence of evil conscience. A persuasion of moral demerit or a consciousness of guilt
has been deeply impressed upon the minds of men in all ages.
With this has been intimately connected the sentiment of responsibility, the conviction of individuals that they were accountable
beings, and that there were unseen powers whose cognizance nothing
eludes, and from whose unerring justice even death can afford no
escape. Here the imagination came in to perform its part, and this
it has done with so much energy as to drive many individuals into
insanity in all ages of the world.

The preparatory circumstances and the foundation of this disease
are not, then, limited in their extent to nations and times in which
religion has existed in any particular form. They belong to the
condition and circumstances of human nature, at least of human
nature in a state not altogether uncultivated and brutalized. Accordingly we are enabled to trace examples of this form of madness
in every period of history, and even before the era of authentic
history. A German writer* whom I have before cited has taken
pains to collect instances in the early fables of Greece. Even before
the Argonauts, Melampus, according to Herodotus, cured by means
of hellebore the daughters of Prœtus, of whom it is said,

> " Prœtides implêrant falsis mugitibus agros."

Hercules, Ajax, Orestes, Athamas, Alcmæon, laboured under religious madness, as well as the famous exile hated of the gods, who is
mentioned in words strikingly descriptive of insanity :

> " Qui miser in campis mœrens errabat Aleis,
> Ipse suum cor edens, hominum vestigia vitans."

Cassandra, the Mænades, the Pythia, are reckoned by Heinroth
as examples of a more exalted and ecstatic period of religious madness, and to these many other instances are added which I shall leave
to the recollection of my readers.

The circumstances in the moral nature of mankind on which these
phenomena depend, have such influence that there is no reason to
hope that their effect will cease. Yet they have been much more
prevalent in certain times and places than in others. It has been
said that in France, since the revolution, the popular influence of
religion has been less than it ever was in any other civilized country ;
and I have been informed by French physicians who have extensive
means of information, that instances have religious insanity have
become in a similar proportion rare. But a question presents itself
whether this change has been on the whole a beneficial one, or may
have produced evils greater than the alleged advantage may be
supposed to compensate. We have to consider this question at
present with reference only to the prevalence of madness, and in

* Heinroth's Stoerungen des Seelenlebens.

this relation the following remarks by a most competent as well as an unprejudiced observer afford a sufficient reply to the inquiry.

"The changes," says M. Esquirol, "which have taken place during the last thirty years in our moral sentiments and habits, have produced more instances of madness in France than all our political calamities. We have exchanged our ancient customs and fixed habits, our old and established sentiments and opinions, for speculative theories and dangerous innovations. Religion now only comes forward as a formal usage in the solemn transactions of life ; she no longer affords her consolations to the afflicted, or hope to the desponding. Morality founded on religion is no longer the guide of reason in the narrow and difficult path of life. A cold egotism has dried up all the sources of sentiment : there no longer exist domestic affections, respect, attachment, authority, or reciprocal dependences; every one lives for himself; none are anxious to form those wise and salutary provisions which ought to connect the present age with those which are destined to follow it."

I shall now shortly advert to an inquiry which has often been agitated, and which I cannot well pass over entirely, whether there are any systems of religion or institutions more favourable than others to the health of the mind, as far as security from religious madness is concerned, and whether in one church or community of Christians there are more or fewer examples of insanity than in others.

It has been supposed by many persons that Roman catholics are less subject than protestants to morbid illusions on subjects connected with religion. Dr. Hallaran declares that in the public lunatic asylum at Cork, which is inhabited by Roman catholics in the proportion of ten to one protestant, "no instance within his recollection has occurred of mental derangement in the former from religious enthusiasm." He adds that several cases of this kind had appeared among the inmates of the same asylum, but that the individuals affected were protestant dissenters.* A similar opinion as to the comparative infrequency of religious madness among Roman catholics is supported by M. Guislain, whose work on mental alienation has communicated much valuable knowledge, especially as to the state of lunatics and lunatic asylums in the Low Countries. It has been observed by Leupoldt that insanity is much more prevalent in the north of Germany than in the southern parts of the same country. This alleged difference is attributed by M. Guislain to the diversity of religion. In the south of Germany the Roman catholic religion prevails. "On approaching the north," says M. Guislain, "we meet with the reformed church and its fanatical discussions. It remains to be proved," he adds, "whether we could not establish the same relation, and deduce the consequences which result from it, in our kingdom. Holland professes generally the reformed worship ; Flanders and Brabant Roman catholicism. This would furnish a very interesting comparison. We should have to deter-

---

* Practical Observations on Insanity, by Dr. Hallaran. Cork, 1818, p. 32.

mine whether Holland affords, in proportion to our catholic provinces, the same number of cases of lunacy, especially of the
religious kind, as Burrows and others have admitted in the reformed
countries of Britain, and as Leupoldt has observed to exist in the
protestant districts of Germany. It would be necessary to obtain
for this purpose the exact numbers of the inhabitants of our houses
for lunatics. As yet we have only on this subject notions too
general to serve as a basis for the comparison."*

Nothing can be more remote from the truth than the impression
which the readers of these statements might perhaps derive from
them, viz., that Roman catholic countries possess an immunity from
the prevalence of madness connected with religious feelings and
ideas. Jacobi, who has devoted much attention to this subject,
observes that Roman catholics are not more protected by the institutions of their church against insanity with religious illusions
than protestants. " Yet," he says, " we must admit that the
character of religious madness in the members of these two communities, and the manner in which individuals become subjected to
them, is for the most part very different. Every person who has
visited the lunatic asylums in catholic Germany must be aware that
many inmates of these establishments belonging to the lower classes
have been brought into a species of religious madness by the delusions of a wild and unregulated imagination, excited by superstitious
phantasms, and through neglect of the culture of the understanding,
and a proportionally overpowering influence of sensual passions ;"
and that the same remark holds good in Italy we learn, among
others, from Chiaruggi, who in his work on insanity expressly
declares that, in Tuscany at least, most instances of melancholy owe
their origin to emotions excited by religion.† History affords us,
indeed, innumerable proofs that religious insanity among Roman
catholics is any thing rather than a rare phenomenon. " I was
much struck," adds Jacobi, " on finding that in the lunatic establishments of Franconia, especially among persons who had been
bred up in the Roman catholic communion, the idea of diabolical
possession, in which individuals not only believe themselves to be
in the power of Satan, but fancied that they conceal bodily a devil
within their own persons, was remarkably prevalent ; while, on the
other hand, at Sonnenstein, as Pienitz has assured me, as well as at
Waldheim, and in the Charité at Berlin, such an impression is very
rarely to be met with." Dr. Jacobi gives the details of one case of
this description, in which cure was obtained by a method adopted
by Dr. Muller, hôfmedicus at Wurtzburg. He then continues his
observations on religious insanity as prevailing in Roman catholic
countries. The following remarks will probably be read with
interest.

* Traité sur l'Aliénation Mentale, &c. par Joseph Guislain, Médicin à Gand.
Amsterdam, 1826, tom. ii. p. 168.
† Chiaruggi della Pazzia in Genere ed in Spezie. Jacobi, ubi supra.

"In returning," says the author, "to the consideration of religious insanity, I must further observe, that although this form of mental derangement is developed in a different manner, and assumes a different aspect among catholics and protestants, when we refer among the former to the lower orders of the people in places where education is neglected, the difference is by no means so considerable, if we advert to places where the state of mental culture is higher, as it is in the better informed classes professing the catholic religion in Germany, and especially among the younger ecclesiastics of that church. Among these religious insanity arises from the same causes which have been already indicated as the most frequent and influential in the excitement of the same disease among protestants, viz., doubts relating to religious controversy, and anxiety concerning the future welfare of individuals. In the hospital of St. John at Saltzburg, there was, among others, a ward especially dedicated to the admission of insane persons of the priestly order, and great as my surprise was in observing this arrangement when I undertook first the direction of that institution, I afterwards found reason to acknowledge its propriety. During the period of my superintendence it happened in three instances that young ecclesiastics in a state of derangement were placed under my care : of these, two appeared in all probably to have become insane in the manner I have just indicated. Although it may be conjectured that a great number of catholic ecclesiastics, and especially the members of some monastic orders, where such still exist, may have been brought into a state of derangement in a different way ; and indeed Chiaruggi, in the four cases of insanity occurring in ecclesiastics, among his 'Century of Observations,' makes no mention of such causes ; yet other physicians, who have had greater opportunities for experience in this kind have found the fact I have stated fully established. We may besides consider this as certain,—that the religious feelings of late awakened in Germany, both among catholics and protestants, and the general practice of reading the scriptures connected with this change both as cause and effect, by powerfully directing the spirit of inquiry to subjects of religion, must have stirred up and excited the minds of many persons to such a degree, and, on the other hand, have thrown others into such perplexing doubts, and into questions of conscience so difficult of solution, that distraction and derangement of the mind have been the consequence. But if this result of the weakness of human nature is to be lamented, in respect to those who fall in such a manner into religious insanity, yet it must not be denounced generally as the greatest of all evils, as every one will be ready to admit who contemplates the opposite extreme, and observes how in France, for instance, while, owing to a general indifference to religion, very few become deranged through anxiety respecting the most important concerns that can engage the human mind, the generality of men have their rational understanding impaired through the influence of lower passions, and of vices which are so much the more prevalent ; and how, in the vast empires of the east, immunity from mental derangement is only the result of a moral and religious torpor, which keeps the human faculties benumbed and stupified."

In order to be justified in forming any decided opinion as to the question whether the catholic or protestant institutions are most favourable to the development of insanity, it would be requisite to compare the state in this respect of large bodies of people inhabiting the same or similar countries, and in other respects living under nearly similar circumstances. It would not be sufficient to compare the people of northern Germany with those of the south, or even the Dutch with the Flemings : differences of habits, climate, and other external circumstances are here added to those of religion, and the former may contribute to any differences that may be found in the proportion of lunatics to the population of the respective countries. If even we should compare the people of Ireland and Scotland in these respects, we could not with confidence ascribe any difference that might be found in the proportional numbers of lunatics to the prevalence of the catholic religion in one and the reformed church in the other, since the habits and characters of these nations are strikingly different in other respects. We must, then, look for some decisive example in a country where the two churches co-exist, and their respective adherents display in other particulars no marked diversity in their character and habits. The most appropriate instance yet adduced, and the most satisfactory means of instituting this comparison, is afforded by the population of the Prussian states on the Rhine, where the number of persons professing the two religions is tolerably well known, and the number of lunatics belonging to each can be more accurately estimated than elsewhere. This comparison has been made, and the results have been published by Dr. Jacobi, in a work which appeared some years later than that from which I have already made citations. The following extract from his statistical table will display the principal data on which conclusions are founded.

The table contains an account of the collective number of insane persons existing in the year 1824, in the lunatic establishments of Düsseldorf, Aix-la-Chapelle, Trêves, Cologn, and Coblentz, or in the Rhenish provinces belonging to Prussia. The total number of the population of these provinces is stated at 2,067,104, and the total number of lunatics at 2,015, which is nearly one to each thousand of the population. These 2,015 lunatics are divided into four sets, according to their religious professions, viz. into Catholics, Evangelicals or Lutherans, Mennonites, and Jews. The following are the numbers in the different provinces :—

	Catholics.	Evangelicals	Mennonites	Jews.	Sum total.
Düsseldorf—					
Population	395,031	239,840	847	5,495	641,213
Number of lunatics	544	241	4	9	
Aix-la-Chapelle—					
Population	320,793	9,382	3	1,782	331,960
Number of lunatics	301	11	—	—	
Trèves—					
Population	301,505	32,804	47	3,451	337,807
Number of lunatics	202	18	—	1	
Cologn—					
Population	323,283	50,001	2	4,049	377,335
Number of lunatics	283	48	—	5	
Coblentz—					
Population	250,613	121,595	333	6,248	378,789
Number of lunatics	236	101	2	9	

The result of this collation is that the proportion of lunatics in the catholic part of the population, compared to that which is discovered in the Lutheran population, is as eleven to ten, or one-eleventh part greater. The Mennonites and Jews give a still higher proportion ; but the numbers of them which are brought into computation are not sufficient to afford the materials of any general estimate or conclusion.

It would seem from this comparison, which is the only document as yet obtained that may be considered as a tolerably fair and unexceptionable comparison of the number of lunatics occurring in a catholic population to that which discovers itself in a protestant population under similar circumstances, that the catholic religion is rather more favourable to the manifestation of insanity than the protestant.

I cannot with perfect propriety conclude this compilation of facts connected with *religious insanity,* without inserting the remarks of the writer already cited on Mr. Tuke's Account of the Retreat, the lunatic asylum belonging to the Society of Friends, near York. Jacobi published a German translation of that work, in which nothing seems to have struck him more forcibly than the fact that the species of insanity now under consideration occurs but in three instances in the list of cases given by the writer, or rather that there are but three cases of derangement out of one hundred and forty-nine which can with any probability be ascribed to anxieties connected with religious impressions. "Equally remarkable it is that in the list of causes, pride, ambition, jealousy, rage, debauchery, as well as extreme penury and care produced by hardships and want of the necessaries of life, causes so fruitful of madness in other establishments, are not even mentioned." The exemptions which this remark implies from the most prevalent modifications of derangement which occur in other communities, are attributed by Jacobi to the strictness of moral education and discipline, for which he says that the Quakers in England are remarkable, to the restraints imposed by them on the imagination and the indulgence of passions, and to the absence of enthusiastical and mystical excitement in connexion with religion.

As several years have elapsed since the Account of the Retreat was published, which drew forth these comments from the distinguished translator of that work into the German language, it seemed to me a matter of great interest to ascertain whether later experience has confirmed the preceding observations, or whether cases of religious madness have occurred of late in so small a proportion as formerly among those which have been admitted at the Retreat. With reference to this inquiry I have received from the intelligent and judicious author of the Account the most satisfactory information. Mr. Tuke says, " In regard to our cases of ' *religious madness*' I may state that we can only enumerate eight since the close of the year 1811 out of three hundred and thirty-four admissions. In none of these cases could it, as I believe, be said that the religious feelings which just succeeded, *or perhaps rather first marked* the commencement of the disease, were excited by any special religious means or occasion. The patients were generally persons of rather weak and of contemplative minds, and several of them were persons who had not been educated in our society."

It seems, then, that religious insanity so termed is a disorder from which the Society of Friends are in a great measure exempt. With respect to the more general question, whether insanity of any kind prevails among the Quakers to a great or comparatively small extent, those writers who have touched upon the subject have been divided in opinion. Dr. Haslam says that insanity is very rare among the members of that society. Dr. Burrows thinks it very frequent among them, and he accounts for the fact by another supposition, viz. that their marriages are confined to the families of their own society, and therefore within a very limited circle. With respect to the first point, which only is relevant to my present purpose, Mr. Tuke has furnished me with some data which are highly interesting. He says that the number of inmates of the Retreat who are members of the religious Society of Friends has of late years been usually about sixty-four. The total number of Friends in England and Scotland does not, as he believes, exceed 22,000 or 23,000. The mean of these sums divided by the number of patients actually in the Retreat gives $2\frac{3}{13}$, or somewhat less than three in a thousand, which is a very high proportion, and considerably exceeding that which is supposed to obtain in the general population of this and other countries.

But there are considerations which render it difficult to believe that such a comparative result is correct, and which seem to lead us almost inevitably to an opposite conclusion, or at least show that some other considerations must be introduced in order to explain facts which turn out so contrary to all expectation from the known circumstances of the case. We have seen that the cases of religious madness so termed, are so few in the Retreat, that the community to

which that asylum belongs may be considered as exempted in a
great measure from that modification of insanity. But the same
observation may be made with reference to several of the most
prevalent causes of mental derangement. Mr. Tuke informs me
that " not more than two cases of disease apparently connected with
intemperance in drinking have occurred in the Retreat among the
members of the Society since 1811." This is well known to be in
many asylums a very productive cause. Extreme poverty and
distress from actual want forms a large article in the tables of cases
given by M. Esquirol and others ; and from this cause of madness
the Quakers are likewise protected by their habits and institutions.
Mr. Tuke says, " We have had a few cases attributed to disappointment of the affections, and several to domestic afflictions, and disappointment in business." Even these are scarcely as numerous as
those referred to the same articles in other establishments. As to the
suggestion of Dr. Burrows, that insanity is rendered frequent in the
Society of Friends by the fact that their marriages are confined
within their own community, we may remark that the numbers of
this community are upwards of twenty thousand. Were this writer's opinion well founded, what would become of the royal
dynasties and aristocracies in Europe ? From all these considerations we are brought inevitably to the conclusion which Mr. Tuke
has drawn. He says, " Unless, then, we have a larger proportion
of imperfect structures amongst us than obtains in the world at large,
we ought to have fewer cases of insanity in proportion to our
numbers than is found in the general population."

But how is this conclusion to be reconciled with the fact that the
proportional number of cases is actually greater than what is calculated to obtain in the general population. Mr. Tuke observes, " If
I were to enter into this subject, I should demur to the data upon
which the estimate of the proportion of lunatics in England rests.
I believe the parliamentary returns to be so *incorrect* as to afford *no*
fair ground for the estimate which is made ; whilst the knowledge
of each other which prevails in our Society, and the character of
the Retreat, brings nearly all the cases which occur among us
into the calculation. I have no hesitation in saying that the standard of sanity is in some respects higher amongst us than in the
general population. Moral improprieties connected with mental
peculiarities are more easily and more frequently stamped as insanity
amongst us than in the world at large, while the care taken of our
poor prevents any individual of that class from being allowed to
roam at large or remain at home on account of the expense of maintaining him in our asylum."

The truth of these observations cannot be illustrated by any
remarks of mine. The more the subject is reflected upon, the more
correct and well-founded will they appear.

In a subsequent chapter I shall advert to facts connected with this
subject, when I proceed to consider the statistical information that is
to be collected in reference to insanity.

Section V.—*Physical Causes of Insanity.*

The physical causes which induce insanity act in some instances immediately on the brain ; in others they affect that organ through the medium of other parts of the system.

1. *Injuries of the head.*

Injuries of the head are much more frequently causes of delirium than of insanity ; but instances are well known in which they induce the latter affection, generally as a remote consequence of delirium. Several cases of this description have occurred within my own knowledge. In some instances madness has been observed to supervene on injuries of the head which appeared to be slight and occasioned at first little or no apprehension. M. Esquirol is of opinion that insanity occasioned by this cause ensues sometimes after an interval of several years. This writer mentions the case of a child who fell on his head when three years of age ; he complained from that time of pains in his head : about the time of puberty these pains increased, and at seventeen years of age he became maniacal. A lady, whose case is given by the same writer, was thrown from a horse, and her head struck against a door. She lay for three months in raving madness, recovered, and died two years afterwards of a brain-fever.

There are instances in which a slight peculiarity of character, not amounting to insanity, has remained long, and perhaps through the life of the individual who has sustained a severe injury of the head. Sometimes this constitutes a kind of moral insanity : the temper is more irritable, the feelings are less under restraint than previously. In other instances there has been greater energy and activity, more of excitement in the general character, which has been thought a change for the better rather than a morbid alteration.*

Cases of this description are sometimes very remarkable. I have been informed on good authority that there was, some time since, a family, not far from this city, consisting of three boys, who were all considered as idiots. One of them received a severe injury of the head : from that time his faculties began to brighten, and he is now a man of good talents and practises as a barrister. His brothers are still idiotic or imbecile. Van Sweiten mentions the case of a girl who was imbecile till she received an injury of the head, and underwent the application of a trephine for the removal of a depressed portion of skull ; she recovered, and became intelligent.† Haller has reported the case of an idiot whom a wound in the head restored to understanding.

* A case analagous to this has been recorded in the instance of Father Mobillon, who is said to have acquired, after the operation of trepanning, a sudden increase of his powers of understanding.—See *Dr. Cox on Insanity,* p. 104.

† Van Sweiten, Comment. in Boerhaavii Aphorismos, tom. 1.

2. *Insolations and exposure to heat.*

Insolation, coup de soleil, or exposure to the ardent rays of the sun, is mentioned repeatedly in Esquirol's tables among the causes of madness. The disorder of the mind is here doubtless the result of inflammation, or of a state bordering on inflammation, in the encephalon.

It has been observed that cooks and other persons exposed, in consequence of their employments, to great heat, are from this cause occasionally affected with mania.

3. *Metastasis.*

The pathological fact that diseases of the brain, and among others that of which insanity is a manifestation, supervene on the cessation of various discharges, on the healing of old ulcers, on the disappearance of cutaneous eruptions, on the cessation of inflammatory disease in membranous and other structures, on the removal of tumours, has been observed with greater or less attention by practical writers on medicine from the time of Hippocrates. Many cases illustrative of this fact are to be found in the works of Hildanus, Tulpius, and Hoffmann ; and Sauvages, among the forms of madness, has reckoned one which he terms metastatic. M. Esquirol says that even a cessation of the usual discharge from the nostrils, of leucorrhœa, of blennorhœa, as well as the disappearance of scabies, of herpes, of gout and rheumatism, has produced madness. In general it may be observed that the suppression of acute eruptions, whether pustular, exanthematic, or erysipelatous, is followed by acute inflammatory affections of the internal organs ; in such cases the brain or its membranes are attacked by phrenitis or meningitis; while the disappearance of chronic disorders of the same class is the precursor of mental aberration. The suppression of more copious discharges, the removal of large tumours, the disappearance in dropsical cases by rapid absorption of deposited fluids without increased excretion, has been followed by determinations of blood to the head, giving rise to fatal apoplexy or severe convulsions.

I have seen some instances of mania supervening on inflammatory rheumatism which had subsided. These have been cases of very acute inflammation affecting the large joints, which had been reduced by too profuse bleedings, a measure which in this disease often gives rise to metastasis.

4. *Intoxicating liquors and other stimulants.*

Among physical causes of madness, one of the most frequent is the immoderate use of intoxicating liquors. There is hardly a tribe of the human race who have not succeeded in inventing some method of producing intoxication. Ardent spirits are perhaps, of all, the most injurious in their effects, particularly on the lower classes in the northern countries of Europe and America.* It has been repeatedly observed that a large proportion of the cases admitted into pauper lunatic asylums arise from this cause. They are in general to be reckoned among the cases most easily cured, for, although this is not uniformly the fact, it often happens that when the exciting cause is removed, the effect begins to lessen, and eventually ceases. When these patients are prevented from obtaining stimulating liquors, and are treated with sedative remedies, they quickly show signs of amelioration and of the subsidence of disease.

Drunkenness is a much more prevailing vice in England and in Germany, than in France, Italy, and Spain. M. Esquirol has declared that this vice is by no means a frequent cause of insanity in France, even in the lower classes. Among 336 lunatics in his establishment, there were only three who appeared to have lost their reason through the habit of intoxication. He adverts to the different habits prevalent in England, where, as he says, the greatest statesmen in the land are not ashamed of the most disgraceful drunkenness. This opprobrium may have been well merited at the time when it was uttered, but the habits of our countrymen have changed much, particularly among the higher classes, during the last twenty years. Intoxication, as it is well known, is still lamentably prevalent among the lower orders, and dram-drinking is a very frequent habit, especially in large cities, even among females, and persons not of the very lowest grade in society. In public lunatic asylums in England, it is generally known that, in a great proportion of the cases, dram-drinking is the exciting cause. I am informed by Dr. Whally that this is particularly the fact in the Lunatic Asylum at Lancaster.

The use of opium and other stimulants is among the exciting causes of madness, though of much less frequent agency than the ordinary means of intoxication.

To the same head we must refer the use of mercury, which sometimes occasions madness in persons predisposed. By such individuals this substance should be used either not at all or with extreme caution.

5. Sensuality.

Sensual vices are frequent causes of insanity, as the tables of physical causes taken from M. Esquirol sufficiently indicate.

This writer has observed that one-twentieth of the female lunatics at the Salpêtrière have been prostitutes. These unhappy creatures, after abandoning themselves to excesses of all kinds, and partly through the effect of misery and despair, fall into dementia, and often into that kind of the disease which is complicated with general paralysis.

---

* See, among other documents illustrative of this remark, M. Esquirol's Memoir on the Statistics of Insanity in the Ann. d'Hygiène et de Médicine Légale. An. 1830.

6. *Intestinal irritation.*

A disordered state of the intestinal canal often becomes a cause of disturbance in the brain, by whatever antecedents the former disease may have been induced. The state of the intestinal canal to which I allude is itself much more frequently of an inflammatory nature than it has generally been imagined, or at least than it was formerly supposed to be. In that condition of the canal which gives rise to costiveness alternating with diarrhœa, and accompanied with indigestion, flatulence and eructations, anorexia and nausea, transient but often acute pains in the hypochondria, livid and yellow suffusions of the skin, viscid secretions in the mouth, or redness of the fauces and palate, with a glazed and dry surface, the whole train of symptoms often depends upon a low degree of chronic inflammation in the mucous membrane of the intestinal canal ; and this is perhaps a frequent, if not an ordinary state, in those cases in which disorders of the nervous system supervene on complaints of the stomach and bowels. This form of disease has been described by Dr. Ferriar, and several other practical writers ; but it is to M. Broussais that we are indebted for a more ample development of its pathology.

The enteric disorder, which lays the foundation for maniacal symptoms, as well as for other affections of the nervous system, is the result in different instances of various and very diverse noxious causes. The most frequent is excess in the use of stimulant and indigestible food. Too great indulgence of the appetite among the more opulent, and among the lower classes long-continued constipation, unwholesome diet, the use of salt provisions, exposure to cold and want, or neglect of warm clothing, give rise to diseases of the same description.

Intestinal worms are one of the results of constipation. Madness produced by the last mentioned cause is probably of very rare occurrence. M. Esquirol has, however, mentioned a remarkable instance of maniacal disease affecting a young man, who was cured at two different periods by the expulsion of a large quantity of worms from the intestinal canal. I shall have occasion to enter more fully into the subject of enteric and other visceral disorders, which are sometimes connected with insanity, when I proceed to the consideration of the morbid appearances discovered by necroscopy.

7. *Causes depending on states of the uterine system.*

States of the constitution connected with irregularities of the uterine functions are well known to coexist or to display themselves in connection with various disorders of the brain. Among these madness is one. Maniacal affections of this class may be mentioned under three heads.

a. Dysmenorrhœal affections.—Some females at the period of the catamenia undergo a considerable degree of nervous excitement : morbid dispositions of mind are displayed by them at these times, a wayward and capricious temper, excitability in the feelings, moroseness in disposition, a proneness to quarrel with their dearest relatives, and sometimes a dejection of mind approaching to melancholia. These are distinct from the cases of hysterical affection connected with the same periodical causes of excitement. The former are sometimes the preludes of a far more permanent disease.

b. Suppressions of the catamenia.—Sudden suppressions of the catamenia are frequently followed by diseases of the nervous system of various kinds. Females exposed to cold, undergoing powerful excitements, experience a suppression of the catamenia, followed in some instances immediately by fits of epilepsy or hysteria, the attacks of which are so sudden as to illustrate the connexion of cause and effect. In attacks of madness the catamenia are for the most part wholly or partially suppressed during the early periods, and in many cases it is not easy to say whether the suppression is the effect or the cause of the disease. There are instances, however, in which the circumstances sufficiently indicate the order of connexion. Dr. Burrows has detailed a case in which suppression brought on by manifest causes was followed by mania. We have already alluded to the case of a young female mentioned by M. Esquirol, who suddenly exclaimed that she was cured of her disorder ; her catamenia had flowed spontaneously, and her restoration to sanity was the immediate consequence. Facts so decisive in their bearings on pathology are not of very frequent occurrence, but their evidence reaches further than the individual cases recorded.

It often happens, that after some weeks or months in the duration of madness, the catamenia, though previously deficient, become restored nearly to their usual state. This, like the other indications of improvement in merely physical health, is only a favourable sign when it is accompanied by some amendment in the state of the mental faculties. Without any such change, it rather gives reason to apprehend that the disorder is becoming inveterate, and perhaps already making its transition from mania into the incipient stage of dementia.

c. Puerperal madness is another modification of the disease connected with the state of the uterine functions. The consideration of this subject is too important to be taken up in a cursory manner, and I purpose to allot to it a separate chapter.

CHAPTER V.

RESULTS OF NECROSCOPICAL RESEARCHES INTO THE CHANGES OF STRUCTURE CONNECTED WITH INSANITY.

Section I.—*Morbid Phenomena discovered in the Head: Researches of Morgagni, Greding, Haslam, Pinel, Esquirol, Georget, Bayle, Calmeil, Foville.*

Few diseases appear to be connected with a greater variety of necroscopical phenomena than insanity. Such phenomena have been sought principally in the head, but morbid changes have been found likewise in other parts of the body ; and there are some pathologists who regard the latter as not less important in connexion with the disease than the alterations of structure discovered within the cranium. This is a consideration on which, at present, we have no business to enter ; it is the office of the anatomist, or the collector of anatomical facts, to record all the phenomena observed, and to regard those as most essential to any given disease which are most generally found to have been coexistent with it. We shall begin with a survey of the morbid appearances discovered in the heads of insane persons, and proceed afterwards to those which have been found in the thorax and abdomen.

The elucidation of this disease, as of most others, by pathological anatomy, may be said to begin with Morgagni. That celebrated writer has, however, related the details of but seven or eight dissections referring to cases of insanity. In these he remarked several facts which later observations have confirmed. He found the substance of the cerebral hemispheres more firm, and that of the cerebellum softer than natural. In one instance the white substance of the cerebrum was hard and of a brownish hue, and its bloodvessels, as well as those of the plexus choroides, much distended with blood : in another there was hardening of the hemispheres and softening of the fornix, fulness of the cerebral vessels, adhesion of the pia mater : in a third, injection of the meninges.

The first author who recorded an extensive series of observations on the appearances of the brain in cases of insanity was Dr. Greding, physician to a public hospital at Waldheim, where a considerable number of lunatics and demented persons are congregated. The following are the most important of the facts which he has noted.

1. In the *cranium.*—" Experience has proved," as he says, " that the skulls of almost all insane persons have a natural shape." In 16 cases only of the whole number examined, viz. nearly 220, the forehead was contracted, the temples compressed, and the occiput large and expanded. In a few the head was elongated and compressed at the temples. Some had a head almost round, or of a square shape : these were epileptic idiots. Two had small heads, quite circular : these were epileptic madmen. Of 216 cases, including those of madmen, idiots, and epileptics, the skull was unusually thick in 167 : this fact was observed in 78 out of 100 cases of raving madness, and in 22 among 30 of idiotism. In many cases the cranium was remarkably thin. Holes were observed in the inner table in 115 out of 216 cases : in other instances bony projections from the inner surface.

2. *Membranes.*—Dura mater firmly adherent to the skull in 107 out of 216 cases ; in a few instances of a blueish black colour, thickened and partially ossified. Pia mater thickened and opaque, more or less, in 86 out of 100 cases of mania ; beset with small, spongy bodies, in 92 out of 100 : these bodies were often united to the surface of the brain, and were in some instances the seats of ossific deposits.

3. *Brain.*—Cerebral substance softer than usual in 118 out of 216 cases : soft and pulpy in 51 cases of mania out of 100, as likewise in 19 out of 24 cases of melancholia, in 8 out of 20 epileptics, and in 16 out of 30 idiots. Those maniacs who had the cerebrum softened had the cerebellum still more soft and pulpy.

4. *Effusions.*—Between the dura and pia mater in 120 out of 216 cases ; in 58 out of 100 maniacs. Between the pia mater and the surface of the brain in 28 among 100 maniacs. Lateral ventricles in 29 very full of serum, in 23 ready to burst ; in 10 among 24 melancholics astonishingly distended. Third ventricle quite full in 57 out of 100 maniacs, and in 16 of 24 melancholics. Fourth ventricle ready to burst in 80 out of 100 maniacs, and quite empty in only 3 : completely distended in every one of 24 melancholics.

Other appearances.—Plexus choroides in a nearly healthy state in only 16 out of 216 cases, thickened and full of hydatids in 96 out of 100 maniacs. Lateral ventricles either larger or smaller than natural in many cases. Softness of parts of the brain, as of the tubercula quadrigemina in some cases.

Dr. Haslam has given the histories of 37 cases of madness with the appearances discovered on dissection. In not one of these cases were the brain and its membranes free from morbid appearances. In almost all either the membranes bore marks of former inflammation, or the vessels which they contained were distended with blood : in 16 cases there was an effusion of serum between the membranes, and in the lateral ventricles in 18. In 9 cases the consistence of the brain was firmer than usual ; in 7 it was softer, but in 20 not perceptibly altered. In 3 cases the cranium was thicker, and in 3 thinner than the natural state. In several cases a peculiar looseness of the scalp was observed.

M. Georget has recorded with great precision the facts which he has himself observed. The following are the most remarkable. Irregular conformations of the cranium, the prominences of which are developed irregularly, those of the right side being generally larger than those of the left ; some skulls having the lateral diameter of equal extent with the antero-posterior, and the cavities of the base irregular in extent ; some skulls, 1 in 20, thickened partially or generally ; more frequently the bones hard, white, with diploë, resembling ivory ; some very light. Dura mater rarely changed ; sometimes adherent to the skull, thickened, containing deposits of bone. Arachnoid displaying in places additional laminæ of a red or grey colour ; sometimes thickened but smooth. Pia mater injected ; or thickened and infiltrated with serum, giving at first the appearance of a gelatinous deposit. Volume of the brain sometimes less than the cavity of the cranium seems to require. Some brains very hard, cut with difficulty ; the white substance glutinous, elastic, and suffering distension ; more frequently the brain is soft, the grey matter being pale and yellowish, and the white substance discoloured, of a dirty white, the colour and consistence of these portions almost confounded. The convolutions separated by serosity and the pia mater thickened. Interior cavities of the brain appearing in some instances very large, in others small, often filled with a serous fluid remarkably clear and limpid ; plexus choroides exsangueous, containing hydatiform vesicles. Partial softenings of the brain; erosions, ulcerations of the surface of the ventricles. Cerebellum generally softer than the cerebrum ; sometimes partially softened. Mesocephalon, medulla oblongata, and medulla spinalis rarely displaying morbid changes of structure.

M. Pinel, after observing that the phenomena displayed by dissection in the heads of lunatics are similar to those which occur in other cerebral diseases, seemed to give up the hope of elucidating the pathology of mental derangement by necroscopical researches. M. Esquirol was inclined, on the whole, to participate in this opinion, although he carefully noted the appearances which were discovered in numerous examinations. His enumeration of these phenomena is in general similar to that of M. Georget. But in the report given by M. Esquirol of the Royal Hospital of Charenton, the mature opinion of this able writer is expressed, and it is by no means calculated to encourage sanguine expectations. He says, " The inspection of bodies of lunatics offers numerous varieties as to situation, number, and kind of morbid appearances. The lesions of the encephalon are neither in relation to the disorder of the mind nor to the maladies complicated with it. Some lunatics whose mental and bodily disease had given suspicion of extensive organic lesions, have presented but slight changes of structure in the brain, while others whose symptoms had been less severe have been the subjects of great and numerous alterations. But what disconcerts all our theories is that not unfrequently, even in the instance of patients who have passed through all the stages of insanity, and have lived many years under derangement, no organic changes whatever have been traced either in the brain or its containing membranes.

" However important may have been the researches of anatomists made during our days into diseases which affect the mind, we may venture to repeat that pathological anatomy is yet silent as to the seat of madness, and that it has not yet demonstrated what is the precise alteration in the encephalon which gives rise to this disease. What shall we, then, think of the rash pretensions of those who assume that they can fix upon the diseased portion of the brain, judging merely from the character of the disease ? But these inquiries are foreign to my purpose, and I shall at present only specify the number of organic lesions which have been discovered in different cavities in 199 bodies examined at Charenton. In these we have found 263 organic lesions of the brain and meninges, 46 alterations in the lungs, the heart, or in their coverings, 113 lesions of the abdominal viscera. Thus it appears that morbid phenomena have been much more frequent in the brain than elsewhere."

M. Esquirol avows that this conclusion is different from that which he had formerly obtained in the examination of bodies at the Salpêtrière. In that hospital females only are the subjects of obser-

vation, who, being less subject to general paralysis than men, are
likely to afford fewer morbid phenomena in the examination of the
brain. M. Esquirol, however, candidly admits that a great part of
the difference in the result of these researches may arise from the
greater care with which the brain is now dissected, and the slightest
changes observed. " Hence," he says, " few bodies of lunatics are
now examined in which they are not proved to exist at the same
time injections or adhesions of the meninges, softenings, and tubercles in the brain, serous effusions in the cavities, &c. while at the
period when we made our earliest investigations, we only kept account of obvious and manifest alterations."

Since the publication of M. Georget's works on insanity, minute
and laborious researches into the morbid changes connected with this
disease have been prosecuted by various writers. M. Bayle availed
himself of the opportunities for observation afforded by the hospital
of Charenton, and on the phenomena which he traced founded his
new doctrine of mental diseases. According to M. Bayle, the
proximate cause of insanity is seated, not in the brain itself, but in
the meninges. From the inflammation of these membranes effusions
follow, and the phenomena usually dependent on compression of the
brain. " The cessation or diminution of maniacal violence, the great
loss of power observed in the intellectual faculties, and the commencement of general paralysis, which take place at the transition
into the last period of the disease, result from compression of the
brain, owing to the exhalation of serosity into the cavity of the arachnoid, the serous infiltration of the pia mater, and an effusion of the
same kind into the lateral ventricles." " The progress of paralysis
and of dementia indicates," according to the same writer, " a corresponding increase of cerebral compression. A state of stupor with
obliteration of the faculties and ideas, and the existence of general
paralysis in its most aggravated form, are the effects of compression
of the brain, resulting from serous effusion now attaining the greatest
degree.*

The opinions of M. Bayle have been directly opposed by M. Calmeil, who has availed himself of the same resources with remarkable
ability and success. His researches into the morbid changes connected
with general paralysis are highly valuable in their results. It must
be observed that this last disease, and not insanity, was the object of
M. Calmeil's investigation. The combination of these two diseases
necessarily occasions ambiguity as to the inferences deduced from the
phenomena, since it is scarcely possible to determine how far these
appearances are connected with either morbid state; and certainly
most of the phenomena traced by M. Calmeil in the paralysis of insane persons are similar to those which other anatomists have regarded
as connected with mental derangement, without reference to the
existence of that disease in its simple form, or as complicated with
paralysis.

* Bayle, Nouvelle Doctrine des Maladies Mentales. Paris.

I shall give as brief an abstract as I can from M. Calmeil's observations.

1. Bones of the skull sometimes very full of blood, which fills the spongy tissue, reddening it, and exudes from the surfaces of the cranium when denuded and separated from the dura mater. This is mentioned merely as indicative of vascular turgescence often connected with it in the encephalon.

2. Vegetations or excrescences arising from the pia mater, with absorption of corresponding parts of the inner table of the cranium. These are granulations growing up from the surface of the pia mater, penetrating the dura mater, and causing absorption of the inner bony surface. As for the pathology of this appearance, it is remarked that infiltrations and thickenings of parts are found almost constantly under these excrescences of the pia mater.

3. Effusions of serosity in the great cavity of the arachnoid, in the ventricles of the brain, and in the cavity of the rachis. This is one of the most striking and uniform symptoms in persons who have died of general paralysis. The quantity of serosity varies. Six or eight ounces are often found in the cavity of the arachnoid. M. Calmeil attaches less importance to this phenomenon than many have done. The following are his reasons. 1. He has observed it to be wanting in some strongly marked instances of the disease. 2. He has frequently discovered similar effusions in the heads of individuals who had perished under dementia, without any symptom of paralysis, even to the last. 3. In cases in which effusions were found of five or six ounces of serosity, the symptoms of general paralysis had been not less intense, or even more intense, than in others displaying effusions of twice that extent. 4. If the compression of the brain was so considerable as many have thought, the structure of its parts would display disorganization of some kind, but the structure of the convolutions, commissures, septum, &c. is uninjured. 5. In cases of chronic hydrocephalus of long duration, the deposit of serosity has been enormous, without loss of locomotive power till the disorder reached its last degree. 6. If compression from such a cause acted mechanically, we should expect paralysis depending on it to affect all nerves equally or indifferently ; no reason could be perceived why the motive faculty should be impaired first in the tongue, then in the muscles of the lower members, and lastly in the upper, as the fact is observed to be in general paralysis. 7. We certainly cannot imagine that, such a cause acting, the upper extremities would still retain its mobility unimpaired, after the total palsy of the lower limbs. For these and other reasons M. Calmeil concludes that the symptoms of general paralysis are not, as M. Bayle supposed, dependent on compression of the brain, the result of effusion, but on the state of the encephalon which gives rise to such effusion, and chiefly to inflammation, of which the thickenings, adhesions, and vascular turgescence of the pia mater, and the peculiar condition of the cineritious substance otherwise afford sufficient proof.

4. Other morbid phenomena occurring in general paralysis with

relation to the state of the membranes are, false membranes, sometimes organized, at others unorganized, between the laminæ of the arachnoid ; encysted concretions with hemorrhages between the same laminæ : these phenomena are referred in like manner to inflammatory action, or to erethism in the capillaries of the meninges ; simple hemorrhages in the great cavity of the arachnoid ; serous infiltrations of the pia mater and the cerebral arachnoid, a phenomenon found in many diseases, but rarely to such a degree as in the paralysis of dementia ; thickenings of the pia mater and the cerebral arachnoid ; a high state of vascular injection of the same membranes.

5. Adhesions, either general or local, of the internal surface of the pia mater to the cineritious portion of the brain. This is not universally observed in cases of the disease described, although strongly marked. It is important as giving an indubitable proof of inflammation affecting the surface of the brain.

6. A curious and no doubt important series of observations refer to the state of the grey and white substance.

The grey substance contiguous to the pia mater is softened, and has the consistence of the pulp of a rotten apple. This ramollissement extends to the depth of a quarter or half a line. This appearance is accounted for by the observations of M. Lallemand, who remarks that permanent accumulations of blood diminish the cohesion of any parenchyma ; even muscular parts, spleen, lung, can easily be crushed when gorged with blood. In brains of persons destroyed by intense cerebral congestion, the corpus callosum, the septum lucidum, and other parts are found relaxed, and their consistence gives way to slight pressure ; it is to accumulation of blood that the loss of consistence in the superficial grey substance in general paralysis is to be ascribed. The same state is further manifested by a violet or red coloration of the pulp and injection of vessels ; varieties of colour resulting from inflammation, the only cause that can be imagined to maintain in the brain a continued vascular plethora. "We conclude," adds M. Calmeil, " that the want of cohesion in the grey substance is the result of inflammation." To phlegmasia, under different circumstances, and in a different modification, he likewise ascribes the hardening of the convolutions observed in some rare instances of the same disease, although he does not agree with MM. Bouchet, Casauvieilh, and Bouilleau,* in maintaining that this hardening is the first degree of inflammation.

This softening of the grey substance peculiar to general paralysis, in which it is separated into laminæ, and the external adheres to the pia mater, is, however, strongly distinguishable from ordinary ramollisement of the brain, in which its substance is really diffluent, and its component particles have lost all their organic texture and relation. Whatever affinity there may be in the pathological causes of these two states, they are distinguishable in appearance and different in results.

The consistence of the white substance is generally normal or

---

* Bouilleau, Traité de l'Encephalite, et Archives Générales de Médecine, t. viii.

natural; in some few instances, as above hinted, it is harder than usual in the convolutions.

Besides the appearances resulting from high vascular injection, there is a discoloration of the grey substance, which is a peculiar phenomenon. This appearance has been observed by M. Lallemand. It is attributed by M. Calmeil, as connected with general paralysis, to inflammation of the cortical substance, which he considers as the proximate cause of the disease.

7. This inflammation extends, as it would appear, to the ventricles, as the rugous or roughened state of the internal membrane, owing to subjacent villosities, indicates. These villosities, and the membrane itself, are often of a bright red colour. The appearance of inflammation is generally more marked in the fourth than in the lateral ventricles.

8. Local and particular lesions in the substance of the brain, such as apoplectic cysts, and likewise partial ramollisement, sometimes found in the medulla spinalis, are considered by M. Calmeil as merely accidental and peculiar to the occasional disorders complicated, in particular instances, with general paralysis.

The conclusions resulting from these observations are very clearly deduced and expressed by the author. He says,

"The changes discovered in the heads of persons who have perished under general paralysis, viz. injection and absorption of the bony structure ; injections of the dura mater ; separation of its fibres ; effusions of serosity into the cavity of the arachnoid ; false membranes, organized or without organization ; cysts filled with blood between its two laminæ ; simple hemorrhages in the arachnoid ; œdema of the meninges ; injections and thickenings of the membranes ; vegetations of the pia mater ; development of their vessels ; adhesions between the pia mater and the convolutions ; disappearance of the grey substance ; softening, hardening, and discoloration of the same substance ; consistence and injection of the white substance ; redness and tumefaction of the ventricular villosities ; serosity in the ventricles, apoplectic cysts, erosions of the convolutions ; ramollisement of the brain, or of the spinal marrow ;—these phenomena do not sufficiently explain the symptoms observed during life. The changes enumerated are so various in their appearance, and so far from uniform in occurrence, that they cannot on this account be immediately connected with the results." M. Calmeil considers them all to be evidences of inflammation. This he infers to be the identical state of the brain, of which the several appearances are diversified signs, only varied manifestations of one and the same disease. "Nearly all these disorders," as he says, "indicate a chronic phlegmasia in the brain, producing an identical modification of which the morbid appearances are only symptoms."[*]

The observations of M. Calmeil must be compared with those of M. Foville, who has more recently pursued the research into the

* Calmeil, p. 416.

state of the brain in cases of insanity.* It will be seen that in many leading particulars they agree, but that M. Foville connects with mental derangement appearances which M. Calmeil regards as restricted to general paralysis.

It was a part of M. Foville's plan to compare in every instance on the spot, healthy brains with those which were the particular subjects of examination. By this method some minute peculiarities of structure seem to have been detected which might otherwise have escaped notice. M. Foville's inquiries were carried on at the Salpêtrière in conjunction with his colleagues. MM. Delaye and Pinel Grandchamp, when that hospital was under the superintendence of M. Esquirol, and subsequently by himself at the extensive hospital of St. Yon, in the department of the Lower Seine, which has been for some years under his immediate care. His observations are arranged under the following heads: 1, morbid changes in the cortical substance ; 2, changes in the white or fibrous substance ; 3, changes in the nerves of sensation ; 4, changes in the membranes ; 5, observations on the skull and hairy scalp ; 6, changes observed in idiots. I shall abstract the most remarkable observations made by M. Foville under several of these divisions.

1. *Changes in the grey substance.*—In the most acute cases the surface of the cortical portion presents, on the removal of the membranes, a most intense redness, approaching to that of erysipelas. This is still more marked in the substance of the grey matter itself ; it is more striking in the frontal region than on the temporal lobes, and in the higher regions than in the posterior parts of the brain. In brief terms the morbid changes observed by M. Foville in *acute cases of madness* are nearly confined to the following : " Red colour, uniform and very intense ; numerous mottled spots, varying from a bright to a violet red, bloody points, minute extravasations of blood ; diminished consistence in the thickness of the cortical substance, coincident mostly with a slight increase of consistence in its surface ; dilatation of the vessels, resistance of their parietes." In acute cases M. Foville has never observed adhesions of the membranes to the cortical substance. Such adhesions are very frequent in chronic cases, and hence, as he conjectures, may be explained the curable nature of recent maniacal affections, and the hopeless and incurable state of those patients who have long laboured under madness or dementia.

Among the chronic changes of the cortical substance, the most frequent is a very perceptible increase of firmness and density in the superficial part, extending to no great depth, but uniform, constitut-

* M. Foville's original and highly interesting Researches into the Structure of the Brain were presented to the Academy of Sciences in March, 1828. They were consigned in an unpublished memoir, of which Dr. Hodgkin has given a most valuable extract in his Catalogue for the anatomical museum of Guy's Hospital. M. Foville's observations on the morbid changes connected with insanity are to be found in his article *Folie*, contributed to the " Dictionnaire de Médecine Pratique et de Chirurgie."

ing a distinct lamina, smooth externally, but internally irregular, of lighter colour than usual, which, when torn off, leaves the remainder of the cortical substance red, soft, and mammillated, somewhat resembling granulations. Something like this external pseudo-membrane of the cortical substance has been noticed in wild animals which have died in a state of confinement, by M. Foville, and is conjectured by him to denote a cerebral disease in them. The pale and almost bleached hue of the surface of the cortical portion is always connected with this increased density in its substance. Sometimes the surface is rough and granulated, containing small grains of a yellowish white.

In conjunction with these changes the volume of the convolutions remains natural, or is less than usual. When it is lessened, there are sometimes linear depressions or irregular pittings on the surface of the convolutions, and in the cortical substance itself there are small yellowish lacunæ filled with a serosity of the same tinge. These lacunæ are supposed to correspond with the minute extravasations observed in acute cases. In other instances, the diminution of volume is a real atrophy of the convolutions, which appear thin and angular, as if pinched up towards their extremities. This morbid change corresponds with what MM. Gall and Desmoulins have termed atrophy of the convolutions. It is very frequent in the frontal regions of the hemispheres. It often comprises particularly three or four convolutions on each side of the sagittal suture, a chasm filled with serosity occupying the place left by absorption of the cerebral substance. Coexistent with this appearance is that species of atrophy in the cranium in which the diploë disappears, and the external lamina approaches the internal, leaving a superficial depression on the head. In these cases of atrophy of the convolutions, the diminution of substance is confined frequently to the cortical or grey matter. What remains of the cortical substance is harder than natural, and sometimes presents, when carefully examined, a really fibrous structure ; it is of darker colour, or seems to separate into layers, of which the exterior is pale and the interior of a rose colour.

Another state of the cortical substance observed in chronic cases of madness is that of ramollissement ; this is entirely distinct from the softened state of the external portion already described. The whole thickness of the grey substance is equally altered in these cases ; its colour is more brown than usual ; its consistence almost liquefied.

This extreme and general softness of the cortical substance does not necessarily accompany a similar state in the white substance ; it is sometimes conjoined with a hardened state of the medullary portion. In such instances the grey may be separated from the white matter by pouring water upon it. Appearances of this kind seem to belong to cases of the last degree of dementia, with general paralysis and marasmus. M. Foville mentions cases apparently of the same nature, in which limited portions of the grey substance had disappeared previously to death. M. Calmeil, in his work on the paralysis connected with insanity, had related two instances of a similar description.

It seems that the grey substance in other parts of the brain is not subject to a similar change ; its morbid alterations coincide with those of the medullary portion. From this remark must be excepted the cortical substance of the cornu ammonis, which is sometimes softened, and at others of a scirrhous hardness.

2. *Morbid changes of the white substance.*—Morbid alterations of the white or fibrous substance in deranged persons are in relation to its colour, its density, and its texture.

The white substance is often the seat of vascular injections; sometimes vessels of a certain size being affected, the appearance of bloody points is produced on the section of the white substance. In other instances a finer injection gives rise to a mottled appearance of a deep red or violet colour. A magnifying glass is required in order to discover the vascular injection which produces this appearance. These injections of the white fibrous substance do not always coincide with similar injections of the surrounding cortical substance.

It is not rare to find in lunatics the fibrous substance of a splendid white; this particular aspect generally corresponds with an increased density of the parts. The hardness of such parts of the brain is sometimes almost fibro-cartilaginous. The induration of the medullary substance is, however, not always connected with this remarkable whiteness ; sometimes the hardened medullary substance has a yellow tinge or a grey leaden colour. M. Foville attempts to account for this hardening of the fibrous portion of the brain by the supposition that each cerebral fibre has contracted morbid adhesions with the surrounding fibres, so as to render their separation impossible. This opinion is offered as more than conjectural with respect to the different planes of medullary substance, of which it is considered as proved that the white substance of the brain consists. The fibrous mass of the hemispheres results, according to this writer, from the super-position of several distinct layers or planes, applied one upon the other, and connected by means of a very fine cellular tissue. These planes are easily separable in the healthy state, but in the state of maniacal induration they are inseparable.

Among lunatics affected with general paralysis, M. Foville has found these adhesions wanting in only two cases ; and in these two instances the cerebral nerves, the annular protuberance, and the medulla oblongata presented an extreme hardness. The same alteration has been found in the brains of old men whose voluntary movements have become uncertain or vacillating ; it has never been seen in lunatics whose muscular powers had remained unimpaired.

The brains of some lunatics are so full of serous fluids, that an abundant serosity flows from the surface of incisions ; sometimes this serous infiltration is so abundant as to deserve the name of cerebral œdema. A change more rare, which M. Esquirol has remarked, was the presence in the brain of a multitude of small cavities, from the size of a millet-seed to that of a nut, containing a

limpid fluid. The section of a brain thus changed is compared to
that of a porous cheese. The cavities are supposed to be the sequelæ
of extravasations.

The changes in the structure of the cerebellum are analagous in
kind to those of the cerebrum, but much more rare.

Tubercles and other tumours in the brain are considered by M.
Foville as accidental in their connexion with insanity.

3. *Morbid changes in the nerves.*—M. Foville is persuaded that
he has traced morbid alterations in the nerves corresponding with
peculiar phenomena of sensation.   In a female lunatic, tormented by
hallucinations of sight, the optic nerves were found hard and semi-
transparent through a great part of their thickness.

4. *Morbid changes in the membranes.*—In acute cases, the only
morbid appearance discovered in the meninges is for the most part
injection of the pia mater.   This injection is generally proportioned
to the degree of inflammation in the cortical substance of the convolutions.   The small arteries and veins, passing from the membrane
and penetrating the grey matter, are seen distended with florid or
black blood : the arachnoid in the mean time preserves its natural
aspect.

The chronic changes in the membranes consist for the most part
in opacity, increased consistence, thickness of the arachnoid, the
formation of granulations and pseudo-membranes on its surface, and
the effusions of serosity into the cellular tissue of the pia mater and
the ventricles.

The arachnoid membrane displays either extensively or in patches
a pearly whiteness.   The opacity never exists without thickening ;
and in those places where the arachnoid and pia mater are naturally
contiguous, they are found to be adherent.   These opaque patches,
as M. Foville supposes, result from the deposition of albuminous
layers upon the arachnoid.

The observations of the same writer on the peculiarities observed
in the skulls of lunatics add little to our previous knowledge on this
subject ; and his remarks on the conformation and texture of the
brain in cases of idiotism do not necessarily belong to the inquiry in
which we are now engaged.   I shall conclude this abstract of his
observations by briefly citing his general inferences.

"The morbid changes which we have surveyed present many of
the anatomical characters of inflammation ; intense, general, diffused
redness; in many cases tumefaction ; and lastly, in passing to the
chronic state, the formation of adhesions between the cortical substance of the convolutions and the contiguous membrane ; besides
this, adhesion of the different planes or layers of the cerebral substance to each other in a certain number of cases.

"If the simple redness, the perceptible tumefaction—if the general
and partial softenings, the increased resistance which we have noted
in acute cases, left any doubt of the true nature of the organic
disorder, the adhesions observed so often in chronic cases certainly
admit of none ; and we are forced to allow that there exists in the

brains of lunatics a state of true inflammation, unless we cease to regard adhesions observed in other parts as undoubted traces of such a state, and refuse to admit that adhesions of the pleura, peritoneum, and pericardium afford evidence of the former existence of pleuritis, peritonitis and pericarditis.

" As the different traces of inflammation are more constant in the brain than in the membranes, it is necessary to conclude that the essential change has taken place in the brain, and that the change produced in the membranes is only accidentally complicated with it." In his remarks on this subject M. Foville plainly means to express his dissent from the opinions maintained by M. Bayle, who, in his treatise on affections of the brain, attributes insanity to disease of the membranes.

Among the morbid appearances of the brain, the varied changes of the cortical substance are the most constant in connexion with symptoms of mental derangement. Although M. Calmiel maintained a different opinion, and was inclined to ascribe paralysis or the loss of muscular power to disease of the cortical substance, the facts on which he founded this inference do not, as M. Foville contends, warrant such a conclusion. In all instances of the general paralysis of lunatics which he has examined by dissection, there was, besides the change in the cortical substance, some alteration, either hardening, serous infiltration, or softening of the white substance; and in most cases, in addition to these appearances, there were adhesions of the principal planes of the cerebral substance to each other. A very remarkable case which occurred in the clinical course of M. Esquirol in 1823, affords strong evidence in favour of M. Foville's argument. The cerebrum of an idiot displayed the grey substance of both hemispheres in the last stage of atrophy and disorganization, while the white portion of the brain remained perfect on one side. In this person the intellect had been entirely defective, but the muscular power on one side only had failed. From this and similar observations M. Foville concludes that the function of the cineritious portion of the brain is essentially connected with the intellectual operations, and that of the fibrous or white structure with muscular action. His two principal inferences are expressed in the following terms:

1st, Morbid changes in the cortical substance are directly connected with intellectual derangement.

2d, Morbid changes in the white substance are directly connected with disorders in the motive powers.

It has been further remarked by M. Foville, that in some affections of the maniacal class, succeeding the action of debilitating causes, as in the puerperal state, nothing has been discovered in the brain more striking than its extreme and general paleness, and that, although there are in these instances some mottled appearances of a light red or rose colour in the cortical substance, such changes are too slight to be considered as idiopathic. The same writer adds that in the small number of cases of this description which he has had an opportunity of examining, the disorder in the brain has appeared to him to be sympathetic and the result of some deeply seated disease of the uterus or abdomen.

Section II.—*Of morbid Appearances in the thoracic Viscera.*

1. *Lungs.*—It is commonly imagined that madness is much more nearly related to diseases of the abdominal viscera than to those of the thoracic ; but this opinion is scarcely borne out by necroscopy. M. Esquirol found in 168 melancholic lunatics only two instances of disease in the liver, while in the same number there were 65 cases of disease in the lungs. The same writer has computed that, in two cases out of eight, mental derangement is accompanied with disease in the thoracic viscera ; and M. Georget declares that he has found in more than three-fourths of the bodies of insane persons examined by him, organic affections of the lungs, such as chronic pnueumonia, suppuration, or a tuberculated state. The same writer, in his work on insanity, reports that phthisis is the cause of death in more than half the lunatics of the Salpêtrière. The disease, he says, is never acute, and it is often so obscure that it is not discovered until the body is opened. In such instances there exists not the slightest indicative sign of pulmonary irritation : the patient neither coughs nor spits, and he makes no complaint ; he wastes, gets weak ; looseness or constipation succeed : he dies : these changes take place slowly. The most remarkable fact is, that, although no expectoration is perceived, cavernous excavations are found in the lungs after death.*

2. *Disorders of the heart.*—Disorders of the heart have frequently been discovered on examining the bodies of lunatics ; it has not been supposed that such phenomena are connected with madness. Such facts were generally looked upon as accidental coincidents until a contrary opinion was maintained by Nasse, in his " Zeitschrift für psychischen aertze."† This writer, in support of his opinion that disorders of the heart exercise a morbid influence on the cerebral functions, has cited the following case. An individual, with a pulse of forty strokes in a minute, had scarcely any appearance of life. When his pulse rose to fifty, he is said to have been melancholic ; when to seventy he was perfectly rational ; and with eighty pulsations he became maniacal. Nasse has also referred to dissections made by Dr. Romberg of Berlin, who, in five out of seven bodies examined by him, found softening of the heart, and in one a complete atrophy of the aortic ventricle. The same writer has maintained that insanity results in some instances from inflammation of the heart ; and he brings forward in proof of this assertion observations made by some anatomists, who have discovered in cases of madness traces of such disorder in that organ, while no morbid

* De la Folie, par Dr. Georget, p. 474.
† Zeitchrift, ann. 1818. Guislin sur l'Aliénation, p. 7.

appearances have been found by them within the cranium. He
likewise mentions the case of a young man who during six years
laboured under the signs of disease in the heart, and at the end of that
period became affected with melancholia.*

The fact last mentioned admits of a different explanation. Hypochondriasis or nervous excitement often produces disorder in the
function of the heart which is mistaken for organic disease ; and
such a state is in frequent instances a prelude to insanity as well as to
other affections of the nervous system. I have observed two strongly-
marked cases of hypochondriasis accompanied and chiefly marked
by disordered function of the heart. They occurred in young men
who had grown rapidly. In both auscultation gave evidence of disease : there was the " bruit de soufflet," with too strong impulse, and
the sound accompanying contraction of the cavities was heard over
the whole chest. Both these individuals were supposed by myself
and others to labour under hypertrophy. Mania in both supervened
on hypochondriasis, and the symptoms of disease in the heart in a
great measure disappeared.

According to the observations of M. Foville, diseases of the heart
must be considered as very frequent attendants on insanity. That
accurate anatomist has stated that in the bodies of lunatics examined
by him after death during three years, five out of six displayed some
organic affection of the heart or of the great vessels. He adds that
this was frequently hypertrophy of the heart.

If it should be established as the result of general observation that
organic affections of the heart are coincident with insanity in a proportion of cases nearly as great as the fact just mentioned would lead
us to suppose, it could no longer be doubtful that some connection
subsists between these disorders. This connection may be either
that of cause or effect. M. Foville supposes that disorders of the
heart, when complicated with mental derangement, are more frequently the results of continued agitation and of the violent efforts
and cries, which in lunatics appear likely to bring on disorders of
the thoracic viscera, than predisposing causes of insanity. Perhaps
this is the most probable conclusion. It is the inference which particular facts and the succession of symptoms have led me to adopt in
those cases which have fallen under my own observation, displaying
morbid states of the heart in connexion with mental derangement.

SECTION III.—*Of diseases in the Abdomen discovered in cases of
Insanity.*

Vestiges of diseases in the abdominal viscera have often been found
in the bodies of lunatics. Perhaps the most frequent morbid phenomena discovered in the abdomen, in individuals who have died
insane, is the appearance of inflammation in the mucous membrane

* Nasse, Archiv. für Med. erfahr, 1817. Guislain, Aliénation, t. i

of the alimentary canal. It has been reported by M. Scipion Pinel that in 269 bodies of lunatics examined, gastro-enteric inflammation, or phlegmasia of the mucous membrane lining the intestinal tube, was discovered in 51. Among these 269 cases there were only 13 of organic disease of the abdominal viscera. M. Guislain has cited some cases from Prost in which the gastro-enteric inflammation above mentioned was strongly marked. Such an appearance, according to that writer, has been many times observed, and is a frequent accompaniment of insanity.

A singular displacement of the transverse colon is one of the most remarkable changes yet observed in the abdomen in cases of insanity. This was first pointed out in a distinct and particular manner by M. Esquirol, who discovered the fact in several instances.* One of them was the case of the famous Téroigne de Méricourt a female who performed a celebrated part in the tragedy of the French revolution. This woman, after exciting the populace and occasioning disturbances, became insane on the suppression of popular ferment by the Directory. She was sent to the Salpêtrière in 1810, in a state of agitation, raving about " *liberty, the public safety, and committees.*" She died, and among other morbid phenomena discovered in her body, the transverse colon was found " *perpendicularly precipitated*" behind the pubis.

This perpendicular position of the transverse colon, descending into the pelvis behind the os pubis, has been minutely described by M. Esquirol in several other cases ; and he affirms that it was found in not less than 33 out of 168 bodies of individuals who had laboured under melancholia. It does not appear to have been the immediate cause of death in these instances. The colon itself was healthy in all the cases alluded to. This appearance has not been satisfactorily explained. It is attributed by M. Esquirol to augmented weight either from increased density, or from repletion of the colon acting mechanically. M. Georget thought it was owing to a relaxed state of the peritoneal folds which support the intestines in their position.†

Nasse's Zeitschrift contains dissections of thirteen bodies of lunatics by Bergman, in which very considerable contractions were found in the colon. In some of these the colon was contracted to a very small calibre through a great part of its length ; in others it was in parts contracted and dilated ; in some it was likewise displaced nearly in the manner described by M. Esquirol. In combination with this state of the colon, Bergman found the following morbid phenomena : —plethora of the abdomen and the encephalon ; hemorrhoidal disease ; tumefaction of the spleen, liver, and uterus ; distention of vessels in the brain. The symptoms during life were in these instances peculiar, viz., hardness and tumefaction, and tenderness of the abdomen ; slow and difficult progression in a bent forward position ; anxiety in the præcordia ; obstinate constipation with vomiting ; coldness and a

---

* Journal Général de Médecine, 1818.   Guislain, de l'Aliénation, t. i. p. 105.
† Georget, art. *Folie*, in Dict. de Méd.

blue colour of the skin ; trembling and agitation ; convulsion, rigor, diarrhœa, ushering in the final catastrophe. The mental phenomena in such instances are chimerical ideas ; the patient thinks he has frogs or serpents in his bowels ; mania and dementia ensue. To these cases of Bergman's, M. Guislain has added others of a similar description from Hufeland's Journal, and from the report of Dr. Muller of Wurtzburg.

M. Guislain attempts to account for the contraction as well as the displacement of the colon in these instances, by attributing them to inflammation. This solution cannot be admitted in the instances of the displacement observed by M. Esquirol, because the intestine is expressly affirmed by that writer to have been in a healthy state. The contraction of the canal, however, may be well imagined to result from a chronic inflammation between the planes of fibres which form the muscular coat of the intestine, comparable, as M. Guislain contends, to the chronic phlegmasia which in rheumatism brings on gradually a disorganization and contraction with wasting of the muscles of the limbs.

The question, which is the primary disease in cases displaying morbid phenomena in the abdomen in connexion with insanity, without excluding the usual vestiges of mental derangement as discovered in the encephalon, belongs to a later department of this inquiry : in the present I am chiefly intent upon a collection of facts. It must be stated, however, that insanity, in most of the instances now cited, in which disease was traced in the abdominal viscera, had been apparently the result of moral causes, agencies which exert their influence in the first instance on the brain and nervous system. This must be concluded to be the fact in nostalgia, of which several instances with dissections have been reported by Larrey, Laugier, Devaux, and Guislain. Although the causes of the malady were mental emotions, different phenomena, indicative of disease in various tissues, were found after death, and among the most prominent of these was inflammation of the mucous coat of the stomach or intestines.

Medical writers formerly attached great importance to the liver in disorders affecting the mind ; later researches have by no means confirmed this prejudice. Esquirol found only two instances of diseased liver in 168 melancholics, while in the same number there were sixty-five morbid changes of the lungs. In sixty cases of dementia, there were only two diseases of the liver ; and Scipion Pinel reports only five organic lesions of that organ in 259 cases of insanity, accompanied with alterations of structure in various parts.*

Notwithstanding the infrequency of connexion between organic disorders of the liver and insanity, there are yet facts on record which seem to prove that disease originating in the liver has given rise to mental derangement. One strongly marked instance of this kind has been recorded by M. Scipion Pinel. A man received a violent blow on the right hypochondre, which was followed by loss of sense,

* Guislain, p. 138.

vomiting, and afterwards by all the signs of hepatitis, jaundice, severe inflammatory symptoms, &c. The disorder terminated in melancholia and death. The brain was found in a natural state ; the liver greatly diseased.

The rare occurrence of organic diseases of the liver in cases of mental derangement is no proof, as M. Guislain has remarked, that pathologists have been always in error when they have conjectured or inferred, from circumstances, that the functions of the same organ have been in a disordered state, and even that such disorder has had a considerable share in evolving the train of morbid phenomena which refer to the mind.

CHAPTER VI.

THEORY OR PATHOLOGY OF MENTAL DERANGEMENT.

SECTION I.—*General Remarks on Opinions maintained by different Writers : Opinions of Heinroth and others, that Insanity is a Disease of the Mind properly so termed.*

FROM noticing the changes of structure found in the bodies of persons who have died insane, the usual progress of investigation would lead us, considering these changes as causes of the symptoms which had been observed during life, to inquire in what manner the symptoms may have resulted from the morbid states discovered. But here we are stopped by an obstacle arising out of the nature of the subject. In other instances of disease, as in affections of the heart and lungs, a discovery of morbid changes often accounts for the impediments which had arisen to the healthy function of organs of which the operation is to a certain extent understood. It is not thus with respect to disorders in the brain giving occasion to derangement of the mind. As we know not by the aid of what organic processes the mental faculties are exercised, we are at a loss to discover a connexion between defects in the structures to the instrumental operations of which they are referred, and the disorders recognized in the exercise of these faculties. And here, if we follow a cautious method of inquiry, doubts interpose themselves, whether the phenomena of insanity are really the results of changes discovered in the brain. May it not be supposed that these changes are the effects of mental disorders rather than their cause? In this latter point of view the subject has been considered by several practical writers, as by Crichton, Cox, and Arnold, who have observed that hardenings of the brain, adhesions, opacities of membranes, and other phenomena of disorganization, have been discovered chiefly and almost solely in protracted cases of insanity, and have been wanting in recent examples of the disease, that is, the bodies of those who have died during its early stage. The inference to which these considerations have led is, that such morbid appearances have been effects produced by long-continued derangement of the mind on the state of the brain, and that the real proximate cause of insanity, or the condition from which its characteristic phenomena in the first place arise, may be some deviation from the healthy state of a very different kind from that which anatomy displays.

In this point of view the morbid appearances connected with insanity have been contemplated by one class of writers, who admit this disease to be essentially an affection of the organized body, but deny that conclusive evidence has been furnished of the fact that its principal seat is in the brain. Others, also, avail themselves of the same argument, who maintain that madness is a disease of the mind in the strict sense of that expression. This last opinion, although it has been abandoned by most enlightened physicians in England, is still prevalent among the public, as we know from the frequent inquiry, whether such or such an example of insanity is the result of bodily disease or an affection of the mind itself. The same notion has found strenuous advocates in Germany, even among celebrated writers; and the arguments adduced by them in its support, although inconclusive, are not without some appearance of reason.

These writers insist strongly upon the evidence which they deduce from the want of any peculiar and distinctive phenomena manifested by anatomy as uniformly connected with insanity. They assert, and adduce many authorities to support the observation, that instances of this disease have occurred in which no disorganization has been discoverable in the brain or in any other structure of the body. They remark that many lunatics have the external appearances of health, that they live for many years with their bodily vigour slightly or in no degree impaired, while their minds are in a state of the utmost disorder.

" The causes," as they further remark, " which are chiefly productive of madness are circumstances which influence the mind. Violent passions, anxieties, grief, joy, the cares of life, are the principal causes of insanity.

" Insanity is cured by moral treatment, or by remedial means suited to a disease of the mind, often without any measures adapted to the removal of physical or bodily disorder.

" The predisponent causes of insanity are, in many instances at least, moral or mental influences. Faulty education, an habitual want of self-control, a fickle over-sensitive character unaccustomed to and incapable of steady pursuits, the dominion of passions, vices of various kinds, are among the circumstances which experience every day proves to be most influential in laying a preparation for this disease." Professor Heinroth, who carries to the utmost this line of argument, insists on the assertion that *moral depravity* is the essential cause of madness.* According to him, sin and guilt, evil

---

* " Aus der schuld entspringen alle seine uebel, auch die stoerungen des seelenlebens."—*Heinroth's Seelenstoerungen*, tom. i. § 179.

conscience, is the real origin of mental derangement. Violent
passions, sinful indulgences, want of mental discipline, give a preponderance to all the evil tendencies of our nature, and render them
so impetuous as to destroy all power of restraint. In the total loss
of restraint, even over the actions of the mind itself, consists that
subversion of the understanding which, according to Professor Heinroth, constitutes insanity.*

This doctrine has been supported by the author with a most imposing array of arguments and learned researches. The whole
theory and the grounds on which it rests have been examined by
Dr. Jacobi in his last work, entitled " Beobachtungen über die Pathologie und Therapie der mit Irreseyn verbundenen Krankheiten,"
in which the reason for entering so fully into the discussion of this
singular hypothesis is alleged to be the influence which it has exercised over the public opinion in Germany.† In referring to Heinroth's dogma, that insanity is the result of moral depravity, Jacobi
has taken occasion to record the case of one individual, selected from
many others, whose history affords sufficient proof that mental derangement is a calamity that may befal the most pious and excellent
persons. Absurd as the opinion of Heinroth will appear to most
English readers, and superfluous as it may be to enter seriously into
a refutation of it, I shall yet insert Jacobi's account of this case; which,
as related by the author, is not without interest.

" The wife of John Caspar Lavater, of Zurich, was a person regarded, by all who knew her, with respect and love. Her mind
was endowed with the highest principles, sensible and intelligent ;
her disposition was cheerful, pious, and benevolent. She had been
tried and proved by misfortunes and sorrows, was the friend, the
counsellor, and the comforter of many. She was induced, by the
sole desire of doing good to her suffering fellow-creatures, to undertake the chief care of several insane persons. It pleased Divine
Providence that, in an advanced period of her life, this excellent
person should herself become insane, and continue for a long time to
be a victim to the deepest melancholy. Towards the close of her
life she recovered from the disease, and her friends had the gratification of knowing that the last few months of her existence were passed
in a state of mind resembling that of her earlier days, and in that
state she died. Now let Professor Heinroth direct his attention to
the character of this excellent individual, and from the point of view
which he assumes, explain how the state of mental darkness to which
she was reduced can be regarded as the result of guilt and evil conscience, connected as it was with long-continued ill-health, and in all
probability depending on a chronic bodily disease under which she
had for a long time laboured."

---

* Heinroth's doctrine is set forth in the first part of his " Lehrbuch der Stoerungen des Seelenlebens," and it is maintained in the annotations subjoined by
the same writer to Hill's German translation of M. Esquirol's treatises.

† Heinroth's doctrine has likewise been criticised by M. Guislain, in the work
which I have repeatedly cited, on mental alienation.

It would be no difficult task to multiply instances of a similar description, but it is scarcely necessary to contend seriously against the docrine of Professor Heinroth. Yet it cannot be denied that this opinion has, in a limited view, some foundation in truth. Vices, inordinate passions, and the want of mental discipline tend in two ways to increase the prevalence of insanity. In the first place, vicious indulgences, intemperance, and other depraved habits have an immediate tendency to bring on diseases of the brain and nervous system of that kind of which madness is a result or manifestation ; secondly, irregular mental excitement produces a state of the moral constitution which renders the mind more subject to perturbations, violent passions and agitations, and these are known to be frequent precursors and causes of derangement. In the former instance, the injurious influences above mentioned come under the head of physical agents : in the latter they must be referred to that of the moral causes of insanity. Minds well disciplined by self-control, and brought by habit to a sedate and moderated state of feeling, are protected against the causes of violent emotion and distraction, which in persons of different habits of mind and conduct tend to increase the natural excitability of the moral constitution, and break down the feeble powers of the understanding. This line of observation can however, only be carried to a certain extent. A great proportion of the cases of insanity which occur arise from causes independent of any moral weakness or defect.

Several writers have entered at large into the discussion, whether insanity is a disease of the mind or of the organic structure of the body. MM. Franck, Nasse, and Guislain have brought forward a variety of arguments in defence of the latter opinion. They conclude that this disease has its seat in the organized body, and that it consists sometimes in a modification of the vital properties or functions, and sometimes in an alteration of the tissues or textures themselves.* I shall have occasion hereafter to add some further remarks upon this subject.

If we consider the fact to be admitted, that insanity is always a disease of the body, an affection of the organized structure or the functions of organized parts, we shall still find it necessary to advert to some contradictory opinions as to its nature and particular seat.

SECTION II.—*Of the Opinions of MM. Georget, Foville, and others, that Insanity is an idiopathic Disease of the Brain.*

Many writers of celebrity, both in Britain and on the continent, have regarded madness as an idiopathic disease of the brain. Of this opinion are Cullen, Cox, Haslam, Foville, and many others. M. Georget is perhaps the most decided and unconditional advocate for his doctrine.

* See Nasse, Zeitschrift, 1824.   Guislain de l'Aliénation, tom. i. p. 31-40.

He says, " Insanity is a disease of the brain ; it is idiopathic ; the nature of the organic alteration is unknown.

" The first proposition results from the following considerations.

" 1. The essential symptom, intellectual disturbance, depends upon a lesion of the cerebral functions.

" 2. It is always preceded, accompanied, or followed by other important cerebral or nervous disorders.

" 3. The disturbances of the other functions are neither constant nor severe : they are, besides, precisely similar to those which accompany any sudden lesion of an important organ : such are loss of appetite, irregularity of bowels, suppression of catamenia, &c. : they are transient, subside after the period of excitement has passed, and leave the essential symptoms yet subsisting.

" 4. The causes are such agents as are known to act directly on the brain and nervous system.

" 5. The natural terminations of insanity are permanent disease of the brain."*

The peculiarity of M. Georget's doctrine respecting insanity is, that he considers all the disorders of physical functions and of parts remote from the brain as only connected accidentally with the idiopathic cerebral disease, or at least as but its consequences ; while other writers maintain that these disorders are of much greater importance, that they lay the foundation for mental derangement, that the disturbance of the brain is merely sympathetic or secondary. Some term the disorder manifested in the state of the mental faculties a *symptom* of the primary disease. In this class of pathologists, who, however, differ very much from each other in particular views, we must reckon Pinel, Esquirol, and Broussais,† and their followers, as well as Nasse, Guislain, and Jacobi.

SECTION III.—*Of the Opinion of Pinel, that the cerebral Disease is sympathetic.*

It seems to have been the opinion of Pinel that the primary seat of disease in cases of insanity is in the region of the stomach and intestines : thence, as from a centre, the disorder was supposed by him to propagate itself, until, reaching the head, it deranges the understanding. The meaning of this is not very obvious, but it has been exemplified and illustrated by the phenomena of some remarkable cases, and particularly by facts recorded by Pinel himself. The first symptom of an attack of furious delirium, according to this writer, is in some instances a strong sense of heat in the abdomen : the bowels are confined, and the patient complains of thirst ; the sense of heat ascends from the epigastrium to the neck and face : the countenance reddens, the eyes become sparkling, the features are agitated, the temples throb, and the mind is excited into delirium or raving madness.

* M. Georget, De la Folie, p. 74.
† M. Broussais, De l'Irritation et de la Folie.

These observations lead us directly to the opinion which was admitted by Guislain, that the state of the brain on which madness immediately depends, whether the causes have primarily affected that organ or have reached it through the medium of the viscera of physical life, is a kind of sanguineous orgasm or erethism, a sudden injection of the cerebral bloodvessels. This is regarded as a temporary condition. Hence the remark of M. Pinel, that we can hardly expect to discover the actual cause of this disease unless by examining the heads of individuals who expire under the paroxysm of raving madness. But this opportunity, as he says, can seldom be obtained, since lunatics sink under diseases of various kinds.

This state of sanguineous orgasm is nearly allied, as Guislain remarks, to nervous excitement: it is more transient than inflammation, but leads to it.* Primary inflammation, as the same writer thinks, rarely subsists in insanity. "When I discover," he adds, "in cases of mental derangement resulting from the influence of moral causes, the symptoms or the traces of cerebral inflammation, I am convinced that the causes have not operated immediately on the vessels of the brain, but that they have in the first instance acted on the nerves, whence this nervous modification, or if you prefer so to term it, this irritation has been communicated to the bloodvessels." The brain is in a state of functional activity in the process of thinking, and it is in this action, when madness is excited by a moral cause, that the disorder has its sphere of existence: the disturbance of the circulation is only a consequence, the result of a change more recondite." He continues, in opposition to the opinions of other writers, to say, " I consider insanity to be a disease which has its seat in the brain ; but when I place it in that organ, I refer to the disease itself, and not to its cause. It has been held by some that insanity may have its local seat in the liver, in the heart, or in any other organ ; but can it be said with propriety that the seat of the disorder is in such organs? and is it not rather the cause of the disorder which has been discovered in such various situations ? To be in a state of derangement is to have the understanding disturbed, and no person imagines the understanding to be seated in the breast or in the abdomen : the viscera may, however, undergo morbid changes which react upon the brain, and give rise to madness. I therefore hold that mental derangement is always a disease of the brain, but that in many cases it has for its cause an irregular condition of some other organ, and in such instances the disorder is termed 'sympathic insanity.' "

Jacobi has made objections to some of the positions maintained by Guislain.† When madness arises from moral causes, as from violent passions, the first morbid action is, according to his opinion, much more frequently seated in remote organs than in the brain. The morbid changes in parts remote from the brain have been generally

* Guislain, Traité de l'Aliénation Mentale, tom. i. liv. 2.
† Beobachtungen : dritter abschnitt.

looked upon as less essentially connected with the disease than they really are ; and, according to this writer, the only way of throwing additional illustration on the causes and nature of insanity is to make a diligent study of all the organic affections which accompany it, and of which, in the view of Jacobi, insanity is merely a symptom. This writer objects still more strongly to the opinions of Georget, who regarded the concomitant diseases of the viscera as results of the disorder in the brain. These writers, MM. Georget and Jacobi, hold the two extremes of opinion in respect to the nature of insanity. The former considered it as in every instance idiopathic inflammation of the brain : the latter views the cerebral disorder as the least essential in the train of morbid changes. Madness, according to him, is, to chronic diseases of the viscera, what delirium is to fevers, in which the main object of attention is often a gastro-enterite or an inflammatory disease of some organ in the abdomen, or perhaps in the chest, and in which the delirium is relieved only or chiefly by remedies directed to the state of the parts originally affected.

SECTION IV.—*Inferences collected in relation to the Pathology of Madness.*

Such a review as I have now taken of the theories maintained by medical writers as to the nature of insanity, and the relations which the disordered states of different organs bear to the derangement of mind, seemed requisite in order to illustrate the present state of opinions with respect to this disease. From considering the diversity and contradictory tenor of these speculations, we might be induced to regard the subject as one beyond the reach of satisfactory elucidation. Yet the nature of the inquiry is not such as to lead us to this conclusion. The writers who have treated on it have perhaps failed at arriving at certainty, owing to the too discursive way in which they have entered upon the investigation, and the too general points of view in which they have contemplated it. By proceeding in a more analytical way, or by beginning from particulars, we are more likely to arrive at some tolerably certain inferences, and at least to perceive how far we can advance on sure ground, and what yet remains in the region of conjecture.

I shall remark in the first place, that in cases such as those described by M. Calmeil, in which not only the brain and its investing membranes display after death the signs of long-continued inflammation, but affection of the power of voluntary motion is combined with the disorder of intellect, and is often either coincident with it in origin or shortly supervening on it, there arises from the alterations observed, and from a comparison of this with other cerebral diseases, sufficient reason for concluding that the whole train of morbid phenomena depends from its commencement to inflammation of the parts in which the appearances described are discovered. We have no reason for hesitation in setting down cases of this description as instances of chronic cerebral or meningeal inflammation.

When again, the intellectual faculties are affected in nearly a similar manner and degree, without disorder of the motive powers, as in cases of mania or monomania complicated with or passing into dementia, or in examples of dementia occurring under other circumstances, we have strong reasons for presuming on the existence of a similar morbid state, since in these cases we find after death the results of long-continued inflammation in the encephalon, and because these cases bear a close analogy in many respects to those which belong to the class above described.

There are many cases of madness in which the nature of the exciting causes, or the circumstances preceding the appearance of the disease, when viewed in connection with its ultimate results, give no room for doubting that the whole disease from its commencement to its termination has been of an inflammatory nature. If we take, for example, an attack of mania, supervening immediately on an injury of the head, or on exposure to a coup de soleil, or to excess in the use of stimuli, or a violent fit of intoxication, which is known in other instances to induce phrenitis ; and if the individual is found, after surviving a longer or shorter period, to display in his brain the phenomena before described, nothing seems to be wanting to the chain of evidence supporting the conclusion.

It must be admitted that in the generality of cases of mania and monomania the existence of inflammation is only a matter of probable inference. The arguments which present themselves in support of this inference may be summed up briefly under the following heads.

1. Analogy with cases in which the evidence of such a diseased state is stronger. If such examples of mental derangement as those above described admit of a tolerably certain inference, it may be extended by analogy to other cases in which the morbid phenomena are similiar, though the causes and results of the disease may be not so clearly marked.

2. The morbid changes found in the encephalon, after the termination of protracted cases, being such as inflammation induces, afford an argument, which, when the subject is properly considered, cannot be set aside by any method of evasion. On this subject I shall add nothing further to what has already been said.

3. The physical causes which excite madness bring us to the same conclusion. These are principally of a description likely to give rise either to inflammation in the brain, or to a full and distended state in the vessels of that organ. Exposure to severe heat or cold, insolation, concussion or other injuries of the head, intoxication, and generally excess in the use of stimuli, are all of this class ; the condition of the brain, which it is the tendency of these agents to promote, is either inflammation, or something bordering upon it.

The metastatis of inflammatory diseases from other parts of the body, among which is included the recession of gouty or rheumatic inflammation, or of cutaneous eruptions, is well known to be followed not unfrequently by the appearance of maniacal symptoms. Suppressions of catamenia and other discharges, giving rise to similar diseases, strongly confirm the same pathological principles.

This argument does not apply fully to cases of insanity induced by moral causes. But many of the moral causes of insanity are circumstances of excitement giving rise to excesses in the action of the brain.

4. The connection of insanity with other diseases known to depend on cerebral congestion or inflammation, the mutual conversions of such diseases and of madness into each other, affords a strong presumption that the immediate causes on which they depend are analogous.

The instances of mental disorder which leave the greatest doubt with respect to the presence of disease in the brain are those of moral insanity, or disorder affecting merely the moral character, the propensities, habits, temper, and feelings, without involving any notable lesion of the understanding. In such cases what proof have we that the brain is disordered ? The complaint is often brought on by moral causes alone ; it lasts for a time, and disappears without the aid of physical remedies, through the effect of time, and by the influence of circumstances which act upon the mind alone.

If we were assured that the brain is what some German physicians term it, the " seelenorgan," or instrument in all the manifestations of mind or the attributes of the soul, we might be at liberty to conclude that disorders in the affections and feelings imply, not less than intellectual disturbances, some disorder in the brain. But this preliminary step has not been gained. However probable it may be thought by some persons that the passions and propensities are seated in the brain, or that modifications which the mind undergoes in respect to these phenomena are connected with instrumental changes in the brain, the fact has never been proved., Variations in the state of the temper and feelings are experienced in connexion with bodily disorders : the fact is one of daily observation. Disorders of the alimentary canal, dyspepsia with flatulence, a torpid state of the abdominal viscera with scanty and unhealthy secretions, are accompanied by lowness of spirits amounting often to despondency : this state constitutes hypochondriasis. An opposite state of feelings, hope scarcely to be depressed, a sanguine expectation of recovery, often with unusual vigour of intellect, prevail almost uniformly in the most severe diseases of the lungs. A highly sensitive state, with excitement of the feelings, in some cases, according to Nasse and others, accompanied by an irascible disposition and even a proneness to commit acts of violence, is attendant on diseases of the heart. All medical practitioners are well aware that disorders of the urinary system are connected with a peculiar anxiety of disposition, a restless and irritable state. Particular conditions of the uterine or genital systems are likewise denoted by particular phenomena in the mind or disposition. In all these instances are we authorised in assuming that particular conditions of the brain are intermediately and instrumentally co-operative, and interposing themselves between the disorder of the organ primarily affected, and then the state of the mind or temper which is traced as its manifestation or accompaniment ?*

But without attempting a solution of this general question of physiology, we may collect some facts which render it probable that moral insanity depends, in some instances at least, on disease of the brain.

1. The characteristics of moral insanity, obliquity of character, perversion of the natural temper and disposition without any aberration of intellect, occasionally supervene on manifest cerebral disorders.

2. Similar phenomena, with eccentricity of conduct and habit, belong sometimes to individuals in 'families in which intellectual madness and other cerebral diseases are hereditary.

3. Some cases of moral insanity are manifestly connected with diseases affecting the bodily constitution, and particularly the brain. Instances, for example, of homicidal propensity will be mentioned in a succeeding chapter, in which this connexion was so manifest that it could not be mistaken.

Cases in which such a connexion is apparent and may be demonstrated are probably by no means the majority among the instances of disordered propensity, but from these we may draw an inference by analogy to the remainder, and this, I apprehend, is all the evidence that can be furnished of the existence of cerebral or other bodily disease in many examples of moral insanity.

I shall close these remarks on the proofs of cerebral inflammation in mental derangement with one observation which will be found important in a practical point of view. If it were allowed that the proximate cause of this disease, or the state of the brain on which it depends in its origin or first accession, is not proved to be, generally speaking, of the nature of inflammation, still we know sufficiently from necroscopy that the results of inflammatory action take place in cases which have any considerable duration, and that the disorganized state of the brain which renders recovery impossible, or generally precludes it in the advanced stage, is produced by inflammation. We have, then, in practice nearly as strong inducement for treating the disease on antiphlogistic principles as if we were sure that cerebral inflammation, in the strict sense of the terms, was its proximate cause.

What has been said in the preceding part of this section refers most obviously to those cases of insanity which are produced by causes acting immediately on the brain, and exciting idiopathic disorder in that organ. I shall now make a few remarks on the instances of sympathic or secondary affections of the brain, which are manifested by derangement of the mind.

It would appear, from the great proportion of cases in which disease of the thoracic or abdominal viscera are discovered in the

---

* There seems to be a remarkable want of evidence in support of this opinion, which is often so confidently assumed.

bodies of lunatics, that cases of the description last mentioned are much more important by their frequency than it is commonly imagined. Pinel seems to have referred nearly all cases of insanity to this class, and Jocobi, though he has stated his opinion in very different terms from those of Pinel, may be considered as an advocate for a similar doctrine. I shall take the liberty of observing that a great part of my work " On Diseases of the Nervous System" was devoted to the development of the history and relations of diseases of the brain, originating from primary disturbances in different parts of the system, and giving rise in some cases to maniacal, in others to convulsive phenomena. On the present occasion I shall treat this subject very briefly.

M. Scipion Pinel has reported in his Inaugural Dissertation some cases which clearly prove the influence of the stomach upon the brain in producing mental alienation. A young man swallowed some cigars : gastritis followed, which, after being relieved, became again severe : melancholia ensued, which terminated in suicide. A soldier in an ague swallowed a glass of brandy containing gunpowder : the consequence was a violent attack of mania, which lasted for some months.   The same writer declares that in two hundred and fifty-nine necroscopical examinations which he has either seen or collected from the reports of MM. Esquirol, Louyer-Villermai, and others, there were fifty-one cases in which chronic inflammation was discoverable in the mucous membrane of the intestinal canal.

It is not difficult to imagine that similar states of disease in the alimentary canal should produce disturbance in the brain, when we observe how much that organ is liable to be modified in its functions by slight causes acting through the medium of the stomach. A full stomach promotes sleep ; various substances taken into the stomach occasion sleep or wakefulness ; others intoxication and temporary madness.   On this subject M. Guislain has collected observations from various authors in the first volume of his valuable work on mental alienation.

The theory of mental disorders arising from morbid states of other viscera is more obscure than what regards the stomach, because these instances are more removed from immediate observation and experiment ; but that diseases of the liver, the lungs, and other viscera are connected under a similar relation with affections of the brain and consequent disturbances in the exercise of the mental faculties, is a position which scarcely admits of doubt.   In all these instances the morbid state of the brain, which, though a secondary or sympathic affection, is the immediate cause of derangement in the mind, is probably of the same nature in itself as the morbid condition which arises primarily from causes acting immediately on the cerebral and nervous system.

CHAPTER VII.

TREATMENT OF INSANITY.

It is usual to divide, under two heads, the various measures which suggest themselves to our consideration as likely to promote recovery from mental derangement. The moral treatment of the insane comprehends all the means which are known to exercise immediately on the mind an influence tending to restore the healthy and natural state of its operations. The medical or therapeutical treatment includes the use of remedies which act upon the body and are designed to remove the disorder of cerebral or other functions, known or believed to be the cause of derangement in the mind, or at least to be intimately connected with its manifestation. As this mode of arrangement is attended with some advantages, and as no practical objection has arisen against it, I propose to follow it in considering the various subjects connected with the treatment of insanity.

Section I.—*Therapeutical Treatment of Insanity.*

The proximate or immediate cause of mental derangement is so much concealed from our research, the phenomena of the disease are so complicated, and the morbid states of the constitution with which they are connected so various, that we might foresee no ordinary difficulty in the attempt to lay down, with respect to this disorder, any general principles or indications of cure. In reality this task has been found to be a more arduous one than even the circumstances adverted to would have led us to anticipate ; and hence many writers have given it up, and rest satisfied with stating as merely experimental results the effects which particular remedies have been thought to produce. We are not driven, in my opinion, to this necessity. The medical treatment of insanity may be referred in a great measure to two indications or principles, which in many cases may be followed more or less fully, and will at least serve the purpose of associating in the mind the different curative attempts which may be made with some hope of success.

ARTICLE I.

First practical indication in the medical treatment of insanity.

The first indication is to remove or lessen that diseased condition of the brain on which we have reason to believe that insanity depends as its immediate cause.

In the preceding chapter on the theory of mental derangement, I have collected various facts of which the consideration appears likely to throw light on the nature of insanity, or rather on the physical conditions of the system on which it depends. I shall not recapitu-

late what has been said, but refer my readers to the arguments which
have appeared to establish the inference that the state of the brain
immediately giving rise to the phenomena of madness is in general
one of increased vascular excitement or fulness, a state which, if it
does not really constitute inflammation, is at least closely bordering
upon that morbid condition, and liable to pass into it,—that from it,
in fact, all the usual consequences of inflammation arise if it continues
for a considerable time. This inference, as a pathological one, may
be deduced with much greater confidence than any practical conclusion that may be founded upon it. From the fact that the proximate
cause of madness is nearly allied to inflammation, it does not follow,
with certainty, that the disease is to be cured by the simple use of
antiphlogistic remedies. The physician who would proceed to treat
cases of madness as instances simply of inflammation in the brain, and
who would expect to cure it at once, like any other local inflammatory disease, by the direct operation of antiphlogistic means, would
very often find himself greatly disappointed. He would meet with
many cases in which no perceptible benefit arises from bleedings,
and evacuations of all kinds generally or locally applied, and combined with the whole series of remedies supposed to be required by
the existence of organic inflammation. Many patients would sink
under such a course of treatment if carried on incautiously : it would
leave the disease undiminished, and exhaust the powers of life. This
depends, perhaps, on the influence of diseased states in other structures and organs, or on disordered functions of other parts which are
complicated with, and in some instances give rise to, the disturbance
existing in the brain. Inflammatory excitement is a part of the disease, but does not entirely constitute it.

Perhaps, however, I may venture on the assertion that there are
few instances in which the practical indication arising from the view
which I have taken of the pathology of madness will not be found
applicable during some periods of the case, though in many its application is very limited. The degrees in which it is admissible are
various.

In recent cases of mania, properly so termed, and of incoherence,
particularly in young and plethoric subjects, and where the disease
has made its attack suddenly, and is accompanied with signs of considerable vascular excitement, much may be hoped from the antiphlogistic treatment, at least from certain parts of it judiciously modified. I shall now consider the different means of which it consists,
and advert to the opinions of some of the most eminent practical
writers with respect to their use in cases of insanity.

1. *Of bleeding.*—Dr. Cullen recommended bleeding in the early
stage of madness. He says that it has been common to employ this
remedy in all cases of recent mania, and, as he thinks, with advantage. He observes that when the disease has subsisted for some time,
he has seldom found bloodletting to be of service. " It is," he says,
" a proper and even a necessary remedy in those instances of madness in which there is fulness and frequency of pulse, and when marks

are observed of increased impetus in the vessels of the head." He
prefers bleeding from the arm, while the patient remains in somewhat of an erect posture, and bringing on a degree of deliquium,
which, as he thinks, is a pretty certain mark of diminished fulness
and tension in the vessels of the encephalon.

Pinel, whose authority could not fail to produce an impression, is
in this respect decidedly opposed to Cullen. He considers the signs
of vascular plethora in the head, or of determination of blood thither,
as very deceptive ; and although he allows bleeding to be in some
instances capable of averting attacks of recurrent madness when they
are anticipated, he carefully abstains from the use of the lancet after
the disease has actually broken out. Care is always taken, he says,
to question the relatives of patients admitted into the hospital over
which he presided, whether bleeding has been practised, and if so,
what were its results. " The reply always proves that the state of
the patient has changed for the worse immediately after bleeding."
Pinel held very firmly the opinion that bleeding, even in maniacal
cases which are accompanied by circumstances supposed to indicate
plethora and local determination to the head, tends to retard recovery,
to render it more doubtful. He was persuaded that bleeding gives
to the disease a tendency to degenerate into dementia. The facts,
however, which this distinguished author adduces as proofs of his
opinion, afford, as M. Foville has remarked, but very equivocal evidence. " Two girls, nearly of the same age and temperament, were
admitted into the hospital—the Salpêtrière—on the same day : one
of them, who had not been bled, was cured in the space of two
months ; the other, who had undergone a copious bleeding, sank into
a state of idiotism, or rather of dementia, and did not recover the
faculty of speech till the fifth month. Her perfect restoration took
place at the end of the ninth month." Now, as most authors fix the
mean duration of madness at the period of several months, and some
at more than a year, this case of recovery at the end of the ninth
month, cannot afford a strong condemnation of the practice pursued.
Another case, which the same author has adduced as affording evidence against bleeding, is not more conclusive in respect to the influence of remedies on the ultimate event of the disease. Yet the
opinion of such a writer, founded as it was, at least by himself supposed to have been, on extensive observation, ought not to be entirely disregarded because he happened to select but dubious illustrations. If bleeding occasions a state of collapse in the system, and is
carried beyond what is necessary to reduce an over-excitement, a
fatuous dejection of mind is likely in some cases to be the result.

M. Esquirol coincides with Pinel in the opinion that the diseased
state on which mental derangement depends, is sometimes changed
for the worse by bleeding. He says that he has seen madness increased after an abundant flow of the catamenia, and likewise after
one, two, or three bloodlettings. In such cases melancholy dejection
has passed into furious madness. Yet M. Esquirol approves of
moderate bleeding in plethoric cases, and where some habitual san-

guineous evacuation has been suppressed. He has often with advantage applied leeches behind the head or to the temples of patients who are subject to sudden determinations of blood towards the head. His favourite remedies in such cases were the use of a few leeches at a time, repeated as often as necessary, and cold applications to the head.

To outweigh the authority of these writers who either condemn the practice of bleeding in madness, or allow of its adoption in so sparing a degree, strong evidence is required.

Dr. Haslam says that bleeding is the most beneficial remedy that has been employed in madness, and that it is equally beneficial in melancholic as in maniacal cases. He limits its use to recent cases and plethoric habits, and directs it to be performed by the application of six or eight cupping-glasses to the shaven scalp. The quantity of blood to be taken must depend on circumstances. "From eight to sixteen ounces may be drawn, and the operation repeated as circumstances may require." When a stupid state has succeeded to one of high excitement, Dr. Haslam considers bleeding as contra-indicated.

But Dr. Rush is the most strenuous advocate for bleeding in maniacal cases. He lays the greatest stress on this remedy, and has perhaps carried its use to a greater extent than any other medical practitioner of high repute. The arguments which he has given in support of the practice of large depletion in madness are the following :—1. The force and frequency of the pulse, the sleepless and agitated state of maniacal patients. 2. The appetite being unimpaired in lunatics, and sometimes even stronger than usual, a plethoric state of the vessels easily arises in such habits. 3. The importance of the diseased organ, the delicate structure of the brain, which prevents it from long supporting morbid action without being exposed to the danger of permanent disorganization. This danger, he says, is much increased by the want of sleep, the cries and exclamations, and the constant agitation of mad persons. 4. The want of any natural channel of discharge from the brain, by which the ordinary results of inflammation might be averted or got rid of, in that way by which serous discharges in other parts relieve the inflammatory state. 5. The accidental cures which have followed the loss of a large quantity of blood. Dr. Rush has seen several lunatics who had attempted self-destruction by cutting their throats or opening the great vessels, cured by the abundant hemorrhages which have followed these attempts. 6. Lastly, he says that bleeding is indicated by the extraordinary success which has resulted from its use in the United States, and particularly at the hospital for lunatics in Pennsylvania.

Dr. Rush advises large bleedings at the first attack of mania. If the patient bears it without syncope, he ought to lose, according to this physician, from twenty to forty ounces of blood. If possible, it should be taken from him while standing erect. Free bloodlettings practised early in the disease have, as he says, a surprising effect in calming the patient, and in many instances are sufficient for the cure, unaided by any other remedies. In most cases, however, bleeding from the arm is to be followed by the application of leeches or cupping-glasses to the head or nape of the neck, by low diet, antiphlogistic remedies, refrigerants applied to the head, and the use of warm or tepid baths.

Dr. Rush was of opinion that the evacuation of blood ought to be carried to a greater extent in madness than in any other acute disease whatever. From a patient, sixty-eight years of age, he caused two hundred ounces of blood to be drawn in less than two months. Another patient of Dr. Rush lost four hundred and seventy ounces by forty-seven bleedings in the course of seven months.

I shall conclude this survey of the conflicting opinions of practical writers on the expediency of bleeding in madness, by citing the observations of M. Foville, which are deserving of the most attentive consideration, and which place the subject in the true point of view. He says, "Without ever having pushed the employment of this remedy so far as Rush and Joseph Franck, I confess that it appears to me to be one of those on the efficacy of which the greatest reliance may be placed. MM. Pinel and Esquirol have proved that the 'expectant method,' assisted by a few simple rules, and a moral treatment wisely directed, have succeeded in a great many cases; but although it is better to confine ourselves to the use of simple means, patiently continued, than to employ unadvisedly the method of interference, I believe that the physician devoted to the study of pathological anatomy can draw from the results which it furnishes, compared with the observation of symptoms, valuable inductions for practice; that he may place reliance on their efficacy, and recommend them with confidence when experience shall have demonstrated their good effects. Are not the anatomical characters which so constantly present themselves in acute cases, and the adhesions which are so frequent in chronic ones, evident proofs of inflammation, and are we not by this consideration authorized to hope for advantages from the use of antiphlogistic means?

"If it be added," says M. Foville, "that in several hundred lunatics, whose bodies my situation for nearly ten years has given me an opportunity of examining, I have never found adhesions in acute cases, while they have been very common in chronic ones; if, with these facts, the results related in the works of MM. Bayle and Calmeil are compared, we may conclude, on seeing these adhesions so frequent in chronic cases, that they are incompatible with the regular exercise of an organ so delicate as the brain, and consequently incompatible with the return of reason. We ought, therefore, in every acute case, to choose the most active means, in order to prevent this melancholy termination of cerebral disease.

"These are some of the reasons which have led me, with several physicians who have been placed in circumstances favourable for making observations, to conclude that bleedings ought not to be entirely proscribed in the treatment of mental diseases. In the greatest number of cases of recent insanity which have been placed under my

17*

care,* I have employed evacuations of blood, local or general, rare or
frequent, abundant or in moderation, according to the strength of the
patient, and the state of the pulse, the redness of the eyes, the heat
of the head, the agitation and want of sleep. I have always preferred
general bleeding, when there existed a state of plethora, which the
force and frequency of the pulse evinced. In opposite circumstances,
leeches on the neck, the temples, behind the ears, cupping upon the
same parts, and upon the shaved head, have produced decided benefit.
Local bleeding having appeared to me to produce a marked effect
upon the brain, I have often prescribed it at the same time with general
bleeding whenever the intensity of the general symptoms has imperiously demanded the latter remedy ; but I have never rested exclusively upon the efficacy of sanguineous evacuations, although in many
cases I have seen all the morbid symptoms disappear, as if by enchant-
ment, under their use.

"I have under my care several patients subject for some years to
attacks of intermittent madness, which, left to nature, would last
three or four months, or longer.

"During three years, that is, since they have been confided to my
care, they have not experienced a single attack of a month's duration.
Often in the space of five or six days all the symptoms have been
dissipated. General or local bleedings, proportioned to the intensity
of the symptoms, warm baths, with cold applications to the head at
the same time, are the means by which I have treated such attacks.

"I have several times prevented the return of these attacks by employing the same treatment, as soon as the redness of the eyes, the
heat of the head, and wakefulness, manifested themselves, even when
there had been no delirium."

My own experience has afforded me sufficient opportunities of
forming opinions on the effect of remedies in insanity, since for twenty
years I have never been without patients labouring under that disease
who were more or less under my care and observation. Long before
Dr. Foville's remarks were known to me, and long, indeed, before they
were written, I had pursued the practice which he has recommended,
having been led to adopt it by similar considerations,† and I entertain
no doubt of its practical advantages. I am very far from approving
or wishing to recommend such detractions of blood as those which
appear to have been practised by Dr. Rush ; but I have been convinced by the evidence of numerous facts, with respect to which I
could not be mistaken, that bleeding, both local and general, is, under
due limitations, serviceable in cases of insanity. To what extent the
use of these measures ought to be carried it is more easy, after a long
practice, to determine in particular instances, than it is to lay down
general rules which may be of service to students or young practitioners ; and perhaps all the remarks which I can offer on this sub-

---

* M. Foville has been for several years physician in chief to one of the most
extensive lunatic asylums in France, that of St. Yon, near Rouen.
† Treatise on Diseases of the Nervous System, chap. i. London, 1822.

ject are only such as common sense and discretion would scarcely fail to dictate.

The circumstances which render bleeding most advisable in the treatment of madness are those which indicate an approach in the disease to the character of phrenitis. The age and constitution of the patient must be taken into the account : if young and plethoric, he will more easily bear depletion ; if the attack has been acute and sudden, it will more decidedly require it. If the vessels, especially the carotids and temporal arteries, pulsate strongly and rapidly, and there is heat of the skin, and principally of the head, much redness of the face and conjunctiva, a contracted pupil, intolerance of light and of sounds, total want of sleep, and much agitation, symptoms of disordered sensation, as spectral appearances, in such cases bleeding from the arm will be practised beneficially ; and it should be done before excitement shall have produced collapse and exhaustion. The abstraction of twelve or sixteen ounces of blood under the circumstances above described is often followed by a mitigation of all the symptoms. It may be repeated with advantage if the good effect is only temporary, or may be followed, if this be incomplete, by the use of cupping-glasses, or leeches applied near the head.

Less frequent are the indications, of which even M. Esquirol admits the evidence as proving the necessity of bleeding. I allude to circumstances connected with the origin of the attack, such as its following the suppression of catamenia, or of some morbid, though perhaps also salutary discharge, the sudden disappearance of eruptions, its coming on after the disappearance of erysipelas or of dropsical effusions. All these observations point to the propriety of bleeding, but they do not authorise it unless the arterial circulation and the heat of the skin be considerable. I have seen mischievous results from bleeding in cases of madness which followed the disappearance of eruptions, when the vigour and excitement of the arterial system were not sufficient to support the consequent collapse.

Insanity occasioned by blows or injuries of the head, as well as madness resulting from intoxication, is relieved by bleeding, and many cases of these kinds require antiphlogistic remedies, including the use of the lancet ; but care must be taken to distinguish insanity the effect of intoxicating liquors or of blows on the head from delirium tremens, and from that species of delirium so much resembling it, which is occasioned by wounds. I know that patients labouring under delirium tremens have been killed almost instantaneously by practitioners who were unaware of the nature of such cases ; and traumatic delirium is a disease which confessedly requires the greatest caution. The latter affection, which has been so well described by M. Dupuytren* and by Dr. Crampton, is known to appear shortly after severe injuries of the extremities and compound fractures: in its phenomena it bears a close analogy to delirium tremens. It is ac-

* Gazette Médicale de Paris, Mars 1832. Fédéré sur les diverses espèces de Folie Vraie. London Medical and Physical Journal, 1833.

companied by profuse sweats, a pale countenance, quick tremulous
pulse, great insensibility of external impressions; while the prevalent state of the mind is terror and agitation. In this disease bleeding is highly dangerous, and the appropriate remedies are stimulants
and frequent opiates.

Mania is the form of insanity which most frequently requires abstraction of blood: but I have in many instances found a decided
benefit to arise in cases of melancholia from one or two moderate
bleedings, either general or local. This has been the fact in cases
accompanied with headach or a feeling of oppression referred to the
head, with a full state of the bloodvessels, and generally with confined
bowels.

The circumstances which chiefly preclude the use of evacuant remedies, and particularly of bleeding, are the indications of weakness
and irritability without strength. All approximations to the state
characterizing delirium tremens are decidedly in this class: a weak
and small, or a frequent, very compressible pulse, with throbbings
without strength in the carotid, while the circulation is feeble in the
extremities: a clammy, cold skin, especially in the hands and feet,
or profuse though warm perspirations; a tremulous state of the
tongue or voice; tremors and agitation in the limbs, are symptoms
which should render the practitioner very cautious in ordering de-
pletive measures, though they do not in all cases preclude at least
local bleedings. In puerperal cases it is now allowed by all that
venesection is to be rarely attempted.

In many individuals of weak constitution, when the indications of
plethora and general excitement of the circulation were wanting, I
have observed the best results to follow the use of leeches to the head
after it has been shaved, or the application of cupping-glasses to the
nape of the neck. I have observed instances in which melancholy
dejection accompanied by sleeplessness and want of appetite has been
relieved or removed by the use of this remedy in a few days, after it
had continued for several months.

I have stated my opinion on the subject of bleeding with the confidence which appears to myself to be the result of long and repeated
experience of its beneficial effect; but I must not omit to remark
that, although a majority of physicians who make insanity an object
of study coincide with me, unless I am greatly mistaken, in this respect, there are others who hold an opposite opinion. Among these
are some who have the very best claim to the confidence of the
public, namely, that of more than ordinary success in the treatment
of insanity. I am informed by Mr. Hitch, that at the Gloucester
Lunatic Asylum, which is under the superintendence of Dr. Shute
and his own immediate care, the use of the lancet, leeches, cupping-
glasses, blisters, drastic purgatives, the practice of shaving the head,
are totally proscribed. Yet among the patients admitted to this hospital, a very large proportion of recoveries, as I have already observed, take place, and *no cases* of sudden apoplexy or hemiplegia
have yet happened.

Experience has afforded in this instance a strong evidence against the necessity and propriety of bleeding, and of other antiphlogistic measures in insanity ; but it is here obvious to remark that circumstances probably exist connected with the general condition and the state of constitution of the patients admitted into the Gloucester Asylum, which may prevent the inference hence arising from becoming universally applicable.

2. *Of abstraction of heat from the head : regulation of temperature : bathing.*—The head should always be shaved when there is much vascular excitement and heat about the scalp. By the coolness afforded on the removal of the hair, more benefit and a greater degree of tranquilization is often produced than is anticipated. Cutting the hair short is not sufficient : the head should be shaved once or twice in a week.

Cold shower-baths, and affusions of cold water administered in various methods, have been extensively tried in maniacal diseases. Dr. Rush considered them to constitute a very important remedy, and recommended, in order to obtain the greatest advantage from them, that they should be repeated two or three times in a day. M. Esquirol used this remedy with advantage in some cases : he chiefly prescribed it for young subjects. M. Foville says that he was a witness to an almost immediate cure of a maniacal girl of delicate constitution and nervous temperament, who was subjected by M. Esquirol to the affusion of cold water at the degree fourteen of the centigrade thermometer. She was placed, with a garment covering her, in an empty bathing-tub, and water was poured in small quantities on her head till it covered her body, and shivering ensued. On a second application of this method, which was for some time resisted, it was followed by deep sleep, accompanied by copious sweating ; and when the patient awoke, she was found to have recovered her reason. I have witnessed the application of this remedy by M. Foville in the manner described, and can add my testimony of its greater convenience and efficacy, when compared with the ordinary methods of applying cold affusions.

The use of the shower-bath is often followed by reaction, when the patient, if excitable, becomes violent. In old cases, attended with a disposition to congestion of blood in the head, its use is precluded by the danger of producing paralysis. It is chiefly serviceable in young persons ; when the constitution is relaxed, and when it is predisposed to hysteric affections.

A method of bathing adopted by M. Foville in the hospital under his management is free from the inconveniences and occasionally injurious results attendant on cold affusions. He places a cap or bonnet, containing ice and closely fitting, on the head of the patient, and keeps the body immersed in a warm-bath for two or three hours, and renews this proceeding twice or three times in a day, according to the intensity of symptoms. On adopting it, as he was accustomed to do at first, only once in a day, he found the tranquillity produced by it followed not unfrequently by increased agitation ; but on repeating the bath, with the ice constantly applied to the head, he has frequently succeeded far beyond his expectation. It has been the apparent means of recovery in many acute cases, and has produced sleep and tranquillity in frequent instances of obstinate restlessness and agitation.

Applications of ice, or, when more convenient, of cold water, are very generally serviceable in cases attended with heat of the head and irritability.

Warm or tepid bathing has been found advantageous in the treatment of madness under a variety of circumstances. A cold state of the skin, languor of the general circulation indicated by coldness of the extremities, a tendency to chronic eruptions, are among the phenomena which suggest its adoption. Sometimes it produces sleep after long-continued agitation. If the degree of heat be not such as to occasion too much vascular excitement, it is generally a useful and safely applicable remedy.

3. *Counter-irritation.*—Counter-irritation, established by various means, such as blisters to the shaved head or nape of the neck, issues or setons in the neck or on the scalp, caustics, actual cautery, irritating ointments, is found to afford in some instances a powerful method of reducing inflammatory disease, or relieving a state of congestion in the brain. The various remedies which belong to this class have been tried in every modification in cases of insanity, but the general result of experience is not favourable to their use. They afford little benefit in ordinary maniacal cases, and often appear to be injurious.

Irritating ointments have been applied in many instances, particularly since their use was strongly recommended by the late Dr. Jenner. Medical practitioners have been generally disappointed in their expectation of benefit from this attempt.

There are, however, instances of mental disease in which these remedies are beneficial, but some care is requisite in order to distinguish them.

M. Esquirol has remarked that blisters, dry cuppings, and other irritating applications, are used successfully in cases which follow metastasis; in monomania accompanied by stupor; in puerperal madness; and in dementia when not complicated with convulsions or paralysis.

I believe that the cases of disease affecting the exercise of the mental faculties in which counter-irritation is principally and perhaps exclusively of service, are those in which torpor and insensibility prevail, instead of excitement and intensity of feeling, or morbid activity. In almost every case of paralysis with a tendency to coma and lethargy in which such remedies have been tried within the sphere of my observation, and these cases have been very numerous, I have witnessed the most decided advantage from their use. In disorders of a chronic form, when means of slow and gentle operation are sought, setons in the neck are most advisable; but when there is great intensity of disease and a state of the brain threatening a fatal increase, issues made by a long incision in the scalp over the sagittal suture are particularly useful. This remedy is not found in experience to be more painful than the more usual application of setons, and it is incomparably more efficacious. In cases of stupor and of dementia following attacks of apoplexy or paralysis, or severe fevers, this method is, according to my observation, more beneficial than any other. I should not advise it with much hope in dementia the result of insanity.

The general paralysis of insane persons, or the "paralysie des aliénés," is so deplorable a disease that it almost precludes expectation of recovery. I have not had an opportunity of prescribing issues on the scalp in cases of this description, but the pathology of the disease so manifestly indicates the propriety of such an attempt, and it has been so successful in disorders in many respects analogous within my observation, that I should not fail to adopt it in any instance of the kind, nor should I absolutely despair of the result until the experiment had failed.

4. *Purgatives.*—No fact in medical practice has been longer established than the utility of purgatives in madness ; witness the fame of Anticyra and hellebore. To confirm a maxim so well supported by the result of constant experience, it seems almost superfluous to adduce pathological facts. It is not, however, difficult to find this species of evidence in its favour. Many authors have remarked that spontaneous cure of madness has resulted from a supervening diarrhœa, in which the intestines have discharged in great quantities a variety of morbid secretions.

M. Esquirol has well observed that purgative medicines ought not to be used indiscriminately in all cases of madness, and that they are injurious when the mucous membrane of the intestinal canal is in a diseased state. This is the case in many instances of insanity. I shall, under another indication for medical treatment, consider the method of practice which is advisable in different states of intestinal irritation, as they occur in madness. At present it will be sufficient to observe that, unless any signs exist of disease in the structure of the alimentary canal, such as inflammation or ulceration of the mucous coat of the intestines, the use of purgative medicines is one of the most important and generally available means in the treatment of maniacal patients. The mildest cathartics are preferable to others in most instances, because their use can be long continued without injury to the structures on which they immediately act. The neutral salts, infusion of senna, rhubarb, jalap, castor-oil, are in the majority of cases sufficiently powerful, and may be used daily or frequently according to circumstances. When there is decided tendency to constipation, or the alvine evacuations are morbid, calomel, scammony, colocynth, or croton oil, may be added, due attention being paid to the cautionary circumstance above pointed out.

5. *Emetics.*—Emetics have been strongly recommended by some practical writers. M. Esquirol says that he has found them useful in most cases of melancholy accompanied by a torpid state of the

system. Dr. Rush considered them to be chiefly indicated in hypochondriasis, or lowness of spirits connected with dyspeptic disease.
Dr. Haslam confirms their utility in cases attended with disorder of
the stomach, merely with a view to the relief of that particular
symptom ; but he declares that, " after the administration of *many
thousand* emetics to persons who were insane, *but otherwise in good
health,* he never saw any benefit derived from their use." " Perhaps no one," he says, " has enjoyed a fairer opportunity of witnessing the effects of remedies for insane persons than myself.; and when
emetics are employed in Bethlem Hospital, they have the best
chance of effecting all the relief they are competent to afford, as
they are given by themselves, without the intervention of other
medicines ; and this course of emetics usually continues six weeks."
" It has been for many years the practice of Bethlem Hospital to
administer to the curable patients four or five emetics in the spring
of the year ; but on consulting my book of cases, I have not found
that such patients have been particularly benefited by the use of this
remedy. When the tartarized antimony given with this intention
operated as a purgative, it generally produced beneficial effects."
The most strenuous advocate, in late times, for emetics in madness
is Dr. Cox, whose work on that disease contains many excellent
practical observations. This author goes so far as to say, that, " in
almost every species and degree of maniacal complaints, from the
slightest aberration of intellect that accompanies hypochondriasis, to
the extreme of mania furibunda, emetics have proved a most valuable
and efficacious remedy." Dr. Wake, physician to the York Lunatic
Asylum, has assured me, that, after extensive experience in the use
of different remedies on the patients of that hospital, he has found
no other class of remedies so frequently efficacious as emetics.
    The use of emetics in madness requires caution. Dr. Haslam says,
that, " in many instances, and in some where bloodletting had been
previously employed, paralytic affections have within a few hours
supervened on the exhibition of an emetic, more especially where
the patient has been of a full habit, and has had the appearance of an
increased determination to the head."   The possibility of bringing
on attacks of apoplexy or paralysis ought always to be taken into
consideration in the prescribing of emetics to maniacal patients. The
use of medicines of this class is precluded by the signs of a plethoric
habit and cerebral congestion ; but, as MM. Esquirol and Foville
have well observed, they are likely to be of service, and this probability is confirmed by ample experience, in cases of melancholy or
hypochondriacal dejection attended with stupor, and where the languid state of the functions, both animal and physical, appears to
require the use of remedies which are fitted to excite new actions,
and to stimulate the secretions of the abdominal viscera. It may be
added, that emetics are sometimes useful during a state of furious
excitement, and produce calmness and a mitigation of violence.
Sometimes under these circumstances their exhibition is followed by
a restoration of sleep and tranquillity.

Insane patients often require large doses of tartarised antimony, as from six to ten grains, before vomiting is excited ; and this is especially the case when the remedy is given during a paroxysm of violent excitement. It is, however, better to begin with moderate doses, and to combine ipecacuanha with the preparations of antimony.

The use of antimony in nauseating doses is generally safe, and very frequently beneficial in controling maniacal excitement and the febrile state of the system which accompanies it.

6. *Digitalis.*—Digitalis has been much extolled both by English and foreign writers as a remedy in cases of insanity. In this country it has been more especially recommended by Dr. Cox, and abroad by Dr. Muller, of Wurtzburg, and Dr. Guislain. Continental physicians have given this medicine in large doses, so as to produce vomiting, and they have witnessed decidedly good effects from its administration in this manner. Muller gave five grains at night and morning, or two grains every second hour. Guislain has reported a remarkable cure, the patient having taken only one grain and a half, which, however, had produced such vomiting and prostrations, that recourse was had to the ceremonies of the catholic church, under the opinion that the individual was moribund. Dr. Cox began with small doses, and gradually increased them. He relates the case of a man who was kept under the influence of this remedy, the state of the pulse being always in relation to the degree of morbid excitement in the mind : when the pulse was at ninety, he was furious ; when at seventy, rational ; at fifty, melancholic ; and at forty, half-dead. He was perfectly cured by keeping his pulse steadily at seventy.

The cases of insanity in which digitalis is most likely to be useful are those accompanied with great arterial action, and displaying the phenomena of high mental excitement. M. Foville has expressed an opinion that little benefit is to be expected from this remedy except in those instances in which hypertrophy of the heart is complicated with insanity. Such instances, as we learn from necroscopic researches, are by no means infrequent. We might probably be not far from the truth in comprehending within the number of cases in which the trial of digitalis is advisable, those in which the circulation is preternaturally increased, though no manifestation of disease may appear in the organic fabric by which it is carried on. In other instances the same remedy, if given so as to produce full vomiting and prostration, may be of use in breaking through a train of morbid actions, and by the great changes which it induces in the general state of the system, in the determinations of blood, and the relative activity of particular organs.

Having mentioned the use of digitalis in this department of curative recommendations, I shall proceed to consider that of the other narcotics, though there may be some doubt whether, in strict propriety, this is the most proper place for mentioning them.

7. *Of the use of opium.*—Opium is far from being a remedy generally admissible in cases of insanity ; yet there are instances in which it is decidedly useful. Its adoption requires care and dis-

crimination. We are not possessed of any precise rules by which the effects which may arise from it can be with certainty predicted.

Opium is always a very doubtful remedy in disordered states of the brain, and is *generally* injurious when the vascular system of that organ is over-loaded with blood. I have seen apoplexy supervene on a moderate dose of opium in such a condition of the system ; and I well remember an instance of acute phrenitis occurring in a man who had swallowed a poppy-head fomentation intended for his legs, and who with difficulty recovered after large depletion. The first effect of opium is undoubtedly accompanied by increased arterial excitement ; its action is in a great degree analogous to that of alcohol and wine : it brings on delirium, and is known to aggravate it when previously existing. Nothing can be more contrary to probability than that a remedy of this description should be serviceable in a state of the brain such as we have inferred to exist generally in madness. It is only under particular circumstances that we find an exception to this conclusion. There is a condition of the living body, produced by long-continued excitement or stimulation, when the powers of re-action are beginning to be exhausted, and what the Brunonians term indirect debility ensues, in which the sudden abstraction of stimuli gives rise to extreme prostration. This, for instance, is nearly the state of the system in delirium tremens, the disease of the habitual and worn-out drunkard, marked by occasional fits of violent delirium, in the intervals of which excessive weakness ensues, with tremblings of the limbs, tremulous movements of muscles, paleness, cold perspirations, a rapid and feeble pulse. In this disease opium is well known to be a most important remedy ; and in analogous conditions of the body occurring under other circumstances, it may be beneficial by sustaining the vital actions in a certain degree of energy until the restorative powers of the constitution can come into play, and exert their usual influence. A state more or less of this description exists in some cases and periods of insanity, and it is probably under such circumstances that opium has been found useful : but it is not an easy matter to make the necessary discrimination.

The state of the vascular system, as M. Guislain has well observed, is a principal guide in determining as to the propriety of administering opium in insanity. In cases of high excitement, strong full pulse, heat of skin, fulness of vessels in the head, opium is injurious ; it tends to increase the symptoms and aggravate the severity of the disease. It is more likely to be of service in delicate and attenuated persons, of feeble constitution, pale, cold, relaxed skin, frequent, small, weak pulse. " If the disease has been of long duration, if the circulation has been losing its force and activity from day to day, if the attack of mental derangement has not been a sequel of suppressed cutaneous eruption or suppressed hemorrhage, causes tending in a high degree to produce an inflammatory state of the brain ; if there are only nervous symptoms to be contended with, I should have no hesitation." says M. Guislain, " in having recourse to opium."*

* Guislain, Traité sur l'Aliénation Mentale, tom. i. p. 350.

The circumstance which most plainly indicates the propriety of using opium is long-continued restlessness, a want of sleep bringing on dangerous exhaustion. Cullen declares that he has frequently employed large doses of opium in maniacal cases, and that, when they had the effect of inducing sleep, it was manifestly an advantage.* Esquirol has given it with advantage to individuals of great sensibility, in that state of the constitution which he terms excessive tension of the nervous system.

It is generally agreed among practical writers that opium should be used, when it is given to deranged persons, in considerable quantities. Van Swieten and Cullen gave it in large doses : the former relates the case of a female maniac, who swallowed by mistake a scruple of opium dissolved in vinegar, and was cured of her disease.† Darwin has reported an example in which he declares that two scruples of solid opium were given in a dose, and one scruple after four hours ; the patient is said to have been cured. Dr. Kriebel, of Berlin, recommended that one grain should be given every hour until sound sleep should be produced ; he is said to have administered twenty-six grains in the course of twelve hours. These facts are interesting as showing what may be expected under extraordinary circumstances, but they are too much out of the usual course of experience to furnish an example for imitation or a rule of practice. It would be more prudent, in all cases, in the use of an ambiguous remedy, to proceed cautiously, to give moderate doses at first, and larger ones afterwards, if the results of such trials and the circumstances of particular cases appear to warrant the proceeding. Two grains may perhaps be the maximum of a first dose.

8. *Hyoscyamus.*—The use of hyoscyamus was recommended by Dr. Willis as a substitute for opium, and it has been very generally adopted, but with uncertain success. Five or ten grains of the extract, or a drachm of the tincture of henbane, will often succeed in producing sleep. This medicine is certainly devoid of many of the injurious qualities which belong to opium. It has no stimulating influence, but diminishes sensibility and irritability without any previous excitement ; it diminishes not the secretions, nor does it produce constipation, but it often leaves a greater degree of languor, want of appetite, and of the general uneasiness which ensues on the use of narcotic remedies than does opium. It is likely to be useful under nearly similar circumstances as opium, but may be administered without requiring so much caution. I have repeatedly given it to patients who suffered for want of sleep in different modifications of mental disease with some advantage, but do not consider it to be a remedy of great importance.

9. *Camphor.*—Camphor has been recommended by Hufeland, Awenbrugger, and other German physicians, for the cure of insanity ; but it has been most extolled by Perfect.‡ This writer appears to

---

* First Lines, 1571.   † Comment. in Boerhaav. Aph. tom. iii. p. 533.
‡ Perfect's Annals of Insanity.—Guislain, Traité sur l'Alienation.

have given it in very large doses to many patients, who recovered
after taking it, though no other remedies were administered ; at the
same time it is not clearly apparent to what means the prosperous
result is to be attributed. These remarks apply to the following
case :—" T. B——, a married woman, of leucophlegmatic habit, became melancholic ; her complexion was pale, urine high-coloured,
tongue dry, pulse contracted, hard, irregular. After bleeding her
and giving an emetic, Perfect prescribed *two scruples* of camphor to
be taken every night and morning. An eruption appeared over her
whole body ; the catamenia, which had been suppressed, became restored ; and she recovered."

Practical physicians, whose testimony is deserving of the fullest
confidence, Dr. Cox, Muller of Wurtzburg, and Guislain, appear to
have given a fully sufficient trial to the use of camphor in insanity, in
various doses and under various forms of the disease. The result is
such as to convince us of its inefficacy.

The journals of Hufeland and Nasse contain various accounts of
cures obtained by means of stramonium and of belladonna. The former
of these narcotics was used by Dr. Schneider with great success in
the form of a tincture, made by infusing two ounces of the seeds in
eight ounces of Spanish wine with one of spirit of wine, of which
the dose was from six to twenty drops. Franck has recommended
belladonna, especially in mania combined with epilepsy. Muller of
Wurtzburg is said to have cured mania by giving the powdered root
of this plant in doses which reached the quantity of thirty-six grains
in a day, taking care to desist when dilatation of the pupils or any
other specific effects of the poison were discovered.*

10. *Mercury.*—The use of mercury has been highly recommended in madness by several writers, and particularly by Dr. Rush.
Mercury is by no means a general remedy for maniacal diseases ; but
in cases of torpor, with suppression of a very scanty state of any of
the secretions, mercury is frequently employed with great advantage.
It should be used in mild alterative doses, and discontinued as soon
as the gums become slightly affected.

11. *Rotatory motion.*—Rotatory motion has been proposed long
ago, and frequently brought into use as a method of reducing the
force of circulation, by occasioning vertigo and nausea with some degree of faintness. The first suggestion of this attempt is to be traced,
as M. Guislain has pointed out, in the works of Cælius Aurelianus.
Darwin, in modern times, made the proposal known. A rotatory
coach, in which the patient was to be turned round with rapidity in
a horizontal position, was the plan recommended by the last mentioned writer. Dr. Cox, who brought the suggestion into actual use,
improved also on the scheme. He used a swinging or rotatory chair,
in which the patient remained seated during the operation. Hallaran and Von Hirsh have recommended a ship-bed or hammock. In

---

* Hufeland's Journal.—Nasse's Zeitschrift, 1823.—Guislain, ouvrage cité
t. i. p. 368.

the hospital of *la Charité* at Berlin, rotatory machines on both principles are constructed ; one for horizontal and the other for perpendicular rotation. The application of this remedy has been still further varied by Dr. Hoven and by Hayner.

In whatever manner rotation may be applied, the effects of the process are nearly similar. Whoever has experienced sea-sickness must be aware of the strongly sedative influence which this state exerts on the nervous system and the voluntary powers. That it must be advantageous to a medical practitioner who has the care of maniacs to have within his reach the means of reducing occasionally the morbid activity of such persons by thus lowering the energy of the physical powers, could scarcely admit of doubt. Experience confirms this presumption. Some writers have, indeed, ridiculed the idea of attempting such a remedy, and others have thought it difficult to imagine on what principle it can be of any service ; but those practitioners who have put the proposal to the test of experiment have, if I am not mistaken, in most instances been convinced of its utility. It was used by Dr. Cox in cases of violent maniacal excitement, and was found by him to be a powerful sedative. The nausea and sickness induced were found to tranquilize the patient and put a speedy termination to his paroxysm. It was not found requisite in all cases to bring on vomiting. Quiet sleep often followed the trial of this process. Many other physicians who have made use of the same remedy have assured me that they have derived similar advantages from it, and consider it as a resource of great value in the treatment of madness. Among them, I shall mention Dr. Bompas, the relative and successor of Dr. Cox, who now superintends the same establishment, and Dr. Wake, physician to the asylum at York.

The rotatory swing is also useful as a method of moral restraint. Its effects are so disagreeable that the threat of a repetition has a salutary influence upon turbulent and untractable patients.

ARTICLE II.

Second practical indication in the medical treatment of insanity.

The principle of medical treatment hitherto considered, which has respect to the physical condition of the brain in cases of maniacal disease, is chiefly applicable to the acute stage and early period of its duration. The pathological fact on which it is in part founded, may be usefully borne in mind in the subsequent progress of the complaint, and acted upon more or less when circumstances allow or require it, but it cannot, when the disorder has become confirmed, be the chief guide of the practitioner. The marks of determination to the head have generally, under such circumstances, in a great measure subsided. In these instances inflammatory action in the brain has probably given way to a state of relaxation bordering on serous effusion, or to other changes which imply rather the consequences than the existence of increased vascular action.

The second indication for the medical treatment of insanity, which has relation chiefly to the more advanced period and chronic aspect of the disease, is to restore and maintain, as far as it can be done, a healthy condition of the physical or natural functions, and to obviate or remove disorders in other parts of the system, which may be connected or coincident with the diseased condition of the brain.

I have already observed that in a great proportion of maniacal cases there are symptoms of disturbance in the natural functions, and that diseases of the thoracic and abdominal viscera co-exist with that morbid state of the brain on which madness immediately depends; —that the former are in fact often the immediate causes of death. The relation in which these diseases stand to the cerebral disorder may be doubtful in many instances ; in some it is the relation of cause, in others that of effect : even in the last instance there is a reaction of the secondary upon the primary parts in the series of morbid changes, and the original disease is aggravated by its complication with an accessory one. By relieving the latter we obtain a proportional mitigation of the former. It is indeed a fact that many lunatics have been cured by a course of remedies adapted to the restoration of their general health. I have repeatedly seen persons who had laboured for some months, or even years, under mental derangement, brought from poor-houses in the country, or from their private dwellings, in a state of emaciation and squalid wretchedness, suffering under various disorders which had become complicated with insanity, or had in some instances preceded it. These persons have been placed under medical treatment; care has been taken to relieve the disorders arising from exhaustion, to restore the functions to a healthy state, to afford good and nutritious diet, and to remove complaints which occurred from time to time by occasional remedies. In many cases of this description, as the general health improved, the mental disorder has gradually lessened, and has finally disappeared. In the course of four, five, or six months from the period of their coming under medical treatment, very many patients of this description have been restored to their usual state of health, and to the exercise of their customary occupations, after having undergone the operation of few remedies except such as are adapted to the indication or principle of practice now pointed out.*

* This is the indication which some practitioners follow from the first in the treatment of insanity. Mr. Hitch informs me that the plan adopted at the Gloucester Asylum is very simple. He says, " We first secure the free evacuation of the bowels, and cleanliness of skin and clothing. We assure the patient that we consider him to be mad, and shall treat him accordingly. We allow him a generous and nutritious diet, bread, meat, and ale, &c. and if there is great anxiety and restlessness, we give him ether (Sp. æth. s. c. ℥ss or ℥i) every fourth hour, conjoined with carbonate of ammonia, and camphor, and other stimulants. We enjoin living as much as possible in the open air ; and if the excited state is unyielding to this treatment, we use the douche. For acts of violence, occasional moral delinquencies, &c. we use with remarkably good effects the bath of surprise." Mr. Hitch assures me that when this plan of treatment has been adopted during the stage of incubation, the disorder has *never* proceeded to actual mania.

The mode of treatment required in following this indication must vary according to the state of the constitution and the modifications of disease which particular cases may present.

In examples of madness complicated with intestinal disorder, care must be taken to relieve the latter by the various remedies and modes of diet and regimen which the condition of the intestinal canal or of its function requires. A torpid state of bowels must be overcome by the use of mild aperients, continued daily, or given occasionally according to circumstances. When constipation has given way to diarrhœa, with tenderness, abdominal distention, with or without occasional symptoms of dysentery, with emaciation, coldness of the skin, general debility, a disposition to eruptions resembling those of scurvy or purpura, the cure can only be promoted by a careful attention to a variety of particulars. The action of the bowels should be restrained by absorbent medicines, combined with slight opiates and mercurial alteratives. The use of leeches and the warm bath, warm clothing, and a warm atmosphere, a mild and nutritious diet, should be enjoined at the same time. Bitters, tonics, and aromatics may afterwards be given to support the strength of the stomach and promote digestion : a liberal allowance of animal food, and sometimes malt liquors, and even wine, are given with advantage in cases of debility and exhaustion when the digestive powers will bear their use.

When the actions of the intestinal canal are irregular in chronic cases of madness, without giving rise to so great a degree of disease as in the instances above indicated, a healthy state of their function is sufficiently promoted by giving mild aperients, with tonics and neutral salts, two or three times in a week, and occasional doses of calomel.

When madness has been the result of, or has been accompanied by, diminution or loss of any other natural function or habitual process, an effort should be made to restore it. If we were possessed of any certain emmenagogue, it is highly probable that its successful application would in many cases promote the cure of maniacal diseases connected with the suppression of the catamenia. When habitual discharges from hemorrhoidal veins have been coerced, or have ceased spontaneously, derangement of the health has ensued similar to that occasioned by uterine suppressions. The want of this latter process seems to be more easily supplied by the powers of art than that of the uterine function. M. Foville has mentioned a case which occurred to M. Esquirol, in which paralysis became complicated with madness in consequence of the suppression of an habitual hemorrhoidal discharge. The application of a single leech to the hemorrhoidal veins every day during a month was followed by a restoration of the flux, and the patient was cured of his complaint.

Attempts to restore the catemenia when defective in maniacal patients, as they very frequently are, seldom produce in a speedy manner the desired result. If any effort is perceptible at particular

times to set up the periodical discharge, it should be promoted by
small bleedings ; by the application of leeches to the inguinal
region or the thighs, or by cupping at the loins, together with the
use of the hip-bath, pediluvium, general warmth of clothing and
atmosphere, warm drinks, with doses of castor, camphor, and other
odorous stimulants. At other times aloë, rhubarb, and aromatic
bitters should be given daily by way of preparation.

Attention to diet and regimen are fully as important for the ful-
filment of the last-mentioned indication as any remedy whatever.
In exhausted subjects, as before hinted, great advantage is obtained
from the use of a liberal diet. A plentiful allowance of animal
food of the most wholesome and digestible kind, is required. The
adoption of a liberal diet is not only free in such cases from any
exciting or too stimulant influence, but even appears to calm the
irritation which previously existed. But no rule respecting diet
can be laid down that must not be subject to modification in particular circumstances, and according to the peculiarity of the case and
the state of the constitution.

Fresh air and exercise, for those patients who are in a condition
that renders them fit for it, are among the most important restorative means. Every asylum for the reception of lunatics ought to
be provided with the means of affording regular employment in
the open air to all the patients who are able to undertake it. Gardening and various agricultural works should as much as possible
occupy their time at stated periods of the day, and by system and
judicious management a great majority among the inmates of these
receptacles may be brought into the habit of devoting themselves
mechanically to such employments. M. Esquirol remarks that the
best effects have resulted from the employment of these methods.
They are followed with the greatest advantage in several lunatic
asylums, both public and private, in different parts of England. I
shall return to the consideration of this topic under the head of the
moral treatment of insanity.

Section II.—*Moral Treatment of Insanity.*

The state of individuals is so very different in the several forms
and varieties of insanity, that no rules referring to the moral
treatment or personal management of the insane can be of universal
application. Any remarks that may be made on this subject will
either have reference to particular classes of deranged persons, or
will require modifications if they are adopted in a more general
point of view. Maniacs, for example, who are under strong excitement, during paroxysms of raving madness, require personal
coercion and even strict confinement of body and limbs in order to
prevent mischief to themselves and others. Such treatment would
be quite improper for other classes of lunatics, or even for the same
individuals at different periods.

In order to render the remarks I shall offer on the moral treatment of insanity more distinct and easy of apprehension, I shall arrange them under the following heads : these will be found to comprise, if I am not mistaken, all the most important considerations to which it is necessary to advert.

1. Of the propriety of secluding or confining the insane, and separating them from society.

2. Of other means of abstracting them from the morbid impressions and associations which may have excited and may foster their mental disease.

3. Of the moral discipline and personal control under which they ought to be placed.

4. Of the treatment of their understandings in relation to their illusions or the morbid impressions on their minds.

ARTICLE I.

One of the most important considerations relating to the treatment of the insane turns upon the propriety of secluding them and separating them from their families and from society. This may be taken up, and, in fact, requires to be treated both as a medical and as a legal or medico-legal question. Legislatures have provided for the arrest of insane persons who disturb or endanger the public tranquillity : they have ordained the confinement of such individuals in receptacles which are appropriated to their detention; and they have enacted a suspension of the rights which those who are sane possess, and can alone with propriety exercise in disposing of person and property according to their inclination. Of all these arrangements the maintenance of public order is the principal object, and the second is the preservation of the property belonging to the lunatic, and the interest of his family. It belongs to medical jurisprudence to determine under what circumstances such proceedings are required for the objects above mentioned : the inquiry comprehends what are termed *medico-legal* discussions. I shall advert to the topics belonging to this inquiry on a future occasion. My present engagement is with a consideration strictly medical, viz. under what conditions and in what manner confinement or seclusion is required in order to promote the recovery of insane persons, or as means of restoring their health.

M. Esquirol has observed that all English, French, and German physicians, who have devoted themselves to the study of mental diseases, recommend the confinement of the insane, and are unanimous as to the utility of this proceeding as means of cure.

" Cullen has pointed out the necessity of confining lunatics, and separating them from their relations and friends. Willis, who acquired so great celebrity by having assisted towards the happy termination of the first attack of madness experienced by George III., unfurnished the king's apartments, dismissed his courtiers and domestics, and had him attended by strange servants. Willis asserts that insane persons from the continent, who came to seek his advice, got well more frequently than his countrymen.

" M. Pinel, in his Treatise on Madness, his best title to the admiration and gratitude of mankind, has pronounced seclusion to be the foundation of all rational treatment of mental diseases."

We here find this statement made in very general terms ; whether any and what limitations are required or were intended will be apparent, when we shall have considered the reasons which have been assigned for having recourse to such a proceeding.

The reasons which indicate the necessity of secluding and confining insane persons are briefly stated by M. Esquirol in the following heads.*

1. The insane ought to be confined for their own security, for that of their families, and for the maintenance of public order. This consideration is not within the scope of our present inquiry.

2. To remove them from the influence of external circumstances which may have produced their disorder, and may be likely to protract it.

3. To overcome their resistance to curative means.

4. To subject them to a regimen appropriate to their situation. And

5. To cause them to resume their moral and intellectual habits.

That the second of these objects, which is the foundation of all curative proceedings, can only be obtained by withdrawing insane patients from their homes, and secluding them from their families and society, becomes apparent on considering the prevalent state of the feelings and affections of lunatics, and the results arising from the erroneous impressions which cloud their understandings.

" The sensibility of the insane," says M. Esquirol, " is perverted : they no longer have any relation with the external world but those of a disordered and consequently painful nature. Every thing irritates them, distracts them, and excites their aversion. In constant opposition to all that surrounds them, they soon persuade themselves that persons are combined to injure them ; and neither understanding what is said, nor being able to comprehend the reasonings that are addressed to them, they misinterpret the most affectionate expressions and the wisest counsels ; they mistake the most candid, serious, and tender language for insults, irony, and provocations, and the most attentive kindness for contradictions. The regimen and the prohibitions which are called for by their situation, and to which their attendants wish to subject them, appear to them cruel persecutions.

" The heart of the insane cherishes no feeling but mistrust ; he is irritated to anger by every thing he sees, and is so timid and fearful that he is troubled as soon as any one approaches him. Hence arises the conviction that every one tries to vex, defame, ruin, and destroy him. This conviction puts the finishing stroke to the

* Observations on the Illusions of the Insane, and upon the Medico-Legal Question of their Confinement, by M. Esquirol; translated by W. Liddell, Esq. Mr. Liddell has conferred a benefit on English readers by his translation of this valuable work, and by many useful notes which he has appended to it.

moral perversion of his mind, and from it arises that symptomatic mistrust which is observed in all the insane, even in maniacs who appear so bold and audacious.

"From mistrust these patients soon pass to fear or hatred ; and in these new moral situations they repel their relations and friends, and welcome stangers, throwing themselves into their arms, calling them their protectors or liberators, with whom they are ready to fly, and abandon their home and family.

"With these moral dispositions, if left in the bosom of his family, the tender son, whose happiness used to consist in living near his mother, and in following his father's counsels, persuaded that they wish to disgust him with his home in order to drive him from it, falls into the deepest despair, or escapes to destroy himself."*

"Another unhappy person becomes, all at once, lord of the world, dictates his sovereign commands to all that surround him ; he expects to be blindly obeyed by all those who have been accustomed to yield to his will through respect or affection. His wife, his children, his friends, his servants, are his subjects ; they have hitherto always submitted to his will ; how dare they resist him now ? He is in his own territory ; his commands are despotic ; he is ready to punish with the greatest severity whoever shall make the least remonstrance. What he requires may be impossible—that is of no consequence : should the commands of the all-powerful meet with obstacles ? The affliction of his family, the chagrin of his friends, the anxiety of all, their deference to his will and caprices, and the repugnance that each evinces to oppose him from the fear of exasperating his fury, contribute to confirm him in his imaginary possession of power and dominion. Withdraw him from his pretensions, transport him far from his house, from his empire,—removed from his subjects, surrounded by new scenes, he will collect his ideas, direct his attention to himself, and place himself on an equality with his companions."†

"Very often the cause of mental derangement is to be found in domestic causes. The malady takes its rise from chagrins, from family dissensions, from reverses of fortune, from privations ; and the presence of relations and friends increases the evil, often without their suspecting that they are the first cause of it. Sometimes an excess of tenderness seizes the patient ; a husband persuades himself that he cannot make his wife happy ; he forms the resolution of flying from her, and threatens to put an end to his existence, since it would be the only means of securing her happiness. Her tears, her melancholy countenance, are so many new reasons for persuading this unfortunate person to commit suicide."

"Sometimes the first disturbance given to the moral and intellectual faculties has arisen in the home of the insane person, in the midst of his relations and friends. All these external circumstances

* Observations, before cited.
† Dictionnaire des Sciences Médicales ; art. *Folie.*

being associated with the first attack and the disorder which followed, will often contribute to keep alive and foster the hallucination,
—a phenomenon which easily explains itself, since ideas recur si-
multaneously with certain impressions, when these impressions and
ideas have often been associated, or even when they have been connected, only once, but with remarkable force and energy. It is
generally remarked that insane persons feel an aversion towards
certain individuals, without the possibility of diverting them from
this feeling. The object of their hatred is almost invariably the
person who before the attack possessed their tenderest affection ;
hence it is that they are so indifferent to their relations, and often-
times so dangerous ; while, on the other hand, strangers are agreeable to them. The presence of strangers suspends the delirium of
the insane, either by the influence of new impressions, which is always useful, or from a secret feeling of self-respect, which induces lunatics to conceal their state of mind. I have seen patients
appear quite calm before their physician and strangers, while they
were at the same time abusing their relations or their friends in an
under voice."

M. Georget, one of the most acute and intelligent writers of our
time, who long devoted his attention to disorders which affect the
mind and the nervous system, has in a similar manner urged the
necessity of adopting the course which is advised by M. Esquirol.
He says that " all physicians who have habitually the cure of insane
persons have recommended their seclusion in almost every case as
the most essential condition and one of the first measures to be
adopted in their treatment." " Lunatics," he adds, " ought to be
separated from the objects which have excited their disease, or
which foster or aggravate it ; from relatives or servants whom they
dislike, whom they pretend to command, and to whom they would
never submit ; from busy-bodies, who only irritate them by useless
arguments or misplaced ridicule ; they ought to be separated from
society, and placed in an appropriate habitation, to ensure both the
safety of the public and their own preservation. Their friends are
always repugnant to put this plan into execution ; a mother, a wife,
or a husband, can with difficulty believe that the object dearest in
the world to either of them can be better placed in the hands of
strangers than under the influence of those who are eager to devote
the most affectionate cares ; they fear likewise that in lunatic asylums the sight of the patients will have a bad effect, and aggravate
the disease : that constraint, severity, and all kinds of ill treatment
will be employed to manage the patient, and that, if once cured, he
will preserve a horrible impression of his abode, and resentment
against his relations who have consented to his confinement. These
last considerations induce rich families to place their deranged relatives in private houses destined to receive a single lunatic, who is
surrounded by servants and inspectors whom he does not know.
Besides that these private establishments are very expensive, they
rarely answer the end proposed ; either some relation chooses to

remain near the invalid, or the latter soon perceives that every thing by which he is surrounded is destined for his service : in either case the objects of seclusion are imperfectly attained. Lastly, many things are often required which are only to be found in public establishments. This imperfect separation, however, is all that can be adopted in some families, and we must make as much advantage of it as we can. In public asylums the seclusion is complete ;, the patients soon know that they are under the authority, and even at the discretion of the director ; they are watched and constrained without difficulty, under the care of regular attendants. They find powerful sources of occupation and of distraction in associating even with the other patients. The greater number of lunatics never discover that they are in the midst of mad people, and find nothing to complain of in this circumstance. When their reason begins to return, they are removed into the department destined for the reception of convalescents, and hence are withdrawn from sights which might make unpleasant impressions upon them. As long as the disease continues, they are angry with those who have deprived them of their liberty ; but as soon as they have recovered their reason, resentment is changed into gratitude. On this account, then, the friends of the insane incur no risk. We do not pretend to deny that this separation and abode among other lunatics has occasionally aggravated the disease, when of recent occurrence, in some individuals : on the other hand, we affirm that the same means have cured many lunatics almost immediately. Besides it is next to impossible to preserve and take care of maniacs or monomaniacs in the midst of their families ; and all the inconveniences of separation disappear under the absolute necessity of its adoption."*

The preceding observations on the propriety of secluding deranged persons from society, and confining them in mad-houses, will be found applicable, perhaps, to all maniacs, and to many of those who labour under monomania. In mania or raving madness, indeed, the condition of the patient is such as to render the necessity of strict confinement obvious to common sense, both on account of the safety of the individual and that of his family, without adverting to the advantages resulting from such a measure in the promotion of recovery, and in the facility of applying remedies. In a great proportion of the cases of monomania the propriety of adopting the same course is almost equally evident. The understanding is in this disease so disturbed, and the moral affections of the individual so perverted, that no alternative seems to be left.

But when the disorder of the understanding is so restricted as to leave the patient, according to appearances, the exercise of a great portion of his reason, it is more difficult to come to a determination. It is often feared that the opposition which the individual is about to experience will deprive him of that portion of intelligence which •

---

* M. Georget, De la Folie, 1820: also art. *Folie*, in Dict. de Médecine.

remains. It seems cruel to deprive him of the attentions of his family, and to separate a miserable being oppressed with grief from the objects of his affections; to remove an individual morbidly prone to terror and alarm from the friends and relatives whom he regards as his natural protectors. We dread the shock which the feelings of such patients may sustain when they see themselves in the midst of lunatics.

M. Esquirol, who is so strenuous an advocate for the seclusion of deranged persons, candidly admits that he cannot assert it to have been *never* prejudicial. He frankly owns that its effects are sometimes injurious : he says that it partakes of the nature of those things, the best of which are not always free from inconvenience ; he draws the conclusion "that the measure of confinement should not be adopted too generally, nor too exclusively, and that it should be prescribed only by the experienced physician."*

It was long ago observed by this highly informed and judicious writer, that the necessity of confining madmen depended principally upon the state of their moral affections. He has lately explained more fully the meaning of this remark, and has furnished us with suggestions for following it out to its particular applications.† When the predominant feelings of the monomaniac are such as are calculated to estrange him from and to set him at enmity with his relatives ; when he is actuated by pride and misanthropy, by jealousy, hatred, malice, confinement is absolutely necessary. If, on the contrary, the illusion of the insane relates to objects of indifference, and excites no strong emotions ; if he has no aversion to his home and the persons with whom he lives, although confinement may be sometimes useful, it is not absolutely necessary. " But if the patient, retaining a large portion of his intellect, has a strong attachment to his relatives, it is to be feared that confinement might aggravate the disease."

If the disorder of intellect displays itself in connection with the domestic habits of the individual ; if the real or imaginary causes of excitement are to be found in the bosom of his family, there is, on this account an obvious reason for removing him from his home, though it does not follow that confinement is necessary.

Those lunatics whose propensities are dangerous to themselves or others, individuals who are prone to self-destruction, as well as the malevolent and mischievous, ought always to be confined and closely watched. They are cunning, and know how to elude the most active superintendence.

In moral insanity nearly the same observations are applicable as in monomania. The state of the feelings in these forms of insanity is the same, and monomania is only moral insanity with the addition of disorder affecting the understanding or the rational powers.

In that variety of moral insanity which consists in undue excitement, a disposition to boisterous mirth, wildness of conduct and

* Dict. des. Sc. Médicales.   † Observations, before cited.

deportment, confinement is necessary. It is the only remedy for this disease, and it often succeeds in bringing about the recovery of the individual. Quiet, seclusion, even solitude, are obviously the most applicable means of bringing him to sober reflection, and enabling the mind to subside into a state of tranquil composure. These means cannot be obtained except by having recourse in the first instance to compulsory seclusion and confinement.

Where the disease is manifested by dejection of spirits, gloom, and melancholy, the propriety of confinement is much less certain, and it must depend upon the particular disposition and character of the individual. Some melancholics, when they are brought into mad-houses, derive benefit from the effect which new external circumstances and the various habits of the inmates have in exciting their attention, and withdrawing it from their own internal feelings. A few are shocked, and experience a sense of degradation. If a patient labouring under melancholia in the early stage, and while it is not complicated with illusions, can be safely taken care of in a private abode, where inducements to exercise and beneficial recreations can be administered, it will often be advisable to adopt such a method rather than that of confinement in a lunatic asylum ; but if the dejection of mind is very great, it is necessary to be on the watch in order to anticipate any attempt at suicide. I was consulted some years ago with regard to a case of this description. The patient was a gentleman who had been an officer in the army : he lived with a friend in the country, where he became melancholic, and gave himself up to despondency. I strongly urged the immediate necessity of confinement : it was neglected, and the next intelligence that reached me respecting the individual was that he had shot himself. In every case of melancholy it is requisite that a keeper should be constantly with the patient, who should be enjoined never to lose sight of him. Yet even such precaution is not always sufficient when the disordered person is otherwise at large. I know a vigilant active woman who had once the care of a female lunatic under such circumstances, and who for greater security slept in the same bed with the patient. The latter took an opportunity when her keeper was asleep, got out of bed, and cut her throat with a pair of scissors, which she had contrived to secrete on the preceding day.

A very troublesome description of cases are those in which there is an invincible propensity to drink intoxicating liquors, and in which fits of drunkenness are followed by accessions of mania. Such persons, when brought into lunatic houses and debarred from the use of fermented liquors, are soon restored to a state of composure : they demand their liberty, and after obtaining it soon return to the habit which occasioned their disease, or rather the aggravation of its symptoms. Confinement in such instances would be the only prophylactic. It is said to be practised in some countries, but in this it is not sanctioned. The consideration of these cases does not, however, belong strictly to the subject which is our chief concern at present.

In the early stages of dementia or incoherence, when that state
supervenes on insanity, and the transition is as yet incomplete, confinement is not less necessary, from regard to security, than in mania
or monomania, but in the advanced degrees it is no longer required
on this ground, and may be dispensed with, provided that the relatives and family of the demented person be in circumstances which
enable them to pay due attention to his comfort.

Demented persons, or individuals labouring under incoherence or
fatuity the result of cerebral diseases, constitute a larger proportion
of the inmates of both public and private lunatic asylums. It
would be much better on many accounts that such persons, if confined at all, should be placed in separate establishments, and not
mixed, as they now universally are, with maniacs. Many reasons
connected with convenience and propriety may indicate, under particular circumstances, the expediency of removing demented persons as well as idiots from private families, but these are different
considerations from that of their confinement in lunatic houses,
and quite unconnected with the point of view in which we are now
contemplating the seclusion of insane persons, as a measure calculated to promote recovery or a condition essential to any attempt
at cure.

A very important consideration connected with the subject of
seclusion refers to the period at which it ought to cease. On this
matter we may observe that it is the opinion of all practical men,
an opinion confirmed by the experience of every day, that too much
care and precaution cannot be exercised in setting patients at liberty
who have been under confinement on account of mental derangement. So strong a predisposition to the disease appears to remain
for some time after its apparent cure, that convalescent patients are
known to undergo relapses when excited by such emotions as they
are almost sure to experience as soon as they are at large, and can
only be protected from by seclusion, continued as long as this extreme
susceptibility remains. M. Pinel has given some important remarks
on this subject, which I shall briefly abstract. He observes that
any sudden alarm, transport of anger, or of grief ; that intemperance, hot weather, or even a sudden change from a state of confinement and restraint to liberty, is liable to produce in convalescent
lunatics a disturbance of which they would not be susceptible in
other circumstances, and to renew the attacks of mania when the
habit has not been long suspended : that some convalescent patients,
who have been taken away too soon by their friends have suffered
relapses, and have been obliged to return several times to the hospitals. A grenadier of the French guards, who was one of the
foremost to mount the Bastile at its assault, gave himself up to the
most unbounded ambition, was disappointed in his brilliant expectations, and fell into the most violent maniacal delirium. He remained four months in this state of fury and confusion after his
arrival at Bicêtre. When he became calm, his mother took him
away before his reason was confirmed : hence he experienced a re-

turn of his attacks in the midst of his family, and it became necessary to remove him again to the hospital. The same imprudence
was renewed twice with the same results. His mother, then in-
structed by experience, was no longer anxious to remove him
unseasonably : he passed two years tranquilly and without any attack, left the hospital at the beginning of the winter, and never again
experienced a return of his disease.

Hot weather, and sometimes the return of cold, although much
more rarely, are liable to produce attacks of recurrent mania ; it is
therefore prudent, at such seasons, to employ some preservatives
for convalescent patients who have left the hospitals.

I have no doubt that many convalescent patients would derive
great benefit from a plan of treatment similar to that which is instituted at the establishment of Gheel, in Belgium. Gheel is a large
scattered village, where five or six hundred lunatics are spread
among the cottages of the peasants. Each patient is obliged to labour in the fields or gardens for a certain number of hours each day.
When not employed, they are allowed to walk about without restraint, and are summoned to their homes by the village bell. The
peasants are bound to treat their inmates with kindness, and they
are remunerated according to a fixed rate for the care they take.
We are informed that " the patients are considered to be under the
especial protection of St. Dymph of Gheel, a holy woman who was
there cured of insanity, under whose coffin each person is made to
pass with great ceremony at certain times."*

ARTICLE II.

*Of other means of abstracting lunatics from morbid impressions
and associations connected with and fostering their mental
aberrations.*

In recent cases of partial derangement, when the state of the
mind is judged to be not such as requires absolute seclusion and
confinement, much benefit has often arisen from changes of scene
and occupation, from travelling, from placing the patient amid objects which may divert his thoughts, and change the course of his
reflections. This, next to the consideration of confinement, is the
most important that can engage our attention in reference to the
moral treatment of insanity. The measures to be adopted in particular cases must depend upon the circumstances of each individual,
his condition as to pecuniary resources, his personal tastes or inclinations, his susceptibilities of amusement by travelling, or by field
exercises or sports, his inclination to society, or habitual fondness
of solitude. This last disposition should be as much as possible
counteracted.

Journeys into foreign countries have often been recommended as

* See the account of Gheel in M. Guislain's work, and particularly that of Sir
Andrew Halliday in his General View.

affording greater novelty. Travelling in the south of France, Italy, and Switzerland, has been enjoined to melancholics as well as to hypochondriacs. The use of mineral waters has been resorted to with advantage in both instances : the influence of hope and confidence in a new remedy is here presented in aid of other favourable external circumstances. In some instances mineral waters are beneficial by their medical properties, and particularly warm sulphureous baths in cases complicated with cutaneous affections.* Ferruginous saline waters are also of service in some cases, when there is disorder and weakness of the stomach and digestive organs.

Exercise is of the greatest importance among the means of restoring the health of lunatics in all curable cases. Walking or riding in the open air, during as great a portion of the day as the strength of individuals will support the fatigue resulting from it, is often of great service. I have known instances in which both insane persons and hypochondriacs have been greatly improved by adopting this rule, and systematically adhering to it. Long walks in fields or woods, in company with a suitable guardian, have aided principally in the restoration of health in some instances in which the relatives of patients labouring under symptoms of mental disorder have refused to send them to lunatic houses. All establishments of this description ought to be provided with the means of affording regular employment in the open air to such patients as can be induced to undertake it. Gardening and various agricultural works should as much as possible employ their time at stated periods of the day ; and by system and judicious management many of the inmates of these asylums may be brought into the habit of devoting themselves mechanically to such occupations. It is said that a farmer in Scotland once obtained a high reputation for the cure of mental diseases. He employed lunatics in his farm, made them work in tillage, fastened them to his plough, and by degrees brought the most violent to a state of quietness and submission. Dr. Horn, of Berlin, has constructed at the hospital of *La Charité* a sort of cart fit to hold four lunatics, which is drawn by thirty of their companions, who take their turn to ride and to be pulled along. This exercise is performed in the alleys of the gardens, and under the eyes of inspectors. The course along which the cart is to be driven is marked out beforehand, and the greatest regularity is observed in the performance, which, according to Horn, has been found a very efficacious resource for exercise and diversion, and has tended to the improvement of many patients.†

* Guislain, Traité de l'Aliénation, t. i. p. 265.
† Guislain, ouv. cit.—M. Fodéré cites with commendation Dr. Wendt's account of the lunatic asylums at Copenhagen, and some others in the north of Europe, recently established or improved. In these hospitals we are informed that all the arrangements of construction are on the most aptly contrived plan, and that the principle of gentleness in the treatment of the patients is carried further than elsewhere. " All violent means of repression are proscribed, such as chains, the rotatory machine, solitary confinement, harshness of manner, and forced abstinence : lunatics are treated in such a manner as to spare them as much as possible the

Exercise is necessary for deranged persons in cold and wet weather, and lunatic asylums should be furnished, and they are often
furnished, with galleries where the patients may walk under cover
and protected from rain, with a free admission of air.

Female patients and men of sedentary habits should be engaged
as much as possible in some regular occupation. This rule is followed with great advantage in some of the hospitals for lunatics in
France, where the females occupy their time in embroidery and
working in various ways. It is found, as before mentioned, that
even in the early stages of dementia, it is not impossible to induce
such patients to work steadily at some merely mechanical employment. Such habits mitigate the disease, or at least its manifestations, and in curable cases they tend strongly to promote recovery.[*]

The opinions of practical physicians are undecided as to the utility
of music as a means of amusement and of withdrawing the attention
of lunatics from the disordered trains of thought which constitute
the phenomena of their disease. M. Guislain says that music is
useful in two respects ; in the first place, when the patient plays on
a musical instrument, his attention is for the time occupied and his
mind beneficially exercised ; secondly, when another person is the
agent, a train of soothing sensations are excited in the deranged
which tend more or less to tranquilize. Dr. J. P. Franck is said
to have found music of great advantage in some cases of mania accompanied with violent excitement of anger or rage. On the other
hand Herberski mentions a case in which the sounds of any musi-

---

conviction of their real state." It may be doubted whether this is always advisable. " Patients, whose attacks abate in violence, are admitted to the society of
the director, take their meals with him ; they are allowed free intercourse and
society among themselves, and care is taken to furnish them all with such occupations as are consistent with their habits and education. The men are occupied
either with military exercises, or they cut wood, or cultivate the soil; the women
wash the linen, knit, spin, sew. Both sexes are taught geography, drawing, and
music." " *On Sundays,*" says Dr. Wendt, "they are allowed to play at cards,
billiards, and in some asylums are made to act comedies. Convalescents have
at their use libraries and reading-rooms, where the public journals are put into
their hands." *Essai Médico-légal de M. le Professeur Fodéré.*

[*] These principles have been followed in the establishment of most of the
lunatic asylums founded of late years in different parts of Great Britain, and it
is much to be regretted that they are not introduced into the old ones. In the
Armagh Asylum there are thirteen acres of ground, which is cultivated by the
patients, and furnishes vegetables to the whole establishment. All the linen
used is woven by the patients, and their clothes made by themselves. "As employment," says the intelligent governor, Mr. Jackson, " is now generally
allowed to be one of the best restoratives, every means has been used to promote
it. Such as are at all capable among the females are constantly occupied at
plain work, spinning, &c. The division in which these works are carried on is
remarkable for its cheerfulness. The patients with few exceptions seem grateful
and happy." In the Richmond Lunatic Asylum, out of two hundred and seventy-
seven patients one hundred and thirty are actively and usefully employed, viz.
eighteen in garden labour, sixteen in spinning, twelve in knitting, eighteen at
needle-work, twelve in washing, sixteen in carrying coals, white-washing the
wards, tailoring and weaving, and twelve in learning to read.—*See Halliday's
General View.*

cal instrument immediately excited a maniacal paroxysm ;* and M.
Esquirol affirms that he has seen deranged persons in whom raving
fits were produced by the same cause. There is no doubt that in
many cases music is too exciting ; it produces too vivid an impression on some persons to be devoid of injury, especially in cases of
mania with a tendency to strong excitement. In an opposite state
of the feelings, when the patient has sunk into dull apathy or
lethargy, or is wrapped in gloom and melancholy contemplation
from which he is with difficulty roused, some advantage may be
derived from this amusement, and Dr. Cox declares that he has witnessed very beneficial effects from it.

The good effects of music in madness have been chiefly extolled
by persons who were themselves devotedly fond of it. A fact
which tends to prove that it affords no important resource for the
treatment of this disease, is that it was formerly much used in the
lunatic asylum conducted by Dr. Cox, and has been discontinued by
his successor Dr. Bompas, who had abundant opportunities of witnessing the trial, and who has too much observation and vigilant
attention to leave any means neglected which had been found really
serviceable.

Dr. Cox has very judiciously observed that when the patient has
been a performer, playing on his instrument should generally be
allowed, as it innocently employs both mind and body, and the indulgence or deprivation may make a part of a system of rewards
and punishments.

ARTICLE III.

*Of the moral discipline and personal control under which luna-
tics ought to be placed.*

It is a great error to suppose that lunatics are not susceptible of
moral discipline, or capable of being brought under the control of
motives similar to those which govern the actions of other persons.
It is very possible to subject them to such rule, and this constitutes
indeed a very important and essential part of the means of cure.

The influence of fear and physical force were formerly almost
the only means by which deranged persons were kept in control.
Of late years it has become the universal conviction of those who
understand the treatment of lunatics, that they ought to be managed
with the utmost kindness. The mildest methods have been found,
in point of fact, the most successful in their cure. An union of
firmness in determination with the greatest gentleness of manner is
the sure way of gaining the respect and promoting the welfare, and,
in curable cases, the recovery of lunatics. " Nothing is better
established," says M. Pinel, " than the powerful influence which
the superintendent of a lunatic hospital exercises, when he sustains
in his office the sentiment of his dignity and the principles of a

* Guislain, i. p. 274.

pure and enlightened philanthropy. I may cite, for proofs of this position, Willis, Fowler, Haslam in England ; Dicquemare, Pontion, Pussin in France ; and in Holland the steward of the lunatic house in Amsterdam."* "Ignorant persons," he continues, "perceive only motives of provocation in the cries, the outrageous expressions, and violent actions of maniacs. Hence the extreme harshness, the blows, and brutal treatment which the attendants have allowed themselves to use, unless when they have been persons well chosen, and restrained by severe discipline. A sensible and enlightened superintendent, on the contrary, views these explosions of madness as the impulses of an automaton, or rather as the necessary effects of nervous excitement, by which he ought no more to be provoked than by the shock of a stone falling by its own specific gravity. He allows to lunatics all the liberty that is reconcilable with their own safety and that of others, conceals from them the means of constraint which he is obliged to employ, and treating them with indulgence, leads them to suppose that they are only submitting to the laws of necessity. At the same time their inconsiderate entreaties must be resisted by strength or eluded with address. The time during which the violent exacerbations of mania continue is thus passed over amidst well directed measures for mitigation, while the intervals of calmness are made use of, to render by degrees these accessions less severe and of shorter duration.†

It is an important observation of M. Guislain's, that the physician ought as much as possible to abstain from inspiring fear or dread of himself in the lunatic, by which he would become the object of aversion and lose the confidence of his patient. Another person should appear to be the agent in all restraints or punishments that may be required, and the physician should be regarded as the protector of his patients, and the dispenser of kindnesses and indulgences.‡

M. Georget,§ who has condensed, in an admirable manner, the discursive observations of MM. Pinel and Esquirol, has remarked that "an active and incessant inspection must be exercised in every lunatic asylum over both patients and attendants. Patients who evince a disposition to suicide should never be lost sight of for a single instant, whatever they may say or do to obtain their wish.

* "A lunatic," says M. Pinel, "in the vigour of his age and of great strength, who had been seized by his family, tied, and brought bound in a carriage, so terrified the persons that conducted him, that no one dared approach to untie him and conduct him to his cell ; the steward sent all the keepers away, talked some time with the invalid, and gained his confidence. After being unbound, the latter permitted himself to be conducted quietly to the new abode which had been prepared for him. The steward gained every day more influence over the patient's mind, became his confidant, and succeeded in restoring him to reason, and to the bosom of his family, of which he constitutes the chief happiness."

† Traité Medico-Philosophique sur l'Aliénation Mentale, par Ph. Pinel, Médécin Consultant de sa Maj. l'Empéreur et Roi, &c. 2d édition. Paris, 1809, p. 264.

‡ Guislain, ouvr. cité, tom. i. p. 328.   § Dict. de Médecine, art. Folie.

It is often necessary to confine violent patients with the strait-waistcoat. Those who are addicted to indecent practices,—a circumstance by no means unfrequent,—should be restrained by similar means. Occasionally it is better to confine them by straps round the legs, fastened down in an arm-chair, or shut up in their rooms, according to circumstances. The use of chains is almost entirely abandoned, and we are indebted to the noble efforts of our venerable Pinel for this improvement in the condition of lunatics." It may be observed that M. Foville ascribes to the Quakers who have managed the Retreat the credit of having been the first to discard these inhuman instruments of restraint.* " At the time of the abolition of chains at Bicêtre, M. Pinel observed that the diminution of the number of furious lunatics, and the accidents which they suffered, was very remarkable. The only measures of punishment that ought to be put into practice are the strait-waistcoat, seclusion in a cell, removed from one division to another, the shower-bath, and some occasional privations. A violent or wicked lunatic, who all at once puts on a menacing appearance, or even commits reprehensible actions, should be immediately surrounded by a number of attendants, approached and seized at the same time on all sides, particularly by those who are behind him. Sometimes great advantage has been obtained by suddenly enveloping the patient's head in a napkin, which completely bewilders him. In other cases, while persons placed before the patient endeavour to occupy his attention, others advancing from behind easily lay hold of and secure him.†

All means of punishment or of intimidation should be used as sparingly as possible, and be of the most harmless kind. Solitary confinement with restriction in the strait waistcoat is sufficient in ordinary cases. M. Foville makes great use of cold shower-baths in the hospital of St. Yon, where I have seen this method put in practice with great address and management. A violent maniac is seized at once by a number of strong men, who fasten his limbs instantaneously, and place him in a tub, which is covered with a lid, having an aperture large enough for the head and neck to be protruded. In this he is placed recumbent, and a man standing over him pours out pitchers of cold water, which are supplied by a bystander successively, till the lunatic, however boisterous and violent, becomes completely subdued ; the water which falls from the pitchers passes through holes in the cover of the tub and flows over the patient's body. Refrigeration thus produced is a powerful sedative. M. Foville employs it occasionally several times in a day, and he assured me that he has found it a most efficacious and at the same time safe and easy way of subduing the violence of the most intractable patients.

The use of the circular swing has been found very serviceable with a similar view, and after it has been once used, a threat of repetition is frequently sufficient.

* Foville, art. Folie, Dict. Pratique de Méd. et de Chirurg.
† Georget, Dict. de Médecine.—Pinel, ouvr. cité, p. 208.

Intimidation is sometimes necessary in order to induce obstinate lunatics to take food. Persuasion should be first tried, and if this fails, threats and harmless punishments should be adopted. It is never impossible, even by force, to oblige patients to swallow a sufficient quantity of nutritive broths or other fluids for the support of life. When compulsion has been used but a few times, voluntary submission generally follows.*

ARTICLE IV.

Of the treatment of the understanding of lunatics, in relation to their illusions or the morbid impressions on their minds.

It is a general rule, long since established as a maxim among physicians who have made insanity their particular study, not to direct the attention of patients to the subjects on which their illusions turn, or to oppose their unreasonable prejudices by argument, discussion, or contradiction, in order to bring them to a correct way of thinking. Such attempts are found to be worse than vain and useless; they irritate the temper of the deranged person, whom it is impossible, under ordinary circumstances, to convince by the most evident proofs. I have mentioned the case of a female lunatic, who declared that her husband was dead, and who, though assured that she was mistaken, refused to believe, and was not convinced of her error when he came to visit her. She then averred that the devil had assumed his form in order to deceive her. There are some cases on record in which a striking and palpable proof, suddenly and unexpectedly displayed, has succeeded in dispelling the illusions of insane persons ; but they are rare, and form exceptions to a very general and almost universal rule.

Other and more numerous instances are likewise related, in which monomaniacs, and chiefly persons originally labouring under hypochondriasis, have been cured of their mental delusion, and, as it would appear, eventually of their entire disease, by some deception founded upon the strength of their illusory opinion or hallucination. I shall recite a few of these examples, which may sometimes afford useful suggestions.

A lunatic refused to eat, assuring his friends that he was dead. To the most earnest entreaties he only replied that " dead people never eat." After every other method had been tried, he was left for a time alone, when persons entered his room, dressed in white shrouds, and after talking in his presence, to persuade him that they were dead men or ghosts, sat down to table and began to eat. When his curiosity was excited by this strange scene, they invited him, as one belonging to their own state of existence, to partake of their repast. At first he expressed astonishment, but at length took his seat among them ; and after eating voraciously fell asleep, and on waking became convinced that he was alive and well.

* Mr. Liddell strongly recommends the use of a stomach-pump, which he says that he has employed with good effects. See Liddell's translation of Esquirol on the Illusions of the Insane, &c. London, 1833.

A celebrated story is that related by M. Esquirol, of a lunatic who fancied that he could not let his urine pass without subjecting the world to the risk of being drowned by a second deluge. He was at length prevailed upon by being told that the town was on fire, and that he could thus save it from being destroyed by flames.*

Gatianar is said to have cured a patient who fancied she had frogs in her stomach, by giving her a purgative and introducing by stealth little frogs into the pan that received the alvine evacuations.† A similar case occurred to Ambrose Paré.‡

Dr. Muller of Wurtzburg cured a man who fancied that he had a demon or goblin in his belly, by the following contrivance. He covered the abdomen with a large blister, and at the moment when the vesicated skin was torn off, contrived that a puppet or figure dressed up should be thrown out of the bed. The man fancied himself delivered of his tormentor. Dr. Jacobi imitated this experiment, but only with temporary success.§

Dr. Franck cured a woman who fancied her bones were luminous and ready to take fire, by rubbing her skin with oil containing phosphorus, and pretending to extract the light.

I have seen many cases not unlike some of the above-mentioned as to the character of the illusion or hallucination, but have not had an opportunity of making similar experiments, which, however, I shall certainly attempt whenever it may be in my power, though without sanguine hopes of success.

With the exception of such singular cases, it appears to be the uniform result of experience that monomaniacs are injured by all attempts to advert or in any way to direct their attention to the subject on which their illusions turn. It is always better to draw them out from themselves, and to engage them as much as possible on external objects, and to excite interest in connexion with things remote from the morbid trains of thought.

ARTICLE V.

On the arrangement and management of lunatic asylums.

MM. Pinel, Esquirol, and Guislain have discussed at great length the various subjects connected with the arrangements and management of lunatic asylums. As it is my design to present my readers with a short and compendious treatise rather than to compile a large and voluminous work, I shall beg to refer those who wish for extensive and particular information on the construction and the mode of conducting these establishments to the authors abovementioned, and on the present occasion I shall merely translate the abstract which M. Georget has given us from the extensive disquisitions of Pinel and Esquirol.

"1. M. Pinel has particularly insisted upon the necessity of

---

* Esquirol, Dict. de Sc. Méd.
† Franck, Prax. Med. Guislain, i. p. 286.
‡ Esquirol on Illusions of the Insane.
§ Jacobi's Sammlungen für die heilkunde der gemüthskrankheiten, bd. i.

classing lunatics, of separating such as are liable to injure themselves or others, and permitting those to associate together who may contribute to each other's cure. A lunatic asylum ought to be composed of several parts more or less insulated. There should be a quarter appropriated to each sex, a division for violent lunatics, a second for those that are tranquil, a third for convalescents, a fourth for lunatics who labour under accidental disorders. It will be very useful to have a division for those who are of melancholy habits, and in a state of dementia, and another for furious and noisy patients, and for some lunatics who are of an untameable character, and are confined by way of punishment. It is above all things necessary to separate the sexes, the convalescents, and likewise those patients who have depraved habits and indecent manners. Each division ought to have a court planted with trees, and, if possible, a garden for the patients to walk in.

" 2. M. Esquirol, who has devoted his attention to the arrangements which these establishments require for the convenience of the patients, to facilitate vigilant superintendence and protection, and to prevent accidents, is of opinion that such houses should be built on level ground ; that the cells destined for violent patients should be spacious, with a door and window opposite each other, and opening from without : that they should be boarded and not paved, furnished with a bed firmly fixed in the wall ; that all the cells should communicate with covered galleries or corridors, in which the patients may walk in bad weather, and by means of which the inspectors and servants may easily traverse the different parts of the establishment ; that all the rooms should be warmed by pipes of hot air ; that abundance of water should be furnished by fountains to wash the dirty cells ; that the privies should be separated in such a manner as to occasion no inconvenience to the patients ; that there should be places appointed for a general work-room, for a common dining-room, for baths and showerbaths. In the plan of M. Esquirol there are dormitories only for convalescents, melancholic patients, idiots, and individuals who are debilitated. For others little cells, with one bed are preferable in almost every case : during the day the patients can go out and associate with others, and in the night they do not require companions.

" 3. Beings deprived of reason, who fancy themselves rational, who incessantly desire and demand things that cannot be granted them, and who are nevertheless sensible to kind as well as to bad treatment, must needs be difficult to influence, to govern, and to cure. As long as each person continues insane, he looks upon the director and inspectors of the establishment as accomplices in the power which has deprived him of liberty, and upon the attendants as inhuman jailors. Even after his cure he is not always very grateful. The director, the inspectors, and the attendants will invariably be objects of prejudice, suspicion, and hatred to the patients ; they will receive abuse and often blows from them. On the other hand, it is impossible for one who has not had for a

long time the care of them, and studied their disease, to know the
mental disposition of lunatics. Without such preparation we
should attribute to wickedness what is the effect of disease, or look
upon lunatics as beings deprived of all sensibility. In either case
we might be induced to treat them with severity. It is almost
impossible to make servants understand that mad persons have the
use of some of their faculties, with the exception of those servants
who have been themselves attacked by the disease. At the Salpêtrière and at Bicêtre great advantage is derived from employing
persons who have been cured to take care of the patients. The
physician of a lunatic asylum ought to be particularly careful to
instruct the individuals who are to have the management of the
patients."

"4. It is absolutely necessary that a judicious arrangement of
authority and subordination be established in lunatic asylums, and
that the physician be invested with a power superior to all with
regard to every thing that concerns the patients."

CHAPTER VIII.

OF PUERPERAL MADNESS.

SECTION I.—*Description and general Account of the Disease.*

PUERPERAL madness is a form of mental derangement incident
to women soon after childbirth. This is the proper sense of the
term, but by some writers it has been extended in its meaning, and
made to include cases which occur both before and after the puerperal period. Symptoms of insanity occasionally display themselves during pregnancy, and under circumstances which indicate
that they are dependent on that state. These cases are rare in
comparison with those which occur after delivery. M. Esquirol
mentions the instance of a young woman of very sensitive habit
who had attacks of madness on two occasions, each of which lasted
fifteen days, having commenced immediately after conception.
The same writer observes also that several women at the Salpêtrière
have become maniacal during the time of their pregnancy. Many
females likewise become deranged during the advanced period of
lactation, especially those of irritable temperament, and such as
attempt to suckle their children too long in reference to the strength
of their constitutions.

Cases of puerperal madness properly so termed, that is, coming
on after childbirth, are by no means infrequent. M. Esquirol has
related that among 600 maniacal women at the Salpêtrière, there
were 52 cases of this description. In another report by the same
writer, there were 92 similar cases among 1119 insane females
admitted during four years into the above-mentioned hospital. M.

Esquirol is of opinion that the proportion is still greater in the higher classes of society, since out of 144 instances of mental disorder occurring in females of opulent families, the symptoms had displayed themselves, in 21, either soon after childbirth or during the period of lactation. Dr. Haslam enumerates 84 instances of puerperal mania in 1644 cases admitted at Bethlem. Dr. Rush, however, reckons only five such cases in seventy received into the hospital for lunatics in Philadelphia.

There is no peculiarity in the phenomena of puerperal madness by which this disease is distinguished from other examples of insanity. Dr. Gooch has remarked that " if a physician was taken into the chamber of a patient whose mind had become deranged from lying-in or nursing, he could not tell by the mere condition of the mind that the disease had originated in these causes."

Those cases which are more properly termed puerperal, as occurring in the first period after childbirth, are generally of the character of mania, attended with excitement of the feelings and mental illusions ; while the disorder which displays itself in women exhausted by suckling is most commonly connected with melancholy depression, a tendency to which may generally be perceived in females who nurse their children too long with reference to the strength of their own constitutions. Cases of the former description occur within a short period, and most frequently within a fortnight after delivery. They appear sometimes to be occasioned by fright or other accidental causes of disturbance ; sometimes by error in diet, or by premature exertions or excitements : in other instances they take place independently of any discoverable external cause. The patient passes one or two restless nights, appears unusually excited and irritable, talks loudly and incessantly, and very soon betrays a disturbed intellect. The attack is often attended with febrile symptoms. This is the case especially, as Dr. Burrows has observed, if it takes place about the fourth or fifth day, when the secretion of milk is producing a new excitement. The state of the pulse is the most important symptom in reference to the nature and treatment of the case, as well as to the prognostic which is to be formed of its result. Dr. Gooch has laid particular stress on this circumstance, and he has extracted a valuable passage which bears upon it from the manuscript lectures of Dr. Hunter. " Mania," said this eminent practitioner, " is not an uncommon appearance in the course of the month, but of that species from which we generally recover. *When out of their senses, attended with fever, like paraphrenitis, they will in all probability die ;* but when without fever it is not fatal, though it (i. e. fever) generally takes place before they get well. I have had several private patients, and have been called in when a great number of stimulating medicines and blisters have been administered, but they have gone on as at another time, talking nonsense, till the disease has gone off, and they have become sensible. It is a species of madness they generally recover from, but I know of nothing of any singular service in it."

Dr. Gooch's comment upon this passage is the remark, supported by his own observation, that there are two forms of puerperal mania : one of them is attended by fever, or rather by a rapid pulse ; the other is accompanied by a very moderate disturbance of the circulation. Cases of the latter kind, which happily are by far the most numerous, terminate in recovery ; the former are generally fatal.

Section II.—*Terminations of Puerperal Madness.*

Puerperal madness terminates, in a great proportion of cases, either in death or in the recovery of reason. Few instances, comparatively, become cases of permanent insanity. It is, however, very difficult to obtain accurate information on this subject. Dr. Gooch has observed that the records of hospitals contain chiefly accounts of cases which have been admitted because they had been unusually permanent, having already disappointed the hope, which is generally entertained and acted upon, of relief by private care : the cases of short duration, which last only a few days or weeks, and which form a large proportion, are totally overlooked or omitted in the inspection of hospital reports. This remark accounts for the unfavourable nature of the results which are obtained from such tables as those given by M. Esquirol and others. By this writer ninety-two cases are enumerated, of which fifty-five recovered, and six died, leaving thirty-one as the number of incurables, that is, one in three. Of the fifty-five recoveries, thirty-eight took place within the first six months. Of eighty-five cases admitted at Bethlem, under Dr. Haslam, only fifty recovered, leaving thirty-five as the number of incurables. Dr. Burrows mentions fifty-seven cases, of which thirty-five recovered, and eleven remained uncured ; of the recoveries, twenty-eight took place within the first six months. These tables, as Dr. Gooch observes, throw but little light upon the real proportions of recoveries, and present a prospect unnecessarily gloomy and discouraging. He adds, " Of the many patients about whom I have been consulted, I know only two who are now, after many years, disordered in mind, and of them one had already been so before her marriage."

The question, on the solution of which there is the greatest reason for anxiety in reference to any particular case of puerperal madness, is, whether it is likely to be fatal, because, if not fatal, there is great probability of ultimate recovery. The most satisfactory way of coming to a conclusion on this inquiry in any individual case, is by the prognostications which the particular symptoms afford, and on this subject I can add little to what has already been said. The principal danger which menaces life in cases of this description arises from extreme debility ; the excitement of the vascular as well as of the cerebral functions is so great as to wear out the strength, already at a low ebb, and neither recruited by nutrition nor by sleep, and the patient sinks from exhaustion. Experience has proved that a rapid circulation is the principal circumstance which tends to bring on this state. A very frequent pulse is the most unfavourable symptom. Long-continued resistance to sleep, and a state of complete restlessness, and the appearance of great weakness and inanition, give likewise reason for apprehension. If these signs are not found, the mental derangement of the patient need not give occasion to very serious alarm.

Medical authors have sought to found a prognostic in puerperal madness on the estimate of the proportions which deaths bear to recoveries. This cannot afford evidence on which so much reliance may be placed as on the symptoms of individual cases. Out of the ninety-two cases mentioned by M. Esquirol, of which fifty-five terminated in recovery, there was, as I have observed, six deaths, and in Dr. Burrows's table of fifty-seven cases there were ten deaths. The former calculation gives one death in fifteen cases, and the latter one in six. But the patients in the Salpêtrière are probably removed thither after the period in which the disease is most dangerous to life. There must have been some circumstances tending to explain the discrepancy in the above-mentioned results. The proportion of deaths given by M. Esquirol's table is probably somewhat too low, but the result afforded by that of Dr. Burrows gives perhaps a greater mortality than the average number afforded by general experience.

SECTION III.—*Causes and Pathology of Puerperal Madness.*

The inquiry into the causes of puerperal madness comes within a narrow compass. The principal question which suggests itself in relation to this subject is, whether the disease is the result of delivery, or arises, according to common opinion, from the irritation accompanying the flow of milk.

Sauvages and other writers have recognized two different forms of mental derangement incident to lying-in women. One of them has been termed "*paraphrosyne puerperarum,*" and is observed to succeed labour, immediately or within a day or two, before the secretion of milk can disturb the system, and independently of any lochial suppression. " These attacks," says Dr. Burrows, who assents to the above distinction of varieties in the disease, " will sometimes go off under the operation of a smart purge and an opiate, and may then be considered as merely accessions of delirium : in other instances they are more permanent, and become fully developed instances of puerperal insanity. Sauvages second species is termed ' *mania lactea;*' and Dr. Burrows is of opinion that maniacal symptoms in reality make their appearance most frequently about the third or fourth day after childbirth, which tends to confirm the notion that they are connected with the lacteal secretion. This writer, however, has very candidly referred to the evidence deducible from the tables published by M. Esquirol, although it is rather opposed to the opinion above stated. From these tables it appears

that in the years 1811, 1812, 1813, 1814, eleven hundred and nineteen insane women were admitted into the Salpêtrière, of whom
ninety-two laboured under puerperal madness : of these—
16 became delirious from the first to the fourth day.
21 from the fifth to the fifteenth day, which generally includes the
    termination of the lochia.
17 from the sixteenth to the sixtieth day.
19 from the sixtieth to the twelfth month of lactation.
19 after forced or voluntary weaning.
    The result seems to be, as Dr. Burrows allows, that the disease is
more frequently a consequence of delivery than of suckling.

    On the whole it appears evident that some cause more general in
its influence than any one particular process must be referred to, if
we would explain the frequent occurrence of madness in pregnant,
puerperal, and suckling females.

    The only attempt to explain the theory of puerperal madness
which deserves much consideration, is that which was suggested by
Dr. Ferriar.   I shall cite his opinion in his own expressions.

    " I am inclined to consider the puerperal mania as a case of con-
version.   During gestation, and after delivery, when the milk begins to flow, the balance of the circulation is so greatly disturbed
as to be liable to much disorder from the application of any exciting
cause.   If, therefore, cold affecting the head, violent noises, want
of sleep, or uneasy thoughts, distress a puerperal patient before the
determination of blood to the breasts is regularly made, the impetus
may be readily converted to the head, and produce either hysteria
or insanity, according to its force and the nature of the occasional
cause."

    That new determinations in the vascular system should ensue on
the removal of one so long subsisting as that to the uterus during
pregnancy, is in accordance with a well-ascertained principle in
pathology.   The natural and healthy determination under these
circumstances is to the lacteal glands, but owing to various causes,
either external or of predisposition, morbid determinations occasionally take place.   Some women become phthisical at a very
early period after childbirth, or rather the symptoms of phthisis
develope themselves at that time in a manifest form.   Other constitutional complaints are apt to arise at the same period, according to
the prevalent tendency of the habit.   When the brain is susceptible, it is likely to suffer in its turn, and become the seat of local
disorder, the manifestations of which are affections of the mind.
If we consider the frequent changes or disturbances occurring in the
balance of the circulation from the varying and quickly succeeding
processes which are carried on in the system during and soon after
the periods of pregnancy and childbirth, we shall be at no loss to
discover circumstances under which a susceptible constitution
is likely to suffer.   The conversions or successive changes in the
temporary local determinations of blood which the constitution
under such circumstances sustains and requires, appear sufficiently
to account for the morbid susceptibility of the brain.

The cases of mental disorder which occur in the later periods of lactation are, as it is evident from M. Esquirol's table, of two kinds. In one the disease supervenes on weaning, and probably has its origin in the subsidence of the lacteal secretion. There are other instances which appear to arise from the continued excitement and exhaustion of the system consequent on suckling. This state of exhaustion takes place at different periods in different constitutions. Some women can continue to give milk without injury for years, but by others morbid feelings are experienced in the space of a few months or even of as many weeks, and do not subside for some time after weaning. I have observed very numerous instances of melancholy dejection with symptoms of insanity more or less strongly marked, which have displayed themselves in the protracted period of nursing, and in females who were evidently suffering from exhaustion. In one case a lady, who on former occasions had complained of feelings termed nervous, and had been much indisposed when giving milk, was persuaded to continue suckling a child until the thirteenth or fourteenth month. She was then attacked by a maniacal disorder, which, though of a mild character, was very decided in its nature. Nearly a year passed before her mind was perfectly restored.

SECTION IV.—*Treatment of Puerperal Madness.*

If we consider that the greatest danger to be apprehended for patients labouring under puerperal madness arises from a state of extreme exhaustion, that many women die from this cause within a short interval from the commencement of the disease, and that, if they survive this period, the healthy state of the mind is in most instances restored, it will be evident that our chief endeavours must be directed to the present support of life. If we can maintain and restore the general health, and keep the natural functions in a state compatible with continued existence for a time, the disease of the animal system will in all probability subside. Antiphlogistic and particularly evacuant remedies must be used very sparingly and with great caution.

1. Bloodletting, as a general remedy for puerperal madness, is condemned by all practical writers on whose judgment much reliance ought to be placed. M. Esquirol is decidedly opposed to it. Dr. Gooch's observations on this subject contain the best exposition of the rules which ought to guide medical practitioners as to the use of the lancet in cases of puerperal madness. He says, " The result of my experience is, that in puerperal mania and melancholia, and also in those cases which more resemble delirium tremens, bloodletting is not only seldom or never necessary, but generally almost always pernicious. I do not say that cases never occur which require this remedy ; no man's experience extends to all the possibilities of disease, but I have never met with such cases, and I would lay down this rule for the employment of bloodletting—never to use it as a remedy for disorder in the mind, unless

that disorder is accompanied by symptoms of congestion or inflammation of the brain, such as would lead to its employment though
the mind was not disordered. Even here, however, great caution
is necessary ; local is safer than general bleeding. In one case
the head was hot, and the face red, and the pulse was said to have
become somewhat hard, yet a bleeding of eight ounces was followed
by extinction of the pulse within three hours, and death in less than
six. The only cases attended by a quick pulse which I have seen
recover were those in which no blood was taken. In the really
inflammatory diseases of the brain, bloodletting of course is essentially necessary, but these, I think, can never be mistaken for puerperal insanity ; they are febrile headachs, more or less acute. Pain
of the head with fever is a much better indication for bloodletting
than disorder of the mind without these symptoms."

2. In cases attended with much heat about the scalp, flushing of
the face, and strong pulsation of the temporal and carotid arteries,
it will be proper to shave the head and keep it cool by means of
cold lotions, or an oil-skin cap filled with ice or iced water, or by
evaporating lotions. If the symptoms above mentioned are very
acute, and the debility of the patient is not in an alarming degree, a
few leeches may be applied with advantage. Blisters to the occiput
or nape of the neck are often serviceable ; they are much recommended by practical writers. When the scalp is not hot, and the
tendency of the disease is rather to stupor than to a high degree of
excitement, blisters are usefully applied over the top of the head.

The lower extremities, which are often cold, should be frequently
immersed in hot water. Dr. Burrows recommends bathing the legs
and feet in a warm infusion of mustard or horse-radish. Heat should
be applied in the most convenient form, and the circulation in the
extremities promoted by other obvious means.

3. Purgatives and emetics are among the most useful remedies in
this disease. The alimentary canal is frequently in a disordered
state, the tongue furred, the breath fetid, the skin discoloured, the
evacuations dark and offensive. A few brisk purgative doses, calomel, followed by castor-oil or rhubarb and magnesia, should be given
in such cases. Emetics of ipecacuanha, with small doses of tartarized antimony, are very valuable remedies in this state of the alimentary canal. Dr. Gooch has remarked that they should be used with
caution when the face is pale, the skin cold, and the pulse quick and
weak ; and in general he prefers ipecacuanha to antimonials.

4. After these evacuant remedies have been premised, great advantage is frequently derived from the use of opiates. Full doses
are generally attended with the best success. Ten grains of Dover's
powders may be given at night, or a grain and a half of solid opium,
or thirty drops of the tincture. Several writers recommend Batt-
ley's solution of opium in preference to the tincture ; perhaps the
acetate and muriate of morphia are the best preparations of opium ;
they may be given in doses of a quarter or half of a grain, and repeated every third or fourth hour until sleep is procured. When
opiates disagree, Dr. Gooch recommends the use of hyosciamus,

mixed with camphor. He says that five grains of each should be
given every sixth hour, and a double dose at night : a dram of the
tincture will answer the same purpose. This writer is of opinion
that narcotics are the most valuable remedy in the cure of puerperal
mania ; he says that " they often produce nights of better sleep and
days of greater tranquillity, and this calmness is followed by some
clearing up of the disorder of the mind." He says that these remedies produce salutary effects much more frequently in the mania of
lying-in women than in maniacal disorders occurring under other
circumstances ; if, however, there is heat in the head, flushing in
the face, and thirst, their use ought to be postponed until such symptoms shall have been removed.

5. In the more protracted cases of puerperal madness, tonic and
stimulant medicines are sometimes requisite, especially when the
appetite has failed. Ammonia is much recommended. It may be
given with infusion of cinchona, or any bitter infusion. When it is
not offensive to the stomach, the rectified oil of turpentine is one of
the best stimulants, especially if it can be taken in the dose of a dram
three times in a day with cinnamon water, or any other aromatic fluid.

6. A rule of great importance refers to the *diet* of women in puerperal madness. It may, perhaps, be safely asserted that the greatest
risk which patients in this disease incur is that of being starved
through the mistaken notions of their attendants, who are too often
disposed to consider the excitement of maniacal disease a reason for
withholding food, when this very state, owing to the exhaustion
produced by its long continuance, renders it especially necessary
to support the strength more carefully. Farinaceous fluids of a nutritive quality, milk, rice, and other such matters should be given at
short intervals, when febrile symptoms preclude the use of animal
food. In most instances broth may be allowed and ought to be
given. In the more protracted periods solid meat, with malt liquors,
should be taken. I have seen very many maniacal patients labouring under great weakness and exhaustion, with cold extremities, a
clammy skin, passing sleepless nights, and under continual agitation,
begin to improve as soon as their diet was changed, and meat with
some ale or porter given daily. The pulse has become fuller and
less frequent, the extremities warm, sleep has been restored, and
convalescence has taken place in a surprisingly short period after
such a system has been adopted.

7. The last observation to be made refers to the *management* of
such patients. We must here advert to the remarks to be found in a
former chapter on the management and moral treatment of insane
patients in general. The general rules only require modification in
some particulars in relation to the peculiar circumstances of puerperal women. The latter for obvious reasons cannot be soon removed
from home. They require in other respects similar management.
They should be separated from relatives and friends, and carefully
attended by persons who are fitted for the occupation by habit. It
will not so often be necessary to send puerperal maniacs to lunatic
asylums as deranged persons of a different description.

CHAPTER IX.

OF IDIOTISM AND MENTAL DEFICIENCY.

SECTION I.—*General Description of Idiotism and Mental Deficiency.*

IDIOTISM is a state in which the mental faculties have been want-ing from birth, or have not been manifested at the period at which they are usually developed. Idiotism is an original defect, and is, by this circumstance, as well as by its phenomena, distinguished from that fatuity that results from disease or from protracted age : the latter, as we have seen, is dementia, or incoherence, and it is impor-tant that this affection should not be confounded with idiotism. The distinction was pointed out by M. Esquirol, and it has been gene-rally adopted. By the same writer, idiotism, or original deficiency of understanding, is likewise divided into two stages or degrees, viz. absolute idiotism, and the condition approaching to idiotism ; which last is denominated imbecility. Imbecility is a state in which the intellectual faculties are not wholly deficient, though manifested in a lower degree than according to the ordinary standard.

Idiotism, however, itself is not the same in all instances : it dif-fers in particular cases, and has a variety of forms. One of the most strongly marked of these is termed Cretinism, a species of idiotism connected with personal deformity, which is well known and fre-quent in the Valais and in some other parts of Switzerland. This disease has been described by many writers, and particularly by M. de Saussure and Professor Fodéré.* Cretinism discovers itself in very early infancy. Josias Simler, the historian of the Valais, who wrote in 1574, declares that in his time midwives were able to pro-nounce, from the appearance of a new-born infant, whether it would prove a cretin or not ; but this is denied by M. de Rambuteau, pre-fect of the department of the Simplon, who, in 1803, addressed a memoir on the subject of cretinism to the minister of the interior, from which M. Georget has published some very interesting ex-tracts. According to M. de Rambuteau, cretinism can very rarely be recognized in newly-born infants.

According to M. Fodéré, who has given a very able and, as it appears, an accurate account of the characteristic phenomena of this affection, " cretins often show in the earliest infancy what they are destined to become : they have sometimes in their first years in-cipient goitre, a puffed, swollen countenance ; their hands and head are large, and out of proportion to the rest of their bodies ; they evince insensibility to atmospheric impressions, an habitual state of stupor and sloth ; difficulty in sucking, as if through weakness of

---

* M. de Saussure, Voyages dans les Alpes. Genève, 1826.—Traité du Goitre et du Cretinisme, par F. E. Fodéré, ancien Médecin des Hôpitaux civils et militaires. Paris, an 8.

instinct connected even with the first wants ; very slow and very imperfect development of the faculty of articulating sounds ; often they are only capable of learning to pronounce vowels without consonants. As their bodies attain bulk, they even display more and more clumsy and stupid awkwardness in all their movements ; the same deficiency or absence of intelligence continues to the age of ten or twelve years, since little cretins of that age are unable to take food into their mouths and masticate it, so that it is even necessary to put their aliment down their throats. As they grow up, they still go with an awkward tottering gait, when they can be induced to move at all : they have never a cheerful countenance, are always stupidly obstinate, with a resisting, mutinous temper, which is only tolerated by maternal tenderness : they show a disproportioned smallness of the head in relation to the body ; their heads are flattened at the summit and at the temples, and the tuberosity of the occiput is less projecting than is natural ; their eyes are small, sometimes deeply sunk, at others prominent ; their look fixed and stupid ; their chests are flat ; their fingers thin and long, with small articulations ; the soles of their feet flat, and sometimes bent : their feet often turned inwards or outwards ; puberty comes very slowly, but with enormous size of the genital organs, obscene and inordinate propensities. It is not until this epoch that cretins generally walk about ; their locomotion is yet very limited, and only excited by the desire of getting their food or of warming themselves by the chimney-corner or in the rays of the sun. His litter is to the cretin the term of his longest and most fatiguing journies, and to it he comes tottering, with his arms hanging down and his body reeling about. In seeking his object, he goes forward, without shunning dangers or obstacles ; he can take no other road than that to which he is familiar. When he has attained his full stature, which is generally from thirteen to sixteen decimetres, the cretin's skin becomes brown, his sensibility continues obtuse; he is indifferent to cold, heat, or even to blows and wounds ; he is generally deaf and dumb ; the strongest and most revolting odours scarcely affect him. I have seen a cretin eat with avidity raw onions, or even charcoal, which proves that the organ of taste is gross or imperfect. Still more so are sight and touch, which are modes of discernment and intelligence, the powers of which must be very limited or very imperfect. The affections of cretins seem to be still more dull ; they have often no sort of gratitude for the good offices rendered to them ; they show scarcely any sensibility at the sight of their relations, and evince neither pain nor pleasure in respect to their physical wants. Such is," says Fodéré, " the physical and moral life of the cretins during a long career : for reduced to a sort of vegetation and automatic existence, they arrive without difficulty to an extreme old age."[*]

The observation that cretins attain old age is contradicted by

* Fodéré Traité, du Goitre, &c.—Pinel sur l'Aliénation Mentale.

other writers. Cretins in general die before they have attained
thirty years of age. The goitre and the other external deformities above described are not universal among them, though very
general.*

The causes of cretinism form a very interesting subject of inquiry,
but one as yet but little elucidated. The opinion that it arises from
the drinking of snow-water has been long abandoned. This notion
was refuted by M. de Saussure, who observed that cretinism is
peculiar to certain local situations : cretins are found only in deep
valleys and on the lower parts of mountains, and do not exist in
places of considerable elevation. The cause of cretinism is apparently some congenital defect of organization depending upon the
physical circumstances of families in which it is engendered, but
of what precise nature this may be it is as yet unknown. Some
very curious particulars, however, have been collected by M. Rambuteau. Cretinism seems to be nearly connected with the causes
which give rise to goitre or the bronchocele of mountaineers.
Wherever there are cretins, goitres are also found ; but goitres exist
in some places where there are no cretins. In approaching the
countries where cretinism exists, one meets first with a few goitres
only : these afterwards are found more frequently, and at length
cretins make their appearance. Women of the Valais are much
more apt to have cretin-children when married to Savoyards, who
are commonly drunken and debauched men, than those who marry
Frenchmen, or mountaineers from the higher Alpine country. The
latter are sober and active in their habits. Parents of healthy constitution and sound organization of body seldom have cretins in
their families. Stammering is common in the Valais ; and parents
who have this defect have more frequently cretin-children than
others. It is generally observed that if the first child in a family
is a cretin, those who are born subsequently partake of the same
infirmity. Cretinism seems, therefore, to be a congenital disease,
and to depend upon some defect in the race propagated in certain
situations in mountainous countries. Like other congenital peculiarities, it depends chiefly on causes which exert their immediate
influence principally on the parents. In these particulars it is
analogous to other forms of idiotism ; a defect which is observed to
be more frequent in mountainous than in other regions, owing likewise, as it may be presumed, to local influences.

The idiots of other countries, though not cretins, are deformed in
person, and have the external marks of imperfect organization. They
are often, as M. Esquirol remarks, scrofulous, or rachitic, or partially paralytic, or subject to epilepsy : their heads are either too
large or too small, ill-formed, flattened laterally, behind or before ;
their features are ill-shaped ; their chests narrow, contracted ; their
eyes are blinking and deeply set : they have thick lips, wide-gaping
mouths : their organs of sense are imperfect ; they see imperfectly,

* M. Georget, Dict. de Médecine.

are deaf or hard of hearing, dumb or drawling and lisping in their speech : their taste and smell are also imperfect, and they eat without selection of food. Their limbs are ill-formed, and their gait awkward and unsteady : their movements and attempts at muscular action of any kind are imperfect. Their reflective faculties are still more imperfect than their powers of sensation : they are incapable of directing their attention to anything. Though sensations take place through the organs of sight or hearing, they are scarcely followed by any perception of objects : they have scarcely any traces of memory, judgment, or imagination : their power of speech; if it exist at all, is extremely limited, and they are only capable of expressing the most urgent physical wants. Many idiots have even the instinctive faculties in a defective state, and appear to be far below the brutes in the scale of animal existence ; for brute animals have in perfection all those impulses to action which are necessary for their individual wellbeing and that of their tribe, and they are endowed by nature with powers adequate to the pursuit of the objects to which these impulses direct them. It is otherwise in both these respects with idiots, which, as the writer before cited has observed, are monsters or imperfect beings, who appear destined to a speedy extinction, if the tenderness of parents or the compassion of others did not interfere to prolong their existence. Yet idiots have the bodily appetites, sexual desires : they are likewise subject to anger and rage. Congenital idiots have large heads, imperfect features, with difficulty take the breast, and have a feeble physical life ; are long before their eyes follow the light, and they often squint. They are puny, lean, of bad complexion, incapable of instruction, do not learn to walk till six or seven years of age, or sometimes not till they attain the age of puberty : they articulate imperfectly, and learn but a few words. There are some idiots who display faint glimmerings of intelligence : their attention is sometimes excited by impressions made upon their senses : " they appear to look at certain objects with a sentiment of pleasure mixed with curiosity : they show appetency for certain objects, go to their food and take it : they come to know the persons who habitually take care of them : they indicate sometimes, by means of cries or gestures, the objects of their desires, and manifest the pleasure or pain which they experience : yet it is necessary to dress them, to put them in bed, and to place them where they are to remain."* Idiots of a higher grade of development are capable of moving themselves voluntarily from place to place. These individuals display very remarkable phenomena : they resemble, as M. Esquirol observes, machines made for the purpose of repeating ever the same movements, and habit takes with them the place of understanding : they move their arms in a particular way, as if to facilitate their progression, laugh mechanically, utter inarticulate sounds, as if to amuse themselves : some even are capable of catching tunes of a simple kind, which they repeat :

* M. Georget, art. *Idiotisme*, Dict. de Médecine.

they become attached to particular places, and grumble and appear
ill at ease if they cannot get access to them.

There is no exact line of demarcation between idiotism and a
degree of weakness which is generally termed imbecility ; they
pass by insensible shades into each other, as imbecility likewise approaches gradually to perfection of understanding ; there is no
possibility of saying where precisely one stage of mental deficiency
ends and the other begins, or where the latter ceases and sound understanding has its place. Imbecile persons are, according to the
distinction laid down by M. Georget, those who have some use,
though a limited one, of speech, who display some indications of
mind, of intellectual faculties, and of feelings or affections : these
individuals show the same varieties of character and inclination as
persons of stronger understanding : the senses of some give rise to
dull and feeble impressions, in others to more lively perceptions ;
the power of recollection is tolerably strong in some, in others
scarcely exists, or is confined in its range to the most ordinary and
frequently-repeated ideas. Some have a limited capability for particular actions ; a disposition and some degree of facility in certain
acts or performances, which they get through tolerably well, while
to other modes of exertion they are quite incompetent. " Custom
or habit has a great influence on all their proceedings, and this gives
to the manner of existence of some imbeciles an appearance of regularity which might be mistaken for the result of steadiness and per-
severance."*   All, however, are deficient in power of thought and
of attention. Left to themselves, they are careless, slothful, filthy,
lazy, timorous. At the age of puberty, they display the effects of
animal instinct in the most offensive gestures and habits. Some
become subject to fits of capricious violence, to hysteric attacks, to
nymphomania or satyriasis ; others grow dejected, melancholy, and
sink under a gradual decay of physical health.

In idiots and imbecile persons in general, the physical functions
are in a comparatively perfect state. They eat and digest food, and
females have the catamenia : they are, however, generally short-
lived, and anatomy sometimes displays, as M. Georget has observed,
great and unsuspected anomalies in the viscera of natural and vital
functions ; but these are by no means so constant as deformities in
the shape of the head and defects in the organization of the brain.

Some individuals, who yet come under the denomination of imbecile persons, display glimmerings of talent in particular pursuits.
Some are fond of music, and cultivate with success this aptitude.
An instance of this kind has fallen under my observation : a young
man, otherwise very weak, has a decided talent for music, and can
compose extempore in a way that has astonished many persons.
Some have even very retentive memories, learn languages, or are
capable of other particular acquirements, while in all other respects
they are defective in mental power. Many facts of this description

* Esquirol.

have been collected by Dr. Gall and his followers, as favourable to the doctrine of phrenology.

SECTION II.—*Causes of Idiotism and Imbecility.*

M. Georget has given a brief statement of the morbid appearances in the brain connected with idiotism. Faulty conformation of the head has already been mentioned : from it arises deficiency in the volume of the brain either general or partial. A similar conse- quence results from preternatural thickness of the cranium, which has sometimes been observed. Chronic hydrocephalus is not a fre- quent cause of idiotism. When the brain is small, the convolutions are less thick, less deep, and often less numerous ; particularly in the anterior lobes, when the forehead is flattened. Induration of the medullary substance of the hemispheres is not very rarely found it is generally partial. M. Esquirol has collected seven or eight cases of atrophy of one hemisphere in idiots who had been hem: plegical with atrophy of the paralyzed limbs. The diseased part was reduced by one-third ; the convolutions were attenuated, com- pressed, and some of them destroyed ; the cerebral substance was softened in some parts and hardened in the centre. This kind of disorganization extended through the brain of a deaf and dumb idiot. Some brains of idiots have been found free from disease, though contracted in volume.

Idiotism depends evidently upon congenital disease in most in- stances, but in others it is the result of maladies affecting the brain in very early infancy. It is often occasioned by severe fits of con- vulsion during the process of dentition, as are other manifestations of cerebral disease. Hemiplegia, for example, arises from the same cause. In other cases idiotism has been observed after the sudden disappearance of eruptive diseases of infants, particularly of those affecting the scalp, as of porrigo with extensive suppuration. In these instances inflammation from metastasis becomes the precursor of a change of structure in the brain. It is possible that in some cases such consequences might be averted by the early use of ap- propriate means.

There are different degrees and varieties of mental deficiency, which scarcely amount to what is termed either idiotism, or, in general language, imbecility. Persons so affected are commonly said to be weak in character, stupid, or of mean capacity. When the degree of intellectual weakness is just such as to render indi- viduals scarcely competent to manage business, or to conduct them- selves with propriety, it sometimes happens that legal inquiries are instituted into the state of their understandings and the soundness of their minds. It is in such cases that the want of a criterion of the presence or absence of mental deficiency is chiefly felt, as well as the difficulty of establishing any certain standard.

In a following chapter, on the legal considerations which are connected with unsoundness of mind, I shall take an opportunity of adverting to the attempts which have been made to supply this want.

CHAPTER X.

ON THE HISTORY OF MENTAL DISORDERS AS DEDUCED FROM STATISTICAL OBSERVATIONS.

SECTION I.—*General Remarks on the Opinion that Insanity is an increasing Disease.—Statistics of Insanity in Britain.— Concluding Observations.*

SEVERAL extensive inquiries are comprehended under the title prefixed to this chapter, such as those which relate to the proportion of lunatics to the general population of different countries, the increase or diminution of their relative numbers, their condition, and that of the classes in the community to which they belong. These particulars, and other subjects connected with them, would furnish by themselves matter for a voluminous treatise. The limits of my work prevent me from entering at large into these investigations ; but I cannot pass them by altogether, because from them many general facts are developed which are essential to the history of mental disorders. I shall, therefore, take a brief survey of this subject, and shall refer my readers to the sources of more extensive information.

Two principal inquiries connected with this subject relate to the proportional frequency of mental disorders in different places and times. It is hence that we may expect to throw some light on the connexion of insanity with the circumstances of climate and local situation on the one hand, and, on the other, with the peculiar moral condition and the states of society.

A very general apprehension has existed both in this country and in France, that insanity has increased in prevalence of late years to an alarming extent, and that the number of lunatics, when compared with the population, is continually on the increase. Different opinions have been held on this subject by medical writers, and much discussion took place in reference to it before data existed that were calculated to furnish any secure groundwork for conclusions. The opinion that mental derangement is an increasing disease was maintained by Dr. Powell, secretary to the commissioners for licensing mad-houses, in a memoir published in the fourth volume of the Medical Transactions. The principal ground on which Dr. Powell argued was an increase of numbers apparent in the London Register of lunatics. This register contains an account of all lunatics confined in private asylums in England ; and in the numbers of these a great augmentation was apparent, as it was shown by a table containing the numbers in the eight quinquennial periods or lustra from 1775 to 1814, the aggregate number in the first lustrum being 1783, and that of the last 3647. But Dr. Burrows, who has examined this subject with attention, proved that the conclusion is by no means supported by the data ; for in the first place the Register has no account of the numbers of lunatics in public asylums, or of those who exist elsewhere, and not confined in licensed houses ; its contents may, therefore, vary according as it may be the custom to send patients either to public or private mad-houses, or to keep them at home or in unlicensed receptacles : and, secondly, the increase in Dr. Powell's table is not regular and progressive, but subject to such variations as plainly invalidate the inference drawn from it by the author, while the augmentations observed at particular times admit of a different explanation from that which he has adopted.

An opinion opposite to that of Dr. Powell has been maintained by other writers, as by Dr. Willan, and afterwards by Dr. Bateman, in their reports on the diseases of London, published in 1801 and 1819 ; and this side of the question had been taken by Dr. Heberden, in his Observations on the Increase and Decrease of Different Diseases. But to establish any general and satisfactory conclusions on the subject, more extensive data were evidently required than those of which the writers above mentioned could avail themselves.

The first attempt to estimate the proportional number of lunatics in England was made by Dr. Powell. The author had no other resources for his computation than a comparison of the number of lunatics entered on the register with the census of the population. By comparing the number registered in 1800 with the census of the same date, Dr. Powell deduced the conclusion that the proportion of lunatics in England is one to seven thousand three hundred persons, an estimate which only shows how vain it was to make such an attempt with means so inadequate.

The public attention was drawn to this subject, and to the necessity of obtaining further information, by the exertions of some active individuals ; and in 1806 a select committee of the House of Commons was appointed for the purpose. In the report of this committee we have the first attempt to obtain an official return of the number of insane poor in England. This return stated the number of lunatics and idiots in England and Wales to be only 2248. The numbers were more than double by returns which were called for by a new committee in 1815 ; but this augmentation appears referable to the incompleteness of the former account rather than to an increase in the number of lunatics. Even the last-mentioned returns were found to be very unsatisfactory, and much larger numbers have been obtained, as we shall observe, on later occasions.

Dr. Burrows pursued the inquiry into the statistics of insanity, availing himself of the returns made to the House of Commons in 1819, which he corrected by inserting the numbers contained in St. Luke's and some other hospitals. He found the aggregate number of lunatics confined in public asylums, hospitals, and gaols at the above date to be 1456, and that of individuals resident in private asylums 2585, making a total for all England and Wales of 4041. To this ascertained number the author added conjecturally, for the number not included in the return, that is, for those existing at large or in private receptacles not registered, one half of the num-

ber ascertained. He thus increased the aggregate number to 6,000,
which he regarded as the nearest approximation that could be made
to the total number of lunatics in Great Britain, and which gives,
on a probable estimate of the population at the time, one lunatic to
2000 people.

We have the results of later and more extensive researches in
two works published by Sir Andrew Halliday in 1828 and 1829.
In the first of these the author proved, by a calculation founded on
the returns printed in 1826, that the number of lunatics in South
Britain was at that time considerably above Dr. Burrows's estimate.
The number of lunatics stated to be in confinement in the different
private and public asylums, as well as in gaols, in England and
Wales, amounted, in 1826, according to the data obtained by Sir
Andrew Halliday, to 4782.

" But there is a number," says the same writer, " if not equally
great, at least nearly so, of whom the law takes no cognizance, and
whose existence is only known to their relatives and friends. These
consist of individuals placed in solitary confinement with persons
who only take one patient. I have been persevering and strict in
my inquiries ; I have laboured unceasingly now for twenty-five years,
and I give it as the result of the information I have obtained, that
the aggregate number of persons actually in confinement in public
and private asylums, and with their relatives, or with individual
keepers, in England and Wales, exceeds 8000." " Yet great," he
adds, " as this number may appear, and I am aware that it greatly
exceeds the average given by some late writers on the subject, I do
not think that the disease has increased among us ; and I have good
authority for what I say on this point, from the returns I have collected at various periods during the last quarter of a century."*

The same writer has added a computation of the number of lunatics in Scotland, deduced from parliamentary returns and other public documents. From these it appeared, as he says, that the public
and private asylums of that country, in 1826, contained 648 individuals, and the public gaols 10, a collective number bearing a small
proportion to the aggregate of insane persons in the kingdom. "On
this point," he adds, " I can speak with absolute certainty, for there
are now on my table distinct returns from 800 of the 900 parishes
into which Scotland is divided, all carefully made up and signed by
the respectable clergyman of each parish. From these it appears
that there are about 3700 insane persons and idiots in this kingdom.
Of these 146 are in private asylums, 50 in the public asylum, and
about 60 in Bedlam, in the county of Edinburgh, and 387 in other
public asylums and workhouses ; 1192 are confined with private
individuals, principally with small farmers and cottagers, and 21 are
in gaols ; making the number of persons actually in a state of con-

* General View of the state of Lunatics and of Lunatic Asylums in Great Britain and Ireland, and in some other Kingdoms, by Sir A. Halliday, M. D. & K. H.
London, 1828. p. 15–16.

finement 1861 ; while upwards of 1600 are allowed to be at large, most of them wandering over the country and subsisting by begging."*

Returns of the numbers of persons in confinement in lunatic asylums in Ireland were likewise made up for the same year ; in these the aggregate amounts nearly to 1600. This number, according to Sir A. Halliday, bears a small proportion to the actual number of insane persons and idiots in Ireland. We have no certain data, says the same writer, from which we can calculate what that number is ; but I do not exaggerate when I state it at 3000.

In the year 1829, Sir A. Halliday published further researches in the same subject, in which he was induced to estimate the total numbers of deranged persons in England and Wales considerably above his former computation. After going through a careful examination of all the English counties separately, he states the total number of lunatics at 6806, and that of idiots at 5741, being altogether 12,547 insane persons ascertained, beyond all doubt, as existing in England.† This, however, is by no means the whole number. Considering the towns which are counties in themselves, and the great number of parishes in some counties which had made no returns when the reports were made up, which are the basis of this calculation, we shall have, as Sir A. Halliday says, on the most moderate estimate, to add about 1500 to the number above stated, which will make the whole number of insane persons in England above 14,000.

From a summary of the insane population of different counties in Wales, we have 153 lunatics and 763 idiots, collectively 896 deranged persons ascertained to exist in the principality. From the facts that so great a proportion of these are idiots, and that very few are in any place of refuge, and that many parishes have made no returns, it is very reasonably supposed that the true amount may be fairly estimated above 1000 persons.

To the numbers actually ascertained, by adding 155, the number of lunatics in the Naval Asylum at Haslar, and 122 in the Military Asylum at Chatham, the aggregate number of 15,720 will be afforded. Having thus ascertained that very nearly 14,000 insane persons exist in South Britain, Sir A. Halliday concludes that it will be no exaggerated estimate to state the numbers not returned at 2500, which will give 16,500 as the entire number of deranged persons in the whole of South Britain.

The same writer estimates the proportional numbers of lunatics to the entire population in different parts of Britain, separately, as follows.

The population of England in 1821 was 11,261,437 persons. In ten years an increase of nearly two millions had taken place beyond

* General View, p. 28.
† A Letter to Lord Robert Seymour, with a Report of the Number of Lunatics and Idiots in England and Wales, by Sir Andrew Halliday, K. H. & M. D. London, Underwood, 1829.

the number existing before that interval ; it is, therefore, fair to allow one million and a half for the increase of the population of England since the last census, that is, from 1821 to 1829, and this will make the number of people in England at the latter period amount to nearly 12,700,000, and the proportion of insane persons to the entire population about 1 in every 1000. This refers to ascertained numbers, and is obviously below the reality.

On a similar principle, the population of Wales is estimated at 817,438 in 1829 ; and as the ascertained number of insane persons amounted then to 896, and the returns are known to be very incomplete, the proportion of the deranged to the entire population of Wales is calculated by Sir A. Halliday at 1 to 800.

Sir A. Halliday states the number of insane in Scotland as ascertained at 5652, which, as he says, gives 1 to 574 of the population.

Some curious facts develope themselves in regard to the comparative frequency of madness and idiotism in different ranks of the community. Of the 14,000 insane calculated to exist in England, or of the 12,547 ascertained, not fewer than 11,000 are paupers, maintained principally at the expense of parishes. A most remarkable difference is found in the proportional number of lunatics in agricultural and in manufacturing districts. Previous to inquiry, we should conjecture that the causes of insanity would have more influence, and the disease be more prevalent, in a manufacturing than in an agricultural population ; but the contrary is the fact. Thus, in twelve counties in England, of which the inhabitants are chiefly employed in agriculture, the entire population being 2,012,979, the insane amount to 2526, giving about 1 lunatic to 820 ; while in twelve counties where the majority of the inhabitants are otherwise employed, including Cornwall, where a great number are miners, the entire population being 4,493,194, the insane amount to 3910, or nearly as 1 to 1200. In Scotland and in most of the Welsh counties the population is chiefly agricultural, and this may, perhaps, account for the greater proportion of lunatics in the population of those parts of the island. In Scotland and Wales, it appears that a great proportion of the insane, or of those included under that denomination, are idiots. In six of the maritime counties of England, the proportion of idiots to lunatics is nearly as 2 to 1 ; and this is likewise the case in the Scottish counties of Inverness and Nairn, Argyll and Bute, and Moray ; but in the six counties of North Wales there are about 7 idiots to 1 lunatic.

A survey of the statements which I have collected suggests two remarks, which place the subject of mental derangement in its relation to the community in a particular point of view. In the first place, it may be observed that this affliction appears to fall in a great proportion upon the lowest classes of society, since, in England, eleven out of fourteen thousand lunatics and idiots are stated to be paupers. Hence it appears that mental derangement must be looked upon not merely as an individual calamity, but as a serious public burden, for such must be the permanent maintenance of

11,000 paupers in a state requiring more than ordinary care and expense. It may be remarked, secondly, that mental derangement, considered generally, or with respect to the great aggregate number of cases, may be looked upon rather as a congenital imperfection than as a disease resulting from external impressions. This appears in part from the large proportion of idiots comprehended in the collective number. Idiots are not so numerous in England as lunatics, but their number is not greatly inferior, the statements published by Sir A. Halliday giving 5741 of the former, and 6806 of the latter. In Wales, as we have seen, idiots are to lunatics almost as 7 to 1 ; and in Scotland they are very numerous. The morbid state of lunatics cannot properly be said to be innate, but the predisposition is original and in-bred in the constitution. In those cases in which it has not been inherited, it is an individual peculiarity of organization, which is ready to become hereditary in the next generation. The relation which cases of insanity bear to those of idiotism, the proportional numbers varying under particular circumstances, indicate some analogy in their nature. On the whole it would appear that both idiots and lunatics are persons born with a defective structure of brain, though manifested in different ways. These defects are generally prevalent in various degrees in different parts of the island, and in different classes or castes in the community. The numbers of both are such as to render them important to the public when viewed in connexion with their remarkable prevalence among the lower orders.

In adverting to the inquiry, whether any means could be adopted that would tend to diminish the extent of this evil, we are struck by the obvious consideration that the numbers of deranged persons in the community might be very much lessened if it were possible to regulate or establish any surveillance over the marriages of the lower orders, or if some measures could be adopted to prevent the propagation of idiotism and an hereditary tendency to madness. Idiots who are at large wander about the country, and the females often bear children. I have frequently seen, in Herefordshire, a female dumb idiot, who was said to have borne several children by unknown fathers. Sir Andrew Halliday has made similar observations. We should hear without surprise of the permission of such things in Turkey or Kafferland, but in a country having police regulations it would not be expected. All pauper idiots and lunatics ought to be kept in proper asylums, where every possible alleviation of their calamitous lot should be afforded them, and the public should thus be protected against such evils as those just pointed out. But, perhaps, the propagation of mental disorders might be prevented. in other ways by some restrictions on marriages. Intermarriages between near relations should be prohibited, and the known prevalence of idiotism or madness in a family should be made, if possible, what at present it is not, at least among the lower classes, a bar to its propagation.

The fact that insanity prevails so much in agricultural countries indicates that its development is favoured by some of the circumstances connected with the condition of agriculturists. The labouring of women in the field during pregnancy is, perhaps, as Halliday suggests, one cause. Hard labour and low diet, to which males may be subjected, may, perhaps, have an influence on the offspring propagated by them ; and in Wales and Scotland particularly this may enter into the number of causes which render idiotism so prevalent.

The congenital nature of these diseases, when considered on an extensive scale, renders it, perhaps, less probable than the notions generally entertained would persuade us, that any great increase in the prevalence of mental derangement, beyond an average proportion to the population, has taken place of late years. It is not easy to conceive that ordinary causes of temporary influence can materially affect the frequency of any congenital predisposition. But although congenital predisposition is so important a circumstance, still it does not include the whole of the productive agencies, and temporary changes in the prevalence of the exciting causes may doubtless affect the frequency of insanity at particular times, though the whole influence of such causes is very much overrated when they come to be regarded as the principal foundation of the disease. It is still a matter of great interest to determine whether the proportion of lunatics to the population is actually on the increase. Notwithstanding all that has been written on this subject, I believe that we yet want sufficient means of arriving, on this question, at any positive result, owing to the still remaining doubt as to the completeness of our latest estimates of the number of lunatics. It is exceedingly improbable that Scotland contains proportionally nearly twice as many deranged persons as England. Can the difference be ascribed to the greater accuracy of the returns from Scotland ? This opinion will, perhaps, be thought the most probable one, if the remarks formerly suggested by Mr. Tuke's statements are well considered. But although our information is yet imperfect, there is no reason, in the nature of things, why it should so remain. If the proper care and attention were devoted to the subject, all the questions connected with this inquiry might in a few years be fully elucidated.

SECTION II.—*Statistical History of Insanity in France.*

Similar apprehensions have been entertained in France as to the increase of insanity, and as far as we can depend upon evidence furnished by registers of hospitals, these apprehensions are too well established. The facts leading to this conclusion were brought before the public in the official memoir drawn up by M. Desportes, which was published in 1823.* From the data adduced it appears,

---

* Rapport fait au Conseil-général des Hospices civils de Paris sur le service des Aliénés. 4to. Paris, 1823.

as the Duke de la Rochefoucauld remarked, that the " general aggregate of lunatics existing in the different receptacles of Paris, at the beginning of 1801, amounted to 1070 persons, and at the beginning of 1822 to 2493. The table which affords proofs of this result is divided by the author into five periods. The mean term of admissions during the three first periods was only 2699, and in the fourth period 3769."* This increase seems to have been nearly progressive, as appears by the following numbers : —

In Jan. 1, 1801, the hospitals contained . . . . . 1070 lunatics.
   „   1806, ... 1225 „
   „   1816, ... 1800 „
   „   1821, ... 2145 „
   „   1823, ... 2493 „

M. Desportes observes that if the same ratio of increase should continue to prevail, the hospitals must contain at the end of 1825 about 2900 persons. These facts induced the compiler of the report to request M. Pariset and M. Esquirol, physicians at that time to the hospitals of Bicetre and the Salpêtrière, to communicate their opinions on the causes which had led to the increase, and he has inserted the replies of these celebrated physicians.

M. Pariset, in his memoir, on this subject, observed that in all parts of France, where insanity is principally treated, there is a perceptible increase in the numbers of lunatics. The houses destined to their reception are everywhere found insufficient. " The same remark," he says, " has been made in other parts of Europe. I can affirm that it is true in respect to various provinces in Spain."
" Is this augmentation real in regard to the whole of France, or only apparent ? We may presume that before the revolution a great number of lunatics existed in religious houses, in private families, in hospitals, and even in prisons. A sentiment of shame, or of self-interest, induced convents or families to conceal their lunatics : the deplorable state of hospitals prevented many from removing thither their deranged relatives : those whom their destitution brought to such wretched abodes found there dungeons and chains, or were confounded with other inmates and escaped attention. Many lunatics suffered from the hands of *justice* the penalties due to crimes ! How many demonomaniacs were burned for witchcraft. ' C'êtaient de pauvres fous condamnés par d'autres fous.' Thus was insanity neglected, dissimulated, or mistaken, and hence, in reality so extensively spread, it was supposed to be so rare.
" During the great tumult of revolutions, while all the elements of social life were confounded and agitated, it is probable that a thousand cases of derangement took place without being recognized. Reverses of fortune, sudden changes which elevated or depressed individuals, so many sources of calamity opened at once inundated our country with unexampled calamities, that madness must have

* Rapport fait au Conseil-général par M. le Duc de la Rouchefoucauld, sur le travail presenté par M. Desportes.

been the result in examples without number, but they have been lost sight of in the mass of more general evils. Those who are aware to what a degree the habitudes, the diseases, the infirmities even of the mind, are transmissible, will not deem it rash to conclude that even children born during that era of sorrow and terror must have felt in their mother's wombs the baneful influence. The wars of a subsequent period have added to these afflictions, since nothing is more fitted to extinguish every social feeling, to pervert the understanding and the will, than the disorderly habits which are the result of a state of war.

" In general, every great and rapid change, whether in the physical or moral order of things, is pernicious to the health and to the reason. The sight of wealth and power, raised and thrown down by accidents equally unexpected, has excited not only astonishment, but in rude minds the most dangerous hopes and illusions. Universal reformers, founders of empires and republics, creators of institutions, have arisen on every side ; simple artisans or even operatives, have thought themselves destined to overturn thrones or to mount into them. Such illusions have engendered the most obstinate of all mental aberrations. Pride and ambition produce incurable forms of madness ; I may add that they are most widely spread, since the diabolical pleasure of ruling over men is, as it would appear, the most fascinating among the guilty delights to which the human race abandons itself.

" Even if it should be demonstrated, what nobody can affirm for want of positive data for calculation, that the number of lunatics in France is, *cæteris paribus*, more considerable now than formerly, it would appear that the increase must be attributed chiefly to the two orders of events above indicated. But will the augmentation continue to be progressive. The solution of this question will depend on the movements of society. I shall conclude with one reflexion. The more there is of liberty in any country, the more numerous are the chances of derangement ; but this does not prevent our allowing that liberty is favourable also to the expansion of human reason."*

M. Esquirol has expressed his opinion that the causes of increase in the number of lunatics in the Salpêtrière are both general and local : the first class are principally as follows. Formerly opulent persons deranged were shut up in convents, or in their own estates. The poor, when monomaniacs, imbecile, or old and demented, remained at home, and raving or mischievous madmen alone were sent to asylums. Since the time when Pinel revealed the true principles of treatment for insanity, that disease is no longer considered as incurable, and most rich families send their relatives to asylums in the hope of cure ; while the better management of hospitals encourages persons of the lower class to follow a similar practice, and even public

---

* I have given but a short abstract of this report, which will afford the reader of the original a specimen of the eloquence and brilliant conception of the author.

opinion would condemn them if they were not to have recourse to it. Lunatics are more the objects of care : they are kept longer in the asylums, and being more the objects of attention, they are more in evidence. We ought, perhaps, likewise to take into account the increase in the population of Paris. Among the local causes are the high reputation of the asylum of La Salpêtrière, to which many constantly apply for admission from distant departments. Hence in the ten years from 1803 to 1813, the average number of admissions was annually 280, and during the six years from 1816 to 1821, the average has been 409. Besides this increase in the admissions, the number of cures not equalling that of the entries, the number of permanent inmates has been ever on the increase. The high repute of the Salpêtrière and of other improved hospitals has drawn to them great numbers of the most severe and incurable cases, just as, in general, physicians of great celebrity are consulted on a large proportion of diseases, for the cure of which ordinary skill has been found unavailing.

M. Desportes, after considering the reports of the physicians, and comparing the facts which had fallen under his observation, came to the inference that the causes of increase in the fullness of Parisian hospitals were the following. First, the improvement of regimen and treatment which have overcome repugnance to admission into the hospitals. This, he says, is really a fact, and to such a degree that indigent persons, and even old ecclesiastics, occasionally simulate madness or epilepsy in order to gain entrance. Secondly, the admission of great numbers of persons who are considered to be in a state of senile dementia, and who in reality are only old persons nearly in their ordinary state, but having their faculties slightly weakened by old age, or apoplexy, or paralysis.* Thirdly, the blending of cases of acute mania, such as were formerly sent to the Hôtel Dieu, with examples of chronic insanity, and the caution against dismissing, as cured, individuals whose condition is still insecure,—the mean term of residence of lunatics who are dismissed cured being now, in the two great hospitals, considerably more than double the space of time during which such persons were formerly retained in the Hôtel Dieu.

M. Desportes concluded this part of his memoir by strongly recommending the establishment of separate hospitals for the treatment of curable and incurable cases.

The considerations adduced by MM. Pariset and Esquirol certainly explain to a considerable extent the comparatively greater number of lunatics in the Parisian hospitals, and materially weaken, if they do not destroy, the evidence which at first sight appears so strong in proof of the increase of insanity. But the question is still left in uncertainty ; and a general suspicion has remained on the

---

* Before the year 1790, among 411 cases of admission only 19 individuals were above fifty years of age. In 2451 admitted between 1816 and 1821, one-third, or 880, were beyond that age. This sufficiently proves the increased admission of the old and demented.

minds of many that such an increase exists. These doubts can
be dispelled in no other way than by means of general returns
of the real numbers of lunatics in different departments, and of
their proportion to the entire population obtained for a series of
years. Unfortunately no satisfactory sources of information on this
subject exist, and France is much behind England and some other
countries in all the materials for statistical researches on the frequency of mental derangement. Some means were adopted to
supply this defect in 1812. It was then ascertained that 2100 insane persons existed in the department of the Seine. The attempts
made to estimate the proportional number of lunatics in France on
this ground, were founded on error, because, as M. Esquirol observes, lunatics are constantly sent to Paris from all parts of the
country. In 1818 M. Esquirol addressed a memoir to the minister
of the interior, on the state of lunatics in France ;* and a commission
was appointed for the purpose of improving the condition of these
persons. By this commission a series of questions were addressed
to the prefects of the different departments, the majority of which
were never answered. M. Esquirol has made such researches in
this subject as the extant documents enabled him to pursue. By
collecting the statements of the different establishments for lunatics
in France, and by inquiries as to the number existing in several departments, he has been enabled to draw the conclusion that the total
number in the whole kingdom is about 50,000, which, taking the
population at 30,000,000, whereas it is said to be 32,000,000, gives
1 to every 1000.† This proportion is less than that believed to
exist in Britain and some other countries.

SECTION III.—*Statistics of Insanity in other Countries: General
Observations.*

Most of the information we possess as to the statistics of insanity
in the Dutch and Belgian states has been communicated by M.
Guislain.‡ This writer has collected all the materials that could be
obtained for calculations of various kinds from the lunatic asylums
of the Belgian kingdom ; but he complains greatly of their insuffi-
ciency, and in many instances of the obstacles that were thrown in
his way in the attempt to make inquiries. He appears to have
despaired of collecting data adequate to a calculation of the proportional numbers of lunatics in reference to the general population.

In the provinces of North Holland, or the Dutch states, the returns
of lunatic asylums give the following numbers :—From 1820 to
1825 there were resident in the lunatic asylums of this country 2157
male lunatics, 2363 females : total 4520.

* De l'Etat des Aliénés en France, et des Moyens d'améliorer leur sort. Paris,
1818.
† Statistique des Aliénés, par M. Esquirol, in the Annales de l'Hygiène Publique for 1829.
‡ Traité de l'Aliénation, par M. Guislain, 2 tomes.

For the lunatic asylums of the Belgian states, M. Guislain has given tables including the numbers resident at those establishments in 1810 and 1812, and the numbers of admissions during succeeding years down to 1823 inclusive. They are as follows :—

Gheel, from 1810 to 1823 (including 113 previously resident) .	401
Meastricht (including 18 previously resident) in the same years	115
Tournay and Mons, from 1812 to 1821 (including 22)	86
Louvain, from 1810 to 1823	177
Antwerp	482
Ghent	608
	1869

In reference to the inquiry whether insanity has increased in the countries to which his documents relate, M. Guislain makes the following observations :—

" We deduce from the subsequent table a progressive augmentation in the number of admissions into our asylums for lunatics. This would seem to depend partly on the general increase in the population which has taken place since the cessation of war, and partly from some universal cause ; since the augmentation to which we refer only began to show itself in 1816, a time of trouble, of famine, and of misery. After that period the number of cases began to diminish, or at least has undergone no perceptible increase."

The table gives for the asylums, of Gheel, Maestricht, Louvain, Termonde, Gand, Velscique, Bruges, and Amsterdam, which, for brevity, we include collectively in the following terms of years :—

From 1810 to 1815	627	admissions
From 1816 to 1819	972	„
From 1820 to 1823	792	„

We are thus brought nearly to the same conclusion, with reference to the state of insanity in the Low Countries, as that which Dr. Burrows and Sir A. Halliday were inclined to adopt with respect to this disease in the British isles, viz. that there is no ground for apprehending a progressive increase; that temporary augmentations are owing to the pressure of circumstances and causes which give rise to unusual distress and misery in the population ; and that, when such causes have ceased to operate, the proportional number of lunatics becomes nearly what it previously was.

There is, perhaps, no other country on the continent of Europe where our information on the statistics of insanity is founded on data so satisfactory as in the Prussian provinces on the Rhine. Documents have been published by Dr. Jacobi, furnishing results of great interest.* The following are statements of the general population and of the numbers of lunatics of several states, in the year 1824 :—

---

* Jacobi's Beobachtungen über die Pathologie und Therapie der mit Irreseyn verbundenen krankheiten.

	Population.		Number of Lunatics.
Düsseldorf	641,213	..	798
Aix-la-Chapelle	331,960	..	312
Trèves	301,505	..	221
Cologne	323,283	..	336
Coblentz	250,613	..	348
	2,067,104		2,015

The estimates of the number of lunatics in each province are not
taken from collective statements of asylums, but from documents
collected with the greatest possible care by order of the Prussian
government. Yet they are considered by Jacobi as far from perfect ; and this accurate writer is of opinion that the estimates of some
districts omit not less than half the number of lunatics actually there
existing, and that the deficiency may amount to scarcely less than
one-third for the whole computed aggregate. He thinks the actual
number of lunatics in the whole of the Rhenish provinces should be
reckoned as greater by nearly one-third part than the sum total
above given ; a circumstance which, as he says, renders it still
more remarkable that this number is already so great when compared with the population. The proportion is very nearly 1 to
1000 without augmentation ; and with this increase it becomes, of
course, 1 : 666⅔.

One of the most complete statistical accounts that exists of the
deranged persons of any country, is that which was drawn up some
years since for the kingdom of Norway. It was ordered by the
government, in 1825, that returns should be made of the number,
age, sex, situation of all the insane in that kingdom. The statistical
account was drawn up by Dr. Fr. Holst, and published by order of
the king of Sweden in 1828. M. Esquirol has given an analysis of
this document. This writer confesses his surprise in discerning
from it that deranged persons are more numerous in Norway than,
proportionally to the population, either in England or in France.
The physical circumstances of the inhabitants are, perhaps, most
like those of the Scots. The people are chiefly employed in agriculture and in rearing cattle : they are herdsmen, whose sustenance
is cheese, salt-fish, and the milk of their cattle. Their country is
mountainous : it has no large, populous manufacturing cities : in
that respect it differs from Scotland, as well as in the inferiority of
intelligence and civilization of its people. The facts which relate
to the proportional number of lunatics when compared with the
entire population, as well as those which refer to the comparative
frequency of insanity and idiotism, are very similar in the two
countries : In Scotland lunatics and idiots are to the entire population as 1 to 573 : in Norway they are as one to 551, there being in
all 1,909 deranged persons in the kingdom, and the population being
1,051,318. Of the whole number of deranged, 680 are reported to
be idiots.

Our information is very defective as to the number of lunatics in most other northern countries. A report which M. Esquirol obtained from Dr. Remann of St. Petersburgh gives the number of 1,437 lunatics treated in the asylum of that city from 1814 to 1821. From all the accounts collected by M. Esquirol from the north of Europe, it would appear that insanity is by no means so frequent as in the southern parts of Germany.

No writer has attentively surveyed the state of lunatics in the north of Germany without expressing a sentiment of abhorrence at the cruelty with which these unfortunate beings are treated in the dominions of Hanover. A frightful and disgusting account of the prison of Celle, where lunatics and idiots are confined together with thieves and murderers, may be found in Sir Andrew Halliday's work before cited.

The southern and less civilized countries of Europe present a contrast to the northern, where the intellect of the people is more cultivated. In Spain, according to the information communicated to M. Esquirol by Dr. Luzuriaga, there existed, at the end of 1817, in the asylums of Toledo, Grenada, Cordova, Valencia, Cadiz, Saragossa, and Barcelona, but 509 lunatics. Only 50 lunatics were in the hospitals of Cadiz, 60 in that of Madrid, and there were 36 in the kingdom of Grenada.

The receptacles for lunatics in Italy have been visited lately by M. Brierre. In twenty-five establishments of this description, among which were those of Turin, Genoa, Milan, Brescia, Verona, Vienna, Venice, Parma, Modena, Bologna, Ferrara, Florence, Sienna, Lucca, and Rome.* M. Brierre found 3441 patients. The population of those parts of Italy which were visited by him is said to be about 16,789,000 inhabitants, which gives 1 lunatic to 4879 persons.†

It has been remarked that in Spain and Portugal, where insanity is comparatively rare, malformation of the brain and consequent idiotism are very frequent.‡ Parallel observations have been made elsewhere.

It appears, from an extract given by M. Esquirol from a publication of Dr. Beck on the number and condition of lunatics in the American United States, that the proportion which deranged persons bear to the entire population in the state of New York is very similar to that which obtains in Great Britain. It is given as follows:—

Population of the state of New York	1,616,458
Number of the deranged	2,240
Proportion	1 : 721

* At Rome iron rings, armed with chains and fixed in the wall, serve to confine the furious and turbulent maniacs, who are fastened by their necks and feet. There is no garden nor any particular walk for convalescents, nor any work rooms. Quiet patients have always before their eyes the spectacle of turbulent and furious madmen. More than 300 lunatics are shut up in this frightful prison.

† Annales d'Hygiène Publique et de Médecine Légale, t. x. part 1.

‡ Sir A. Halliday's General View, p. 62.

It has often been observed that insanity is comparatively rare in semibarbarous countries, but it is not immediately obvious to what countries this term applies. Where the people are industrious, and have the arts of life and motives to exertion of mind and body, and the cares and anxieties which are consequent on such a state of society, cases of insanity appear to multiply. In India it seems that there are many lunatics. Numerous asylums have been established in various parts of the Anglo-Indian empire, of which an account may be seen in Sir A. Halliday's work. In China, M. Esquirol believes madness to be of rare occurrence ; but our accounts of that country are defective. In Turkey and in Egypt it is probable that there are few lunatics in proportion to the number of people. M. Desgenettes is said to have found only 14 in the hospital of Grand Cairo, a city containing 300,000 inhabitants ; but it must be remembered that it is not the custom in such countries to confine all lunatics in hospitals. M. Hamont declares that lunatics are by no means unfrequent in Egypt. He says that those who are dangerous are chained and conducted to Cairo, where they are kept in a horrible receptacle ; they eat, sleep, and satisfy the calls of nature in the same spot, of which the stench is intolerable. The only attempt made to cure them is by giving broth of serpent's flesh at every new moon. Lunatics who are harmless wander about the country, some of them quite naked : they are looked upon as saints and prophets, and held in the highest veneration.*

In savage countries, I mean among such tribes as the negroes of Africa and the native Americans, insanity is stated by all scientific travellers, and by naturalists or other persons who have had means of correct information, to be extremely rare. Dr. Winterbottom declares that among the African tribes near Sierra Leone, " mania is a disease which seldom if ever occurs." He adds, that he could not make the natives of that country comprehend the meaning of the term, though they were not unacquainted with the delirium of drunkenness. Idiotism was, likewise, a rare phenomenon among them.† Among the negro slaves in the West Indies, it has been observed by many that insanity is scarcely known.‡ It scarcely exists in the native races of America. This observation was made by Von Humboldt, and it has been confirmed by travellers who in late times have made the most accurate researches into the history of the tribes in the interior of the continent, and particularly by the scientific men who were sent by the government of the United States, in 1819, on the expedition from Pittsburg to the Rocky Mountains.§

I have brought before my readers the most prominent and important facts connected with the statistical history of mental dis-

---

* Lettres de M. Hamont sur l'Egypte, Annales d'Hygiène Publique, &c. Janvier, 1830.
† Winterbottom's Account of Sierra Leone, vol. ii. p. 25.
‡ Sir A. Halliday's General Account.
§ Expedition to the Rocky Mountains. Guislain, tom. i.

cases, from which, if from any thing, inferences may be formed as to the various points of inquiry before suggested, and if, on this groundwork, it is still difficult to construct any system of positive opinions, the difficulty is still such as time and more continued observation may dispel. The period is so recent from which accurate knowledge has been obtained in any country, that we are scarcely authorized in determining that insanity is, or is not, anywhere an increasing evil ; and the reasons pointed out by MM. Pariset and Esquirol in France, and suggested by Halliday and Burrows in this country, explain the apparent increase, or at least prevent our taking the multiplied number of lunatics and of lunatic establishments as a full proof that there has been a real augmentation in the numbers of deranged persons. Yet the apparent increase is every where so striking, that it leaves on the mind a strong suspicion, and this suspicion, that cases of insanity are far more numerous than formerly, can only be removed by a series of observations that may prove the negative. It is encouraged by the reflection that the state of society is, in most countries, such as appears likely to multiply the exciting causes of madness.

From the facts which we have surveyed, sufficient evidence has arisen to confirm in a great measure the remark made, many years ago by M. Esquirol, that insanity belongs almost exclusively to civilized races of men : it scarcely exists among savages, and is rare.in barbarous countries.* To what principle of explanation are we to refer this general fact ? Is it because the exciting causes of madness are not present in the savage state ? Passions and anxieties, doubtless, find their sphere of action wherever men are. We might rather conjecture that congenital predisposition is wanting in the offspring of uncivilized races. If there were as great a proportion of individuals predisposed to insanity in a nation of negroes or Americans as in England or France, it is difficult to suppose that the disease itself would either not exist or be a rare phenomenon : nor could the existence of idiots have escaped the observation of travellers, who were scientific men and physicians, if there had been as many in Guinea or Louisiana as there are in Wales and Scotland. It is an obvious and probable conjecture that the circumstances of the civilized state of mankind, as they give rise to other variations of structure, so, likewise, produce or multiply morbid varieties of organization. Hence a great number of constitutional diseases are common in civilized nations which are rare among savages. The brain receives a different development in the progeny of uncultivated races, or of those whose mental faculties have been awakened: it has a more ample expansion, as the countenance itself, and the shape of the skull, often testify : with greater variations of structure it has new morbid varieties, and while, perhaps, in the majority of persons its organization attains

* The series of observations from which this general result follows is stated in an extensive and striking way by Professor Fodéré, " Essai Médico-légal sur les divers espèces de Folie, à Strasbourg, 1832, pp. 116 et seqq.

greater perfection and completeness of development, in some
the efforts of nature, if we may use the expression, are not fully
successful. I offer these remarks merely as a conjectural solution
of a difficult problem, which seems to me probable from its coincidence with many facts in the physical history of mankind ; but I
do not attach any importance to it.

CHAPTER XI.

OF UNSOUNDNESS OF MIND IN RELATION TO JURISPRUDENCE.

SECTION I.—*General Observations : three Sources of Unsoundness.*

MENTAL unsoundness is a disordered or a defective state of the
mind, impeding in such a manner the exercise of its faculties as to
render an individual incapable of performing correctly the duties
of life, and of maintaining over himself those restraints which are
necessary for the intercourse of society. Unsoundness of mind
impairs or destroys moral responsibility, and calls for interference
in the exercise of personal rights. Various questions connected
with this subject have been discussed among writers on medical
jurisprudence, such as, " what constitutes soundness and unsoundness of mind ?"—in other words, by what distinguishing circumstances are we led to pronounce on the presence or absence of such
a state of the understanding as renders a man incompetent to the
management of his affairs, and absolves him from moral responsibility ?—Is this state of the understanding absolute, or when it
exists at all, extending to all cases and varieties of circumstances,
or does it admit of degrees and modifications ? In furnishing a
solution to these and similar inquiries, both lawyers and physicians
have their part. It belongs to the latter, as observers of nature, to
take note of the phenomena displayed by the human constitution
under disease, and from the relations of these phenomena to deduce
such results as common sense, aided by the habit of reflecting on
similar subjects, may enable them satisfactorily to establish. On
these results, which are the conditions given, legal regulations are
to be constructed. They must be made to accommodate themselves
to the conditions, and they doubtless will be so accommodated when
the latter shall have been set forth in a manner unexceptionable, and
commanding general assent. These arrangements and the elucidation of their principles belong to lawyers and the framers of law.
Physicians are expected to supply to them information as to the
nature of those causes on which unsoundness of mind depends, as
to their extent and duration, their distinguishing characters, and
ultimate results. The entire assemblage of such facts, including the
practical regulations which are founded on them, constitutes a
branch, and by no means an uninteresting one, of medical jurisprudence.

Writers are not wanting who have treated on these subjects in different countries. Germany has produced the most numerous and the most voluminous ; of whom Metzger, Pyl, Hoffbauer, and Heinroth are the most celebrated. In this country the able and well-known works of Dr. Haslam and Dr. Conolly are principally devoted to the same subjects.* The French have no systematic writer on the whole theory of medical jurisprudence as applied to persons of unsound mind, for the commentaries of Professor Fodéré, and the later occasional publications of MM. Marc, Georget, and Esquirol, can scarcely be looked upon in this light. An attempt has been made to supply the defect by means of a translation of Hoffbauer's treatise, to which notes and illustrations have been appended by M. Chambeyron, the translator, and by MM. Itard and Esquirol. This work has not been very well received among the French, who complain of its want of clearness and precision. Notwithstanding this objection, which has not been alleged altogether without reason, the work of Professor Hoffbauer is of great value. It is the most comprehensive in its scope, and the most systematic of any that are known to me, and displays at the same time the results of much reflection and accurate observation on the subjects to which it relates, and to which the author is known to have long devoted his attention.† In going through the different articles which belong to this part of my work, I find that I cannot pursue my object in a better method than by following the steps of Hoffbauer, and, considering the various topics which offer themselves for discussion, nearly in the points of view in which that writer has surveyed them.

Professor Hoffbauer observes that various defects and disorders of the mind are incidentally specified in the Roman law and in the legal code of Prussia, and that in the latter the terms adopted are in some instances defined. In the French code a course has been

---

* To Dr. Conolly's work I have not made so frequent references as might be expected, considering its high value and importance, and the just celebrity of the able and accomplished author. It is a work that does not admit of analysis or condensation, and in the brief essay which I have to give on this subject I have preferred to survey it under a different arrangement.

† Herr Hoffbauer was a doctor of laws and professor in the University of Halle, who made psychology and diseases of the mind the particular subject of his studies. He is the author of several works on insanity and the inquiries connected with it. The first, entitled " Untersuchungen über die krankheiten der Seele, u. s. w. was published in 1802–1807. He afterwards published, in conjunction with Reil, the celebrated author of Researches into the Structure of the Brain and Nerves, a work entitled " Beyträge zur Beforderung einer Kurmethode auf psychischen Wege." His most popular work, entitled " Die Psychologie in ihren hauptanwendungen auf die Rechtspflege nach den allgemeinen Gesichtspunkten," &c. has been translated into French, with notes by the editor, M. Chambeyron, and additional comments by MM. Esquirol and Itard. Hoffbauer likewise translated the work of Crichton on Insanity into the German language. Professor Hoffbauer shows, in many instances, a want of practical knowledge of insanity, but he has discussed admirably the legal relations of mental deficiencies. A critical analysis of his works has been given by Professor Heinroth, in his " Lehrbuch der Störungen des Seelenlebens," th. 2.

followed which in the opinion of this writer indicates the correct
judgment of the legislator ; occasional references are made to various classes of persons whose states are distinguished respectively
by the terms madness, dementia, and imbecility; but the law no
where determines the precise import of these expressions. "In
fact, all legislation ought to proceed on the ground that the objects
to which it refers are well known and understood ; but this knowledge failing, it is much better that the law should leave things
undefined than that it should define erroneously, and thus introduce
mistakes which would be perpetuated by its authority."

The triple division recognized by the legal code of France corresponds with actual facts or with the distinctions established by the
observers of nature. Among the disorders and defects of the understanding we discover three very different states, all of which imply
mental incapacity. These are, first, idiotism or congenital defect,
depending on an originally imperfect formation or development of
the brain, under which article must also be comprised the different
degrees and modifications of weakness of mind or imbecility, though
the latter may be distinguished from absolute idiotism ; secondly,
madness or insanity in its various forms; thirdly, dementia, intellectual decay, or, as I have termed it in the preceding pages, from its
characteristic feature, incoherence.

The English law is less accurate in the distinction of mental disorders than the Roman jurisprudence and the modern systems which
are founded on its principles. The only classes of incompetent persons recognised by the former are idiots, who are properly *idiotæ
ex nativitate*, idiots from birth, and lunatics or madmen, styled
" *non compotes mentis.*" The latter are " persons who *have had*
understanding, but by disease, grief, or other accident, have lost the
use of their reason." " A lunatic," says Blackstone, " is properly
one that hath lucid intervals ; sometimes enjoying his senses, and
sometimes not, and that frequently depending upon the state of the
moon." This indeed would reduce the classes of incompetent persons recognized by law within very narrow limits indeed. " But
under the general name of *non compos mentis,* which Sir Edward
Coke says is the ' most legal name' for a madman, are comprised not
only lunatics but persons under frenzies, or who lose their intellect
by disease ; those that *grow* deaf, dumb, and blind, not being *born*
so ; or such, in short, as are judged by the Court of Chancery incapable of conducting their own affairs.* To these as well as to idiots
the king is guardian." It seems from this that demented persons,
including dotards, or individuals labouring under senile decay and
loss of memory and intellect, are, by the English law, comprehended
under the class of *non compotes mentis,* or lunatics.

An idiot in the English law, to be considered as such, must be
" *purus idiota,*" a mere or absolute idiot. By the Roman law, if a
man by notorious prodigality was in danger of wasting his estate, he

---

* Blackstone, Comment. book i. cap. 8.

was looked upon as *non compos*, and committed by the præter to the care of curators, or tutors. "But in England, when a man on an inquest of idiocy hath been returned an *unthrift*, and not an idiot, no further proceedings have been had, and the propriety of the practice itself," says Blackstone, "seems to be very questionable. It was doubtless an excellent method of benefitting the individual and of preserving estates in families ; but it hardly seems calculated for the genius of a free nation, who claim and exercise the liberty of using their own property as they please. " 'Sic utere tuo ut alienum non lædas,' is the only restriction our laws have given with regard to economical prudence." The propriety of acting on this principle with respect to the imbecile and those morally insane would be less subject to doubt, if such individuals suffered only in their own persons and interests, and were not liable to involve their families and relatives in misfortune and disgrace.

Whatever may have been the decisions of courts of judicature or the opinions of lawyers on this subject, certain it is, as a matter of fact, that idiotism, or mental incapacity depending upon congenital formation, is not a thing to be pronounced absolute and complete within a definite degree. It exists in various shades and modifications, from the last stage of fatuity which places human beings far below the brutes in regard to the manifestations of mind, up to an almost imperceptible inferiority in comparison with the ordinary powers of understanding. There are some idiots whose degradation is of so decided a character, and whose defect is so strikingly displayed by their expression of countenance and manners, that no person could hesitate for a moment to pronounce upon their state, but the number is much greater of those whose affection is of such a kind as to leave room for doubt, and to require attentive examination ; yet it is not less really the fact that these individuals are by nature incompetent to govern their conduct by their own wits, or if left to themselves amid the collisions and accidents of life, to prevent the ruin of their families or relations. Whatever the law of prescript or of custom may be with respect to such unfortunate persons, common sense and humanity indicate most plainly that they ought to be protected, and that the provision of the Roman law and the laws of the most enlightened nations on the continent are wise and humane in this respect, and also in accordance with justice and propriety. The course which the Roman law has adopted is doubtless that to which the legal regulation in this particular, of all countries, will be ultimately brought, and to which they would speedily arrive, if only the indefiniteness and ambiguity connected with the existence and degrees of mental deficiency could be removed, and some clear and distinct principles recognized, which might guide or assist the opinions of arbiters in pronouncing judgment in particular cases. The want of some rule by which the various degrees of incapacity may be measured, and the exigencies of each stage and condition determined, has long been felt. Professor Hoffbauer has made an attempt to supply this desideratum. He has divided the defects of the understanding into several stages, and has endeavoured to describe each by its appropriate phenomena. His arrangement has met with great approbation among his countrymen; by foreigners it has been variously estimated. I believe that it will be found useful as furnishing a scale to which approximations may be made in particular instances, though it may sometimes be found difficult or even impossible to refer individual cases to the description of any one particular stage in the series.

The scheme of Hoffbauer seems originally designed to distinguish the varieties of mental weakness in persons who are by nature deficient, and who have sustained no loss of reason by disease. The state of these individuals is different from that of demented persons, or those who have become incoherent and fatuous. In a medical point of view, and for purposes of nosological accuracy, this distinction ought carefully to be maintained, but as both imbecile and demented persons are liable to be examined as to the powers of the understanding and the extent to which the fault or disorder in either may reach, and as the decision to be formed will depend in either case on nearly similar considerations, there seems to be no reason in propriety why both should not be referred to the same scale. Demented persons in the last degree are as completely beyond all doubt or question as to their incapacity as the merest idiots : in the lower or less strongly characterized stages their cases admit, like those of idiots, of a variety of degrees. For these reasons it seems not improper to comprise the degrees of congenital weakness, or approaches to idiotism, and those of dementia under the same scale.

SECTION II.—*Of mental Deficiency in its different Modifications and Degrees. Hoffbauer's Stages of Silliness and Stupidity.*

Mental deficiency includes all the degrees of intellectual weakness, from the slightest appearance of inferiority in understanding to absolute fatuity. Different modifications of mental weakness are comprehended under this head, whether arising from natural imperfection in the organ of intellect or the consequences of disease; they are arranged according to the degrees in which the mind is found to be defective in its operations.

But though I include at present under one head kinds of deficiency different in respect to their causes and their pathological nature, I must, before I proceed to the arrangement of gradation established by Hoffbauer, distinguish, with that writer, two marked varieties in the character and phenomena of mental weakness. One of these modifications of defective understanding is termed *bloedsinn*, or imbecility, and the other *dummheit*, or dulness : I shall adopt the expressions silliness and stupidity, as the most appropriate glosses for these German words which I can find. The former, in Hoffbauer's phraseology, is said to consist in a defect of *intensity*, the latter in a want of *extensity*. By intensity M. Hoffbauer describes the energy with which a sound mind applies itself to judge with accuracy on the objects of reflection, or on the data already furnished by the senses and by perception ; extensity is a similar energy directed externally to sensation and apprehension, or to the acquisition of ideas. The former defect renders the intellect unable to examine with sufficient exactness the data on which judgment is to be exercised ; the latter renders it liable to suffer some of these data to escape. There is in fact, if I am not mistaken, a marked diversity among men as to the relative degrees of energy in their internal and external faculties, meaning by the former the powers of judgment and reflection, of reason, the faculties by which the mind decides on truth and falsehood, right and wrong, and in general of relations ; and by the latter the ability for external perception and apprehension. When the whole constitution of the mind is weak so as to render the individual barely competent to the business of life, these differences are the more striking and conspicuous. Many persons whose power of judgment is very deficient have a tolerable share of quickness in apprehension ; others, on the contrary, and these often appear much more defective than the former class, are slow of perception, and let many things escape them which would be observed by ordinary men, yet they make occasionally shrewd remarks, and give tokens in their conduct which indicate a sagacity much beyond the measure of intellect which common observers ascribe to them. M. Hoffbauer is correct in distinguishing two classes among weak and half idiotic persons. One of these may be described as *silly* or defective in judgment, in the powers of reason and discrimination, while the other or *stupid* class show their deficiency chiefly in obtuseness or slowness of perception and apprehension, and in a consequent ignorance of external things and relations.*

That form of intellectual weakness which is distinguished by the term silliness or imbecility differs in several respects from stupidity or obtuseness of the mental faculties.

" In reference to the faculty of judgment, it may be observed that the stupid or obtuse person is more liable than the imbecile to form erroneous decisions ; the latter experiences great difficulty in bringing himself to any conclusion. Secondly, the stupid person sometimes judges very correctly on subjects to which his attention has been strongly applied ; occasionally he comes even more directly to a right conclusion than those who are possessed of superior intelligence. When he errs, it is through neglect of some of the considerations which ought to have formed the groundwork of his judgment, and he will say, in order to excuse himself, that ' he should never have dreamt of this or that circumstance.' To the silly the most simple act of judgment is difficult : for instance, a lady who said that she was twenty-five years of age, and had been married six years, could not, after many efforts, tell how old she was at the period of her wedding. Thirdly, the stupid man may often be induced to

* Hoffbauer has explained his ideas on the nature of ' *blödsinn*' and ' *dummheit*' more fully in his Untersuchungen, th. i. s. 9.

correct his mistake, some particular circumstance being suggested to him which leads to its detection. The imbecile man can scarcely rectify his error, being unable sufficiently to concentrate his attention on any particular subject. The stupid man has not this defect, but he views every subject on one side only, and is embarrassed by every complex idea.

"In relation also to memory, there is a decided difference between stupid and imbecile or silly persons. The latter appear to be almost entirely defective in this faculty : the former recollect after a long interval of time some insulated circumstances or transactions. The reason of these peculiarities is the total want of attention to present objects which is characteristic of the one state, and the partial but concentrated attention to them which is observable in the other.

"Weakness of intellect displays itself in both these classes of persons, when their defect is in a high degree, by a propensity which they have to talk to themselves. This is most observable when the affected individual is alone or supposes himself to be so. In reality, we employ words not merely for purposes of intercourse, but as an instrument of thought, and the weakest intellects require their aid in the most perceptible manner. When the mind is morbidly weakened, the silent and unperceived or the mental employment of words is insufficient : they must be repeated more or less audibly. This practice is not uncommon with imbecile and stupid persons, but when in society they generally perceive its incongruity and abstain from it. If, however, such individuals talk to themselves, knowing themselves to be in the presence of other persons, it is a proof of greater deficiency.

"Another distinction between the stupid and the silly is that the former imagines himself to be at least equal to other men in intelligence, whereas the imbecile is ever conscious of his state, and even exaggerates his defect.

"This difference between them is easily explained, as well as the results which it induces in their conduct. The stupid act rashly and without reflexion ; the imbecile can never come to a determination. Hence, also, the imbecile become cautious, timid, and even misanthropic, unless when assured of their security by finding themselves under the protection of persons of whose kind intentions towards them they are well convinced : to the guidance of such persons they give themselves up with blind confidence.

"The pusillanimity and misanthropy of the imbecile lead them to a species of devotion, if such it may be termed. Supposing themselves to be despised and ill-treated by men, they are led to apply for support to the common resource of the unfortunate. The stupid, more confident in themselves, fancy that they acquire merit by their devotions, or confer a favour on the divinity."

This account of the phenomena of mental weakness might suffice for ordinary purposes, but the deficiency exists to different degrees, and one stage in the approach to idiotism has results, in respect to social relations, which do not belong to a different grade in the same scale. M. Hoffbauer has for the first time made the attempt to define the gradations of mental deficiency as a basis for suggestions on the legal bearings of this state in particular degrees. It was hardly to be expected that he should accomplish this undertaking at once in a manner wholly free from error, and requiring no correction or improvement. The outline which he has sketched is drawn with great ability, and is evidently the result of extensive observation, assisted by no ordinary talent for generalising phenomena and tracing their connections. The subject is so important that I shall incur the risk of being thought somewhat prolix, and give an abridged extract of this author's description of the five stages or degrees into which he. divides the affection of *blödsinn*, imbecility or silliness, and the three degrees of *dummheit*, or stupidity.

" The *first* degree of imbecility or silliness manifests itself in the incapability of forming a judgment respecting any new object, even when the necessary data are furnished, and the question is one which in itself presents no difficulty : in this degree of the affection the individual can very well judge respecting objects to which he is daily accustomed, and in familiarity with which he may be said to have grown up ; he often shows, in the pursuit of his daily concerns, a minute exactness which appears to him a matter of absolute necessity. His memory is very limited : not that he absolutely loses the remembrance of things, but because he cannot apply his recollections according to his wishes. He scrupulously observes whatever he thinks becoming in his situation, because he fears to give offence in neglecting it. When he gives himself up to avarice, there is observed in him rather an apprehension of losing than a desire of accumulation. The propensity to talk alone, and the species of devotion to which we have alluded, is seldom to be met with in this instance, the former because the routine of daily occupations, above which the individual seldom raises himself, makes but small demands on his intelligence; the latter because his infirmity is not so remarkable in society as to render it a subject of general observation, and entail upon him frequent annoyance, and thus make him feel the necessity of seeking support elsewhere. He is very subject to gusts of passion, which nevertheless are as easily appeased as they are excited."

The preceding description will be found to coincide accurately with many cases of mental defect arising from original or congenital weakness of the intellectual faculties. I could furnish instances from my own observation which strikingly exemplify it.

" In the *second* degree of imbecility the patient still judges and acts consequently with respect to subjects that are familiar to him, but even on those subjects it often happens that he is deceived, because, through a distraction which is a second nature to him, he forgets places, times, and circumstances. He observes so little what takes place or what passes around him, that he often fancies himself in a different spot from that in which he really is, mistakes strangers for persons of his acquaintance, confounds the present with the past, but more often with the future, and believes himself at home when he is at the house of another person.

"The individual effected with imbecility in the *third* degree is unfitted for all matters which require more than a mechanical mode of action, but he preserves sufficient intelligence to be aware of his weakness and the superiority of others with respect to the mental faculties. We may likewise remark in him that propensity to devotion and to misanthropy which we have mentioned above. His mind is not completely inactive, although it cannot raise itself to any high pitch ; hence he has the propensity to talk to himself. He has not the power of seizing any idea so clearly as to impress it on his mind ; hence a very marked defect of memory, and a propensity to pass rapidly from one topic to another. He is very irritable and suspicious, fancies a design to insult him where it is impossible, because his state yet permits him to feel and resent injuries ; of which susceptibility those around him often take advantage to his annoyance.

" The *fourth* degree of imbecility is marked by a clouded state of the understanding and the memory, with a great insensibility, which nevertheless leaves the patient a confused idea of his weakness. He eagerly seeks excitement by various stimuli.

" In the *fifth* degree of imbecility there is a nullity of intelligence ; the attention cannot be directed to any object : all the faculties of which the activity depends upon the intellect are destroyed or oppressed. The phenomena which depend upon attention are wanting, and those which imply its absence take their place. The imbecile in this degree is insusceptible of passions, of joy, of grief, of pleasure, in a word, of every kind of moral feeling. He is even but little sensible of pain and other physical inconveniences. He only takes nourishment because it is given to him, like an infant ; the natural wants, such as hunger and thirst, have no effect upon him. He has no memory, he has neither devotion nor the desire of talking to himself, which is observed in other imbecile persons, but which implies in them to a certain degree of consciousness of their state."

The fifth stage of imbecility thus characterised by Hoffbauer is precisely the last degree of dementia, or the fatuity which is the consequence of cerebral diseases.

" Stupidity, generally speaking, is a defect less severe than imbecility, according to the definition which we have given of both. The slightest degree, however, of imbecility indicates an imperfection of the intellectual powers less severe than the greatest degree of stupidity.

" We admit in stupidy *three* principal degrees.

" In the *first*, the individual is incapable of judging and of self-determination, only when it is necessary to weigh opposing motives. Then he feels his incapacity, and has recourse to the intelligence of others, unless pride happens to prevent him, which is often the case. If he acts absurdly, it is often because he applies to his actions a rule good in itself, but the application of which requires other considerations.

" The subject of the *second* degree of stupidity forms a judgment accurately and often promptly upon things by which he is daily surrounded ; but he commits serious errors whenever it is necessary to exert a certain vigour of judgment : he embarrasses himself in any train of reasoning, however simple it may be. His memory is perhaps faithful, but it is slow ; he cannot, without great difficulty, express a complex idea, if it is the result of his own reflections, and has not been received from another. When his faculties have been somewhat developed by education, he is an obstinate partisan of any thing which is, as we say, good in theory but useless in practice ; because he cannot observe the circumstances which distinguish particular cases, and appreciate them according to their just value. These two conditions are, however, indispensable, in order to make with propriety the application of general rules.

" In the *highest* degree of stupidity the individual cannot go beyond one single idea ; and he must completely lose that one before he can pass to another. He is hence less capable of judging than the imbecile, because the comparison of several ideas is necessary to form a judgment. Individuals who are afflicted in the third degree of stupidity often express themselves in half-uttered words, return incessantly to the same subject, make known their ideas by sentences, short, incoherent, and unfinished, like children who can retain words but do not know how to connect them together ; they express often the subject and the attribute without connecting the one to the other by an affirmative or negative. If they wish to say ' the rose is beautiful,' they will say ' rose beautiful,' or only rose, or beautiful, according as the subject or the attribute strikes them most. Often they reverse the natural order of words, and say, for example, ' rose beautiful is ;' and when they perceive an omission which they wish to repair, they become still more perplexed.

" With respect to legal relations, the first degree of imbecility may be assimilated to the second degree of stupidity, and the highest degree of the latter to the third degree of the former."

M. Esquirol has made objections to the minuteness and attempted accuracy of these distinctions. He thinks it difficult, if not impossible, to determine the exact limits of each stage. The endeavour to lay down rules with accuracy scarcely attainable in practice may sometimes impose unnecessary difficulties. This is undoubtedly true, and perhaps it may be admitted that the modifications and degrees of which Hoffbauer's arrangement consists are more numerous than they ought to be. Yet the necessity of adopting some method of this kind is obvious, unless we determine to regard mental deficiency as an absolute state. and admitting of no gradations ; and experience proves more and more the error of such a proceeding.

I proceed now to the practical application of these distinctions.

" In matters of criminal accusation all legal culpability is annulled when it is proved that the party labours under imbecility amounting to the third degree, or even nearly approaching it. Imbecility in the first and second degree may either annul or weaken culpability, or leave it unaffected under different circumstances. Ignorance of the law and of the illicit nature of actions may sometimes be alleged as excuses in criminal accusations in the instance of imbecility amounting to the first degree. But this plea can only be allowed to be valid under one of the two following conditions :—1st, when the law which has been violated by the imbecile neither forms part of general relations which concern himself as well as other members of society, nor belongs to his own particular habits or circumstances : 2dly, when the action forbidden by the legislator is not contrary to the law of nature.

" The second degree of imbecility may lessen or destroy culpability in cases in which the first degree leaves it entire.

" In the first degree of imbecility, inattention or absence of mind, want of foresight, &c. are not considered as excuse when they have regard to objects universally known, as to fire, or to those which are familiar in use to the imbecile, as the tools, &c. of his profession. In all other instances his fault loses the degree of culpability which belongs to it, according to the expression of jurists, *in abstracto.* This is also the case when the act is the result of sudden anger or fear, to which persons are prone.

" The imbecile in the second degree has less responsibility than in the first. His incapacity is greater, as likewise is his proneness to sudden emotions.

" Similar considerations affect the responsibility of persons labouring under stupidity, when it passes the middle degree above described. In fact, the latter being incapable of extending their thoughts to several objects at the same time, must omit many considerations of which intelligent persons never lose sight. Such an individual is so much the less responsible for his actions, as he is known to be incapable of the reflection which might lead another to rectify his mistakes.

" The principles established in reference to criminal law, on the ignorance of the parties, are applicable in civil law to the question— whether an individual is in a condition to recognize the illicit nature of an act by which he has trespassed on the right of another. In imbecility in the first or second degree, ignorance of the law may be pleaded as excuse under circumstances analogous to those before alluded to.

" All the arrangements which the law authorizes or prescribes in regard to imbecile persons are founded either on their own interest or on that of others, and have for their object the personal security of either party. These arrangements refer, 1st, to the appointment of a *tutela* for the administration of the property of the weak or idiotic man, and of a *curatela* for the care of his person ; 2dly, to seclusion, when it is required for preventing dangers likely to accrue to society or to the individual from his unrestrained enjoyment of personal freedom. All the measures judged necessary for his security and for the protection of society must be taken with as much mildness as possible.

" An imbecile person, whose affliction reaches the third degree,

can no longer be judged competent to the care of his own property :
this may be observed *a fortiori*, if his disorder passes that degree.
But in the appointment of a tutela, regard must be had to the necessity greater or less of such protection, and especially to the particular
character, habits, inclinations, &c of the individual. It must be considered whether he is likely to commit actions which, though indifferent in themselves, may occasion public offence, or whether an
excessive liberality or ruinous prodigality may not expose him to
dissipate the property that may be left at his disposal.

" The administration of his property should be left to the imbecile
in the second degree, and a curator should only be appointed for him
under particular circumstances, as for example, when his character
calls for such an arrangement, and when some interests are at stake
which require practical intelligence, and especially constant attention.
With such exception it is unjust to deprive him of the management
of his affairs. The inconveniences to which he may contingently be
exposed cannot be compared with the certain annoyances connected
with a tutela, and some reliance may be placed in general on the
vigilance which self-interest calls forth even in defective minds.

" Persons imbecile in the second degree are more subject to act
without reflection than those whose defect belongs to the first or the
third stage. The former are rather irresolute and timid than precipitate in action, and the latter too negligent and inactive. Hence,
though in the second degree imbecility does not generally authorize
the appointment of a *tutela* it often requires that individuals should
be subjected to an especial *surveillance*.

" The imbecile whose infirmity does not exceed the first degree
cannot justly be subjected to a tutela, or to any particular surveillance, except under circumstances in which his inclinations or habits,
his family, relations, or fortune, or the affairs under his management,
require such an arrangement.

"What has been observed in respect to the degrees of imbecility
may be applied to stupidity, on the principle above laid down. Only
it must be remembered that this last infirmity renders individuals
more liable to rash and hasty actions than does imbecility.

" Imbecile persons in the third degree are evidently incapable of
making wills ; as their state renders them competent only to actions,
which, if not unreasonable, are without reflection. The case is not
so in the instance of imbeciles in the first and second degree, even
though under certain circumstances, before adverted to, they may
occasionally be subjected to a surveillance or even to a *curatela*.
The object of this curatela is to protect them from injuries which
they might bring upon themselves if left to their own discretion, and
to prevent engagements which they might contract and be unable to
fulfil. These considerations are not, however, reasons for depriving
them of the power of making a will. By a testament they might
deprive those who would inherit *ab intestato*, but they prejudice no
formal right. Besides a testament does not require the same intelligence as the administration of property ; it only depends upon a

single arrangement, for which the testator has sufficient time for deliberation."

To this last opinion of M. Hoffbauer it is objected by M. Chambeyron, that by the simple appointment of a tutela the imbecile person is assimilated to a minor and declared incapable of any civil act,
except under some particular circumstances, and when the authentic
consent of the tutor may authorize him to contract. Why then, it
is inquired, should there be any exception for the right of testating?
The author has given a satisfactory reason why this right should be
preserved inviolate in certain instances, namely, that individuals may
and do retain the requisite degree of intelligence for entering into
the arrangements in question, though in other respects in a state
which renders the appointment of a guardian or some especial *surveillance* advisable. The incongruity pointed out by M. Chambeyron has respect to positive institutions, and the observation of M.
Hoffbauer is founded on general principles.

I shall here terminate the consideration of mental weakness or defect, and now proceed to the second division of the subject, namely,
disorders of the mind.

Section III.—*Of Disorders of the Mind considered in relation to Jurisprudence.*

1. *Of intellectual derangement or mental illusion. Monomania and Mania.*—Professor Hoffbauer adopted an ingenious
though erroneous idea as to the nature of these diseases. On this he
has founded some practical conclusions, of which the validity is very
doubtful ; they deserve, however, for reasons which will appear, a
few moments' consideration. Mental illusion (wahnsinn) consists,
according to him, in a loss of that due proportion which, in the sound
state of the mind, the powers of sense and perception bear to the
influence of imagination. The influence of imagination may become
excessive in two ways ; first, by increased intensity or exaltation of
this faculty, the other powers remaining the same ; or, secondly, by
depression of the latter, while the faculty of imagination remains un-
changed. The former is monomania, in which, as the author supposes, the mind is not destroyed or generally affected. The latter is
mania, and in this the powers of the understanding, perception,
apprehension, are greatly impaired.

No practical error is likely to arise from this opinion, as far as it
respects the nature of mania. Persons who are generally deranged
or in raving madness cannot be supposed by any one to be accountable for their conduct, or capable of managing their affairs. No dispute
exists among jurists or physicians on this subject. The state of maniacs is in general too manifest to admit of any doubt. The lunatic
perceives the objects and persons who surround him, but his imagination transforms them, and they are mistaken by him as to their
nature and identity. "Hence in civil law the acts of such an individual manifestly lose all their consequences, and can neither convey

any right to another, nor place the agent himself under obligation. In criminal law he is discharged from all responsibility, and consequently from all culpability ; since what he wills to do in his imaginary situation is not what he would do in his real situation, were he only aware of the latter. This state of disease fully justifies the placing an individual under a tutela, and the disposing of his person in that way which shall appear most conducive to his recovery, or in hopeless cases, to his security and comfort."

It will be apparent to those who entertain a correct opinion as to the nature of monomania or partial derangement of the understanding,that a great part of this reasoning applies almost equally to persons affected by that form of disease. But here we find Professor Hoffbauer's theory leading him into error, an error which is not peculiar to him. As his opinion is common to many, and the inference to which it has led him is by no means a matter of indifference, I shall cite some of his observations, and presently add the comments of a practical physician, the powers of whose acute and penetrating mind have been directed to this subject.

Hoffbauer supposes that, in partial insanity characterized by hallucinations, the representations of unreal objects, or the illusory transformations of existing ones, such illusions can only pervert the judgment when the affected train of ideas is brought into play ; and that on matters unconnected with this illusion the individual is to be considered as a sane man. " In this relation, therefore, insanity cannot be recognized by the law. In civil law all the acts of the party preserve their validity, and in criminal law their culpability." In fact, there is no reason why a man who thinks he has legs of glass, and in other respects is in possession of all his faculties, should not be capable of contracts, and responsible for illegal acts which have no connexion with the subject of his madness. Such a species of insanity seldom prevents a man from managing his own affairs, or undertaking any legal relations for others. Swedenborg, so celebrated by his visions, who was confessedly a madman, fulfilled the duties of his office in so distinguished a manner, that the king of Sweden ennobled him. The author knew a doctor in laws who had taken it into his head that all the freemasons had entered into a league against him. This person, who in other respects was perfectly sane, held with high credit a chair in a university.

In general, in relation to the insane, the ruling idea or illusive opinion characteristic of their disease, considered with respect to the imputability of their actions, ought not to be regarded as an error, but as a truth ; or, in other words, their actions ought to be considered as if they had been committed under the circumstances in which the patient believed himself to be. At Brieg, a soldier killed a child because he thought he saw the Deity near him commanding him to do it. Dr. Glanwitz, in his report, came to the conclusion that the man should be confined in a lunatic asylum.

" When the question relates to consent to some particular matter, regard must be had to the prevailing idea, inasmuch as upon its truth or falsity depends the reality of the consent. If, for example, in a civil affair, as a contract, we suppose that the contractor would not have given his consent without a previously existing illusion, this idea is looked upon as an error, not imputable to the person concerned. As to the question whether the results of the act are cancelled or not, this must depend upon what the laws have decided with respect to involuntary errors.

"In practice it is difficult to decide whether an affair undertaken by a person labouring under madness with a fixed illusion is valid or not, on account of errors likely to result from this fixed illusion. For as long as this person enjoys his rights, it is not the business of another to examine if his act is valid or not. And besides, the person himself neither could nor would acknowledge his error."

"From what has preceded, we apprehend how important it is to determine, in cases of permanent illusion, the paramount idea ; to know whether it brings on a derangement more or less complete of the intellectual faculties, or only prevents the perfect use of the judgment in relation to certain objects ; to discover what influence it has, on one side, upon the notion which the patient has of himself and of his relations with his equals, and, on the other, upon his actions in general. When the prevailing error draws with it a total incoherence of ideas, the case approaches to one of imbecility.

" When a patient attacked by madness with one fixed illusion has a false notion of himself and of his relation to others, this circumstance ought to be taken into consideration. For in criminal justice actions ought to be regarded as if the person really was in the state and in the circumstances in which he believed himself to be. Thus the crimes committed by madmen fancying themselves kings and princes, ought not to be punished according to their nature and heinousness ; the culpability is lessened or destroyed.

" We ought above all to have regard to the illusion under which the patient is carried by his paramount idea to commit actions which he considers as matters of duty. In religious madness, for example, the acts which a person afflicted with this form of the disease commits, ought still less to be punished ; because no kind of human suffering could have any effect upon a lunatic of this description ; divine punishment, or the hope of eternal reward, weighs much more strongly upon his mind than the fear of any thing within the power of man."

Similar opinions have been advanced in a manner less restricted by a high legal authority in France. The following observations are understood to convey the sentiments of the advocate-general, M. de Peyronnet, as they were delivered in a process on the " Affaire de Papavoine."* " The advocate-general," says the report, " proceeds to examine whether every kind of insanity ought to absolve from culpability, and after distinguishing in the clearest manner partial

* Discussion Médico-légale sur la Folie, &c. par le Docteur Georget. Paris, 1826. See, also, Examen Médical des Procés criminels des nommés Léger, Feldtman, Lecouffe, Jean-Pierre, et Papavoine, &c. par le docteur Georget. Paris, 1825.

from total derangement, sustains and demonstrates that the last can alone extricate a criminal from the penalty of the laws. This reasonable distinction thus laid down by the public authority, throws the strongest light upon the questions of mental alienation, the most intricate question in medical jurisprudence, which some physiologists have solved in a manner as unfavourable to accusation as injurious to morality, and alarming to society. M. de Peyronnet here cites some passages from Lord Hale. Of these I should prefer to cite the English text, but as the advocate-general has given to some of the expressions a more definite turn, in a manner which displays fully his own way of thinking, I shall crave permission to deviate from my usual course, and cite the exact words of M. de Peyronnet.

"'Il est une démence partielle et une démence totale ; la première est relative à tels ou tels objets. Quelques personnes qui jouissent de leur raison pour certaines choses sont sujettes à des accès d'une démence spéciale, à telles discours ou tels sujets, où bien elle est partielle dans ses degrès ; telle est la condition d'une foule d'insensés ; et surtout des personnes mélancoliques dont la folie consiste la plûpart du temps à témoigner des craintes, des chagrins excessifs, et qui cependant ne sont pas entièrement privées de l'usage de la raison. Cette démence partielle *semble ne pas excuser* les crimes que commettent ceux qui en sont atteints, *même en ce qui en fait l'objet principal;* car toute personne qui s'arme contre lui-même ou contre d'autres, est jusqu'à un certain point dans un état de démence partielle, lorsqu'elle se rend coupable.............. Je suis en outre forcé d'admettre qu'il est une importante distinction entre les cas civils et les cas criminels. Dans les premiers, dès qu'il est prouvé que la raison de l'homme est altérée, la loi annulle ces actes, *quoiqu'ils n'aient aucune rélation avec les circonstances qui causent sa démence, et qui auraient pu influer sur la conduite. Mais lorsqu'il s'agit de décharger un homme de la responsibilité de ses crimes, et surtout de crimes atroces, on ne peut point réclamer l'application de cette règle, incontestable pour une question de propriété.'*

"After having laid down principles so precise, so positive, so satisfactory to the jury," continues the reporter, " the advocate-general applies them to the cause." The same writer cites further the following passage, which leaves no doubt as to the views of M. de Peyronnet. " The pretended insanity of the accused is a pretext had recourse to in despair of the cause ; certain it is that this derangement cannot have been total : it is likewise proved that it could not be partial, and in this last supposition, if even allowed, *it could not serve for an admissible excuse.*"

M. Georget, possessing much more correct knowledge of the real nature of monomania or partial illusion, considered the joint opinion of these lawyers as highly objectionable. He expressed his astonishment at the sentiments of Lord Hale. " This writer," he says, " appears professedly to consider property of higher value than human life ! There is then no excuse for an unfortunate lunatic, who in a paroxysm commits a reprehensible action, even although it should

appear to be the result of his particular illusion ! And yet the civil
acts of this same individual are to be annulled, although they have
no relation to the insane impressions which might have influenced
his conduct ! And even M. de Peyronnet could cite such maxims
as these with approbation; we do not at least find he has objected to
any part of them. All monomaniacs, according to this statement,
are liable to become criminals in spite of the sixty-fourth article of
our penal code, and may undergo the penalties recorded for atrocious
offences."

M. Georget has refuted these opinions on grounds which must be
conceded by the jurists of all countries, viz. on those of experience
and correct knowledge as to the real state of monomaniacs. Such
persons, as he has clearly proved, though they reason correctly on a
variety of subjects remote from the particular one on which their
illusion turns, are yet more fully deranged than they appear to be,
and are ever liable to display perversities both in feeling and action.
Cases like those of Swedenborg and the German professor mentioned
by Hoffbauer, very rarely occur. Even in these instances, had we
been enabled to follow the individuals affected into private life and
to observe their personal deportment, it is almost certain that something would have been discoverable in their moral character and
habits different from those of ordinary men. M. Georget's observations have led him to form nearly the same opinion as to the nature
of monomania or partial derangement as that which I have expressed
in a former part of this work.

The facts of a remarkable case of this description which came
out in evidence some years ago before an English court, confirm in
a striking manner the character here ascribed to this disease. For a
full account of this I must refer to a " Report of the judgment in
Dew vers. Clarke and Clarke," delivered by the Rt. Hon. Sir John
Nicholl, in the Prerogative Court of Canterbury. It was there
proved that the individual " in the ordinary transactions of life conducted himself and his affairs rationally ; was a sensible, clever man;
amassed a considerable fortune by his profession ; took good care of
his property; and that several of his friends and acquaintance, some of
them medical persons, never even suspected that he was deranged in
mind." It was stated by those who wished to prove his sanity, that
" he was a man of irritable and violent temper, of great pride and
conceit, very precise in all domestic arrangements, very impatient of
contradiction, entertaining high notions of parental authority, rigid
notions of the total and absolute depravity of human nature, of the
necessity of sensible conversion, and of the necessity or expediency
of confessing to other persons the most secret thoughts of the heart."
It was proved that this person, such as he is above described, having
a daughter " amiable in disposition, of superior talents, patient under
affliction, dutiful and affectionate, modest and virtuous, moral and
religious," was in the habit of " tying this daughter to a bed-post,
flogging her with the most unmerciful severity, aggravating her sufferings by the application of brine, flogging her repeatedly with a

horsewhip, pulling her hair out by the roots, and compelling her to perform the meanest drudgery. It is scarcely necessary to add that the able and enlightened judge before whom the investigation of this case was brought, declared the individual to be " non compos mentis."

If such is in general the real character of partial insanity, and if cases which come near to the idea usually entertained of this disease, are, when and if they occur, rare exceptions to the general fact, it will be allowed that criminality should be attached with extreme caution to any individual in whose case the existence of insane illusion has been proved, however limited in its extent this particular phenomenon of the disease may appear to be. The same considerations ought to weigh in an equal degree in questions which respect the exercise of personal rights.

The only remaining topic connected with illusion which I shall at present consider, is the subject of *lucid intervals.*

Hoffbauer has well observed that much depends upon the duration of lucid intervals. In some instances these intervals are very short; in others they are of equal length with the periods of disease, and sometimes they last much longer than these periods. In the former case the individual has consciousness of his actual state with relation to external circumstances, but not with relation to his former periods of existence. His life is only, in his view, in insulated fragments; his knowledge of himself is inaccurate and confused. This observation can only be applied in a more limited manner to cases in which lucid intervals are nearly of equal duration to the periods of disease. I cannot follow M. Hoffbauer into the inferences which he founds upon this observation.

We must likewise take into consideration the circumstances that repeated attacks of disease weaken the understanding, and that, when they are frequently recurrent, the individual generally falls into a state bordering on dementia, in which the remembrance of persons and relations becomes very defective. In such instances it must become a subject of inquiry to what form and degree of MENTAL DEFICIENCY, as before distinguished, his particular case belongs.

In all examinations respecting insane illusions, it will be necessary to bear in mind the well-known fact that many lunatics display great artifice in evading questions relating to their morbid impressions, even while these impressions are strongly fixed in their minds. Hoffbauer is incorrect in attributing this dissimulation to the supposed fact, that the lunatic during a lucid interval has perceived his hallucination to be absurd. I know that such dissimulation and evasion has been practised in cases in which no lucid intervals have occurred, especially when the lunatic has been frequently interrogated upon the subject of his erroneous convictions. A striking fact, exemplifying this observation, is mentioned by M. Chambeyron.

The statement of what the English law has positively determined with reference to insanity comes within a comparatively short compass. *Lunacy,* when proved to exist, absolves from guilt in criminal

cases. " For," as it is observed by Sir Edward Coke, "the execution of an offender is for example, ' ut pœna ad paucos, metus ad
omnes perveniat ;' but so it is not when a madman is executed; but
should be a miserable spectacle, both against law and of extreme
inhumanity and cruelty, and can be no example to others. But if
there be any doubt whether the party be *compos* or not, this shall be
tried by a jury. And if he be so found, a total idiocy or absolute
insanity excuses from the guilt, and of course from the punishment
of any criminal action committed under such deprivation of the
senses : but if a lunatic hath lucid intervals of understanding, he
shall answer for what he does in those intervals, as if he had no
deficiency. Yet, in the case of absolute madness, as they are not
answerable for their actions, they should not be permitted the liberty
of acting, unless under proper control ; and in particular they ought
not to be suffered to go loose to the terror of the king's subjects."*
The question is, what will be considered as *lunacy?* In the penal
code of France, it seems, from M. Georget's statement, that partial
insanity is a sufficient plea against responsibility for offences : this
we rest upon the sixty-fourth article. It would appear, however,
from the passages cited above from Lord Hale, (which, however, the
reader ought to compare with the original text of that lawyer,) that
partial insanity is not considered in English law as entirely cancelling
responsibility for actions, or consequently culpability, or what the
Germans more correctly term *(strafbarkeit)* punishability.

It is observed by Professor Hoffbauer, that in case of partial illusion it is extremely difficult to ascertain how far the influence of the
insane error extends, and what trains of thoughts and acts of the understanding are within or without the limits of its sphere. If this
be borne in mind, and it be also fully made known to juries that
monomania generally involves a morbid perversion, and sometimes
occasions a total change of the moral character of the individual
affected, the cases of punishable criminality occurring under circumstances of mental disease will probably be reduced to a very small
proportion.

The exercise of civil rights is suspended when a lunatic is proved
to be such : he is neither capable of entering into marriage, nor of
any other contracts. These disqualifications, however, only subsist
during actual derangement : in a lucid interval a lunatic resumes the
exercise of personal rights.

The chancellor, on receiving information as to the state of a deranged person, issues a writ " de lunatico inquirendo," and on lunacy
being established by the verdict of a jury, appoints committees to
take care of the individual as to his person, and to administer his
estate.†

* Blackstone, book iv. c. 2 and 3.
† For further particulars as to the modes of proceding respecting lunatics, see
the Appendix to Dr. Cox's work on Insanity, and Paris and Fonblanque's Medical
Jurisprudence, vol. i. p. 289 & seq.: also Blackstone, book i. c. 8, s. 18. Item,
c. 15, 4. Book ii. c. 19, 1. Book iii. c. 27. Book iv. c. 2, 2.

SECTION IV.—*Of Moral Insanity, in its Relation to Criminal and Civil Law : Observations on the Criterion of Insanity according to English Physicians and Lawyers. Statement of a different Opinion.*

In the preceding pages of this work I have described a form of mental derangement, under the title of moral insanity, consisting in disorder of the moral affections and propensities, without any symptom of illusion or error impressed on the understanding. The question whether such an affection really exists or not is very important in connexion with medical jurisprudence, and I think it indispensable to make some remarks on this subject on the present occasion.

I must first observe that no such disorder has been recognized in the English courts of judicature, or even admitted by medical writers in England. In general, it has been laid down that insanity consists in, and is co-extensive with, mental illusion. English writers admit only that form of insanity which the Germans term *wahnsinn ;* they know nothing of moral insanity either as requiring control in the exercise of civil rights, or as destroying or lessening culpability in criminal ones. Thus in a report of judgment issued not many years since by one of the must distingushed lawyers in this country, it is laid down that "insanity is deluded imagination, the substitution of fancies for realities." In the same report I find the following remarks :—

"As far as my own observation and experience can direct me, aided by opinions and statements I have heard expressed in society, guided also by what has occurred in these and in other courts of justice, or has been laid down by medical and legal writers, the true criterion is—where there is delusion of mind there is insanity ; that is, when persons believe things to exist which exist only, or at least in that degree exist only in their own imagination, and of the non-existence of which neither argument nor proof can convince them, they are of unsound mind ; or, as one of the counsel accurately expressed it, ' it is only the belief of facts which no rational person would have believed, that is insane delusion.' This delusion may sometimes exist on one or two particular subjects, though generally there are other concomitant circumstances, such as eccentricity, irritability, violence, suspicion, exaggeration, inconsistency, and other marks and symptoms which may tend to confirm the existence of delusion, and to establish its insane character."[*]

The right honourable and learned judge afterwards cites some authorities, both medical and legal, in support of his opinion. The former are principally the sentiments of Dr. Battie and Dr. F Willis. Dr. Battie says that " deluded imagination is not only an indispensable, but an essential feature of madness."

---

[*] Report of the judgment in Dew v. Clarke and Clarke, delivered by the Right Hon. Sir J. Nicholl. Lond. 1826.

Dr. F. Willis, in his treatise on mental derangement, which was the substance of the Gulstonian Lecture delivered before the College of Physicians in 1822, thus pointed out the difference, according to his apprehension, between an unsound and a sound mind :—

" A sound mind is one wholly free from delusion.   Week minds, again, only differ from strong ones in the extent and power of their faculties ; but unless they betray symptoms of delusion, their soundness cannot be questioned." " The man of insane mind from disease, having been once compos mentis, pertinaciously adheres to some delusive idea, in opposition to the plainest evidence of its falsity, and endeavours by the most ingenious arguments, however fallacious they may be, to support his opinion."

Lord Coke and Lord Hale are referred to for a similar opinion.

It seem, then, to have been the prevalent judgment both of medical and legal writers in this country, that *delusion*, or as medical writers express themselves, illusion and hallucination constitutes the essential character of insanity, and hence, unless the existence of this characteristic-phenomenon should be proved, it would be very difficult to maintain a plea on the ground of insanity in this country, with a view to the removing culpability in a criminal accusation.

It would be doubtless of advantage to have an opportunity of resorting at once to a criterion so decisive and intelligible, and *in general* so easily brought into evidence, if it were only true in point of fact that insanity always involves that particular circumstance which is supposed to be characteristic of it.   Unfortunately the reality is otherwise.   I am fully persuaded that the time is not for distant when the existence of mental disorder unaccompanied by illusion or any lesion whatever of intellect, will be generally recognized.   I shall not recapitulate the evidence which I have already adduced on this subject in the second chapter of the present work, but shall merely refer my readers to it, and observe that the conclusions which I have there endeavoured to establish will be confirmed and illustrated by facts to be cited in the following pages.

I have already considered the subject of moral insanity in a pathological point of view ; I have now to offer some remarks upon it in its relation to moral delinquency and to criminal jurisprudence.

The precise limitation of insanity and eccentricity of character is very difficult to discover, and I shall not attempt to sift this matter to the bottom on the present occasion.   My readers will find many excellent observations upon it in the work of Dr. Conolly.   Some remarks have been offered upon it in the preceding parts of this volume.   I shall not attempt to refer all examples of extreme oddity or eccentricity to mental disease, but am satisfied with maintaining, as I am fully persuaded, that some instances of this kind really constitute cases of madness.   It is perhaps sufficient, in order to prove this position, to remark that such moral phenomena as those which are designated by these terms, actually arise in many instances, and make their appearance for the first time, after an attack of insanity of a most decided character, from which recovery has been supposed to have taken place ; secondly, that the same traits frequently are met with in families predisposed to insanity ; thirdly, that they often take their rise from obvious and even from physical causes. Eccentricity of character, in order to become at all the object of medical or legal consideration, must assume an aspect threatening evil to society, or at least to the affected individual himself, and his family. Even when such persons are complete pests to society, which sometimes happens, it is, under the present arrangements of the law, very difficult, if not impossible, to interfere with them.

The conclusion that eccentricity of habits or character is not, as implied by common expressions, allied to madness, but actually constitutes in many instances a variety of mental derangement, is of some consequence in respect to one point of criminal legislation. Various cases are on record in which homicides and other atrocious acts have been committed by persons of morose and wayward habits, given up to sullen abstraction, or otherwise differing in their propensities and dispositions from the ordinary character of mankind. In the investigation whether such acts of violence are attributable to insanity or not, it will be important to note the fact that the peculiarities of conduct for which the perpetrators had been otherwise remarkable are sufficient to afford in themselves a strong suspicion of insanity.

This consideration, had it been fully entered into, would have led to an important result in the case of John Howison, who was executed for the murder of Widdow Geddes, at King's Cramond. No well-informed person who reads the account of this unfortunate man's trial, as given in Mr. Simpson's late work " On the Necessity of Popular Education," will entertain a doubt that he was mentally deranged. His case constitutes a very characteristic case of moral insanity. He fell a victim to ignorance.

The principal consideration in which the subject of moral insanity is important in criminal jurisprudence, is that of insane propension to such acts of violence. Homicide, infanticide, suicide have been committed in numerous cases under circumstances which gave room for suspicion as to the sanity of the agent. This plea has been set up in many trials, and has often been rejected by juries, while it has been the opinion of medical persons that there were ample grounds for maintaining it. The questions connected with homicidal insanity require all the elucidation that can be afforded to them, and I shall devote the next section to this subject.

Section V.—*General Observations on Homicidal Madness.*

Homicidal madness is of two very different kinds. Cases are well known to take place in which lunatics, under hallucinations, without any malignant or destructive propensity manifested in their temper or dispositions, have attempted to put men to death for the sake of conferring on them some great fancied benefit, or under an impression that they are fulfilling the commands of an angel or of the

24*

Deity.. M. Esquirol mentions the case of a military officer confined
at Charenton, who talked reasonably on various subjects, but was
often intent on inflicting mortal wounds on those who conversed
with him. He used to invite them to approach him in a tone of
calmness and even of kindness, and say, " Let me cut off your head ;
I will immediately make you alive again, and you will be purified.
I will perform the same office for every body." This individual
gave no sign of anger or malice, and only testified his regret in the
privation of liberty, because it prevented him from performing the
commands laid upon him by the Almighty.

In this and in a great number of parallel instances evident hallucination has existed, and the disease has been intellectual insanity or
monomania according to the sense in which that term was first used
by M. Esquirol ; but there have been many cases of a different kind
in which no lesion of intellect has been discovered : the individual
affected has experienced no other mental change than a powerful
impulse to commit an act destructive of life on some particular
individual, against whom, even at the time of commission, it has
sometimes appeared that he has entertained no malicious feeling.
The fact seems improbable, but it is established by ample and
unquestionable evidence. I shall cite some strong examples.

The following instances were published by M. Marc, and have
already been alluded to by several writers. The facts display, as the
author observes, a contest in the mind of the individual between the
instinctive desire which constitutes the whole manifestation of disease, and the judgment of the understanding still unaffected and
struggling against it.*

" In a respectable house in Germany, the mother of the family
returning home one day, met a servant, against whom she had no
cause of complaint, in the greatest agitation ; she begged to speak
with her mistress alone, threw herself upon her knees, and entreated
that she might be sent out of the house. Her mistress astonished,
inquired the reason, and learned that whenever this unhappy servant
undressed the little child which she nursed, she was struck with the
whiteness of its skin, and experienced the most irresistible desire to
tear it in pieces. She felt afraid that she could not resist the desire,
and preferred to leave the house." " This circumstance occurred
about twenty years ago in the family of M. le Baron de Humboldt,
and this illustrious person permitted me to add his testimony."

" A young lady," continues M. Marc, " whom I examined in one
of the asylums of the capital, experienced a violent inclination to
commit homicide, for which she could not assign any motive. She
was rational on every subject, and whenever she felt the approach of
this dreadful propensity, she entreated to have the strait-waistcoat put
on, and to be carefully watched until the paroxysm, which sometimes lasted several days, had passed."

---

* Consultation Médico-légale pour H. Cornier, femme Berton, accusée d'homicide, par M. Marc, &c. Chez Roux.

"M. R——, a distinguished chemist and a poet, of a disposition naturally mild and sociable, committed himself a prisoner in one of the asylums of the Fauxbourg St. Antoine." "Tormented by the desire of killing, he often prostrated himself at the foot of the altar, and implored the divine assistance to deliver him from such an atrocious propensity, and of the origin of which he could never render an account. When the patient felt that his will was likely to yield to the violence of this inclination, he hastened to the head of the establishment, and requested to have his thumbs tied together with a riband. This slight ligature was sufficient to calm the unhappy R., who, however, finished by endeavouring to commit homicide upon one his friends, and perished in a violent fit of maniacal fury."

"A servant maid, twenty-six or twenty-eight years of age, whose bodily functions were perfectly natural, nevertheless experienced at each period of the catamenia a sort of excitement which did not apparently affect her judgment, but which rendered her extremely dangerous, since, without provocation, she menaced every person with her knife ; and one day having realized her menaces, she was sent to a lunatic hospital."

The following instances of propensity to infanticide are given by Dr. Michu. In both cases the individuals were afflicted by the consciousness of their state, confessed it, and recovered without any sinister event.

"A countrywoman, twenty-four years of age, of a bilious sanguine temperament, of simple and regular habits, but reserved and sullen manners, had been ten days confined with her first child, when suddenly, having her eyes fixed upon it, she was seized with the desire of strangling it. This idea made her shudder ; she carried the infant to its cradle, and went out in order to get rid of so horrid a thought. The cries of the little being, who required nourishment, recalled her to the house : she experienced still more strongly the impulse to destroy it. She hastened away again, haunted by the dread of committing a crime of which she had such horror ; she raised her eyes to heaven, and went into a church to pray.

"This unhappy mother passed the whole day in a constant struggle between the desire of taking away the life of her infant, and the dread of yielding to the impulse. She concealed, until the evening, her agitations from her confessor, a respectable old man, the first who received her confidence, who, having talked to her in a soothing manner, advised her to have recourse to medical assistance.

"When we arrived at the patient's house, she appeared gloomy and low, and felt ashamed of her situation. Being reminded of the tenderness due from a mother to her child, she replied, 'I know how much a mother ought to love her child ; but if I do not love mine, it does not depend upon me.'

"At Bures, the wife of a butcher, forty years of age, of a nervous constitution, the mother of several children, of a mild amiable character, endowed with good sense, who had always enjoyed good health, experienced anxiety of mind in consequence of the derangement of her affairs, of which her husband was a chief cause.

" One night she had a dream, and thought she perceived a cord, which she tried to seize in order to hang herself. On awaking, she was silent, and had confused ideas which soon fixed themselves in a project of strangling her children. She mentioned to her husband, shedding tears, this dreadful design, and requested that her children, and even the knives belonging to the trade, might be put out of her way."

M. Esquirol has repeatedly declared his conviction that there exists a species of homicidal madness, in which " *no disorder of intellect can be discovered ;*" the murderer is driven, as it were, by an irresistible power ; he is under an influence which he cannot overcome, a blind impulse without reason : it is impossible to divine the motive which induces him, without interest or disorder of the intellect, to commit acts so atrocious and so contrary to the laws of nature.

The preceding examples are sufficient to prove the reality of this singular phenomenon in the mental economy. It is an important point to establish the connection of the impulse with certain physical states of the constitution. The facts which I shall now recite will be sufficient for this purpose.

The following case occurred under the care of Dr. Hawkins at the Hitchin Dispensary ; I extract the account of it from Dr. Johnson's Medico-Chirurgical Journal.*

" E. B., a young and hitherto healthy woman, the mother of two children, in humble life but not indigence, applied at the Hitchin Dispensary, in consequence of the most miserable feelings of gloom and despondency, accompanied by a strong and, by her own account, an almost irresistible propensity or temptation, as she termed it, to destroy her infant. This feeling first came upon her about a week before, when the child was a month old, and she was now sunk into an extreme state of dejection. She begged to be continually watched lest she should yield to this strange propensity. The appetite is bad ; bowels loose ; stools dark and offensive ; has occasionally discharged portions of tape-worm from the bowels. Pulse natural ; sleeps ill. This account is taken from the Dispensary report-book, October 1824 ; and the treatment need not be mentioned as the symptoms continued without alteration until March 1825, when the patient took the small-pox. During the eruption the mind was serene and happy, and she was free from the dreadful temptation by which she had been previously harassed : but upon the subsidence of the small-pox, the disease returned with its former horrors. About the middle of April, the disease, without any apparent cause, began to decline, and she was at the end of the month discharged from the dispensary by her own request. Her child was now six months old. She nursed it herself from its birth, and continued to do so until it was twelve months old. She remained free from any disorder till the spring of this year (1828), when she had another child, and about a month after the birth of it she was assailed by this propensity to destroy it. The symptoms continued until the child was half a year old ; and from that time have gradually declined. Occasionally, for a few days, a sort of metastasis takes place ; the propensity to destroy the infant entirely subsides, and the place of it is supplied by an equally strong disposition to suicide. It is worthy of remark, that during the most distressing periods of her disease, she is perfectly aware of the atrocity of the deed she is so powerfully impelled to, and prays fervently to be enabled to withstand so great a temptation. She has repeatedly told Dr. Hawkins that the inclination to destroy her child has been so powerful, that she should certainly have yielded to it, if she had suffered herself to use a knife even at her meals ; for the knife is the instrument which she feels necessitated to employ in the perpetration of the act. Whilst this extraordinary state lasts, the bowels are uniformly relaxed, and the stools of a dark colour and offensive odour. She has suckled all her children for twelve months ; she has had three children, but this dreadful state of mind has supervened on the birth of the two last only. It may be proper to observe that, when suffering from any bodily indisposition, the mind is serene and free from any kind of morbid feeling. This poor woman is by no means deficient in affection for her infant, even in the most trying period of her disease."

The influence of bodily disease is equally obvious in the following case, which has been cited by M. Esquirol.

" A peasant, born at Krambach in Swabia, and of parents who had not very robust health, twenty-seven years old and unmarried, was subject, from nine years of age, to frequent fits of epilepsy. Two years ago his disease changed its character without any apparent cause ; instead of a fit of epilepsy this man found himself from that time attacked with an irresistible desire to commit murder. He felt the approach of this attack sometimes many hours, sometimes a whole day before it seized him. From the moment in which he felt this presentiment, he desired with earnestness that he might be tied down, that he might be loaded with chains, to prevent his committing a horrid crime. ' When the fit takes me,' he said, ' I am impelled to kill or strangle even an infant.' His father and mother, to whom he was tenderly attached, would be the first victims of this murderous propensity. ' My mother,' he cries out with a fearful voice, ' save yourself, or I shall be obliged to murder you.' "

A remarkable case detailed by M. Pinel as an instance of *instinctive fury*, which has been cited by many writers as strikingly characteristic, is equally to my present purpose as evincing the origination of homicidal propensity in some evident disorder as to the physical state of the constitution.

" A man who had previously followed a mechanical occupation, but was afterwards confined at the Bicêtre, experienced, *at regular intervals*, fits of rage ushered in by the following symptoms. At first he experienced a sensation of burning heat in the bowels, with an intense thirst and obstinate constipation ; this sense of heat spread by degrees over the breast, neck, and face, with a bright colour ; sometimes it became still more intense, and produced violent and frequent pulsations in the arteries of those parts, as if they were going to burst ; at last the nervous affection reached the brain, and then the patient was seized with a most irresistible san-guinary propensity ; and if he could lay hold of any sharp instru-ment, he was ready to sacrifice the first person that came in his way. In other respects he enjoyed the free exercise of his reason ; even during these fits he replied directly to questions put to him, and showed no kind of incoherence in his ideas, no sign of delirium ; he even deeply felt all the horror of his situation, and was often penetrated with remorse, as if he was responsible for this mad pro-pensity. Before his confinement at Bicêtre a fit of madness seized him in his own house ; he immediately warned his wife of it, to whom he was much attached ; and he had only time to cry out to her to run away lest he should put her to a violent death. At Bicêtre there appeared the same fits of periodical fury, the same mechanical propensity to commit atrocious actions, directed very often against the inspector, whose mildness and compassion he was continually praising. This internal combat between a sane reason in opposition to sanguinary cruelty, reduced him to the brink of despair, and he has often endeavoured to terminate by death this insupportable struggle. One day he contrived to get possession of the cutting-knife of the shoemaker of the hospital, and inflicted a severe wound upon himself in the right side of his chest and arm, which was followed by a violent hemorrhage Strict seclusion and a strait waistcoat prevented the commission of suicide.

Another remarkable feature in these cases is the tendency of the impulse to spread by imitation. This has been noticed by M. Esquirol, who cites an observation to the same effect from M. Dela-place. He says, " In two cases this affection resulted from the change produced by puberty ; in four the propensity manifested itself after the individual had heard the history of a woman who had strangled an infant and separated its head from its body. This principle of imitation is one frequent cause of madness. ' Some individuals,' said M. Delaplace, 'possess, from their organization, or from bad ex-ample, fatal propensities, which are excited by the description of a criminal action, when it has become the object of public attention. Under this idea the publicity of crimes is not without danger.'

" When the affection has continued for some time, and the indivi-duals possessed with the desire of committing murder have been observed, we have seen that this state is, like the delirium of lunatics, preceded and accompanied by headach and pains in the stomach and bowels ; these symptoms have preceded the impulse to murder, and have become more severe when this dreadful propensity is ex-asperated."

The influence of imitation or sympathy in exciting this strange propensity is illustrated by the results of Henriette Cornier's trial. This was a very remarkable case of infanticide, which underwent much discussion, and became the subject of very general conversation in France. Many females of respectable classes, who were strongly impressed by the relation and the horror occasioned .by it, were seized with a similar propensity. M. Esquirol has detailed the circumstances attending several of these cases, on which he was privately consulted.

SECTION VI.—*Continuation of the same subject. Allusion to some remarkable Cases exemplifying Homicidal Madness, and the character of Moral Insanity.*

Several remarkable cases of homicide have been brought before the tribunals of justice in France during late years, which have excited much discussion. Among the physicians of Paris there are many who by their great talents, their expanded views, and disinterested attachment to the cause of science, as well as to that of enlightened philanthropy, do honour to their profession and to humanity. Some of them, struck forcibly with the conviction that the cases alluded to were examples of insanity, laboured assiduously to convince the public of this fact. They could not prevent the sacrifice of several unfortunate beings, already smitten by the hand of the Almighty with the most deplorable of earthly calamities, to the proceedings of what among civilised nations is still termed justice. But the discussion which these cases underwent, and particularly the powerful writings of the late M. Georget on the subject, have had the effect of changing public opinion materially in France as to the real nature of actions, which are either atrocious crimes, or the dreadful effects of disease. It is almost certain that a more rational and humane proceeding will be followed in cases that may occur hereafter, and that means will be more generally adopted for the prevention of similar evils by taking due care of individuals who indicate by their conduct such fearful propensities. The most remarkable of the cases referred to were those of Leger, Feldtmann, Lecouffe, Jean Pierre, Papavoine, and lastly Henriette Cornier, who was spared. An account of these was published by M. Georget, from which I shall abstract a few particulars.

Antoine Leger, vine-dresser, old soldier, was tried before the assize court at Versailles, in 1824. In an extract from his accusation, it is stated that he appeared, from his youth, "sombre et farouche," loved solitude, and shunned females and boys of his own age. In June, 1823, he fled from his home, and concealed himself in a forest, where he lived for weeks, sleeping in a cave, and eating wild fruits. He one day caught a rabbit, which he killed and devoured raw. In his lonely abode a desire seized him, according to his own account, to eat human flesh and to drink blood. Seeing one day a little girl near the margin of the wood, he seized her, murdered her, sucked her blood, and afterwards buried her body. Three days afterwards he was apprehended : at first he denied the charge, and invented absurd stories, but at length, being confronted with the body and interrogated, he avowed the fact. He afterwards acknowledged with calmness all the horrible details of the accusation. " Ici l'act retrace les détails relatifs au voil, à la mutilation des organes genitaux, et à l'arrachement du cœur." Before the audience his countenance displayed profound apathy, even an air of gaiety and satisfaction, but after hearing the deposition of the mother he was affected, and said, with tears, " Je suis faché de l'avoir privée de sa fille ; je lui en demande bien pardon." He then resumed his indifference : in the same state of mind he heard his sentence of death. MM. Esquirol and Gall examined his head : the former discovered morbid adhesions of the pia mater to the brain. M. Georget, after examining the facts of the case, concludes as follows. " Leger n'était donc pas, comme on l'a dit, un grand criminel, un monstre, un cannibale, un anthropophage, qui avait voulu rénouveler l'example du festin d'Atrée. Cet individu était, suivant nous, un malheureux imbecille, un aliéné qui devait être renfermé à Bicêtre parmi les fous."

Feldtmann was a tailor, fifty-six years old, who, according to his own account of himself, had been " comme fou" in his youth from the effect of an injury of his head : he was occasionally idiotical or deranged, but in general industrious and honest. After attempting to gratify an incestuous passion for his own daughter, who had invoked the aid of the police to resist his attacks, he stabbed her to the heart, wounded his wife and another daughter, and then gave himself up willingly to a crowd who surrounded him, exclaiming, in reply to their reproaches, " C'est bien fait." In this case the existence of insanity was not fully established by facts, but it seemed evident that the miserable wretch, who suffered for his offence, had scarcely intellect enough to comprehend its nature, and to perceive the turpitude of his conduct, though he foresaw the destiny which awaited him. M. Breschet considered his brain to be in a condition different from that of health, and M. Georget's opinion was that Feldtmann was a man whose weak intellect was overwhelmed by a passion constituting in itself a real disease, which *ought to have been cured by separating the unfortunate wretch from society,* without resorting to the barbarous expedient of extinguishing it together with his life.

Louis Lecouffe was an epileptic from infancy, had often been deranged, had seen visions, and had been accounted by all who knew him to be deranged or idiotic. At the instigation of his mother, he was induced to rob and murder a woman against whom he entertained no malicious feelings. He was executed. This was a case not strictly of moral insanity, but of imbecility, which rendered the accused a victim to the evil influence of other persons possessed of greater intelligence.

The case of Jean Pierre was one of simulated madness.

L. A. Papavoine was a solitary, morose wretch, who was considered by all who knew him to be half crazy and melancholic. Wandering in the wood of Vincennes, he saw a lady walking with two young children. He went to a village and bought a knife ; returning quickly, he accosted the lady with pale looks and agitation, and stooping suddenly, stabbed one of the children : while the affrighted mother attempted to remove it, he killed the other. He took flight, but was overtaken and brought to trial ; and though he was proved to have been insane, and it was manifest that he had perpetrated the horrible act without motive, and under the influence of disease, was put to death according to law. Papavoine afterwards declared that he could not assign any motive for his act ; that it arose from a spontaneous impulse. The circumstances of the case were very perplexing ; and though the opinions of physicians leaned to the probable existence of insanity, they were not decided. M. Georget says, " Comme médecin nous ne pourrons que rester en doute sur cette question grave : c'est dire que comme juré nous aurions voté pour l'acquittement."

In a subsequent publication by the same author, we find particulars of the trial of Henriette Cornier, which excited so much attention in France that many females, by sympathy or imitation, or by the mere influence of imagination, became severely agitated by the desire or the dread of committing similar outrages. The details of this horrible affair are similar in many respects to those of the cases already cited, except in the circumstances that Henriette, after perpetrating the act influenced by no imaginable motive but an insane impulse to destroy the life of a child of which she had always appeared fond, made no attempt whatever to escape or defend herself, but after confessing that she had determined to kill it, sat down and awaited her arrest with perfect indifference. A copious extract from this singular history has been given in the Cyclopædia of Practical Medicine, under the head of Soundness and Unsoundness of Mind ; and I shall omit to repeat it at present for the sake of brevity. The woman was condemned to imprisonment with hard labour, after the subject had undergone much discussion, and the trial had been deferred in consequence of doubts which the public in France had begun to entertain as to the real nature of similar cases.*

Professor Fodéré of Strasburg has expressed a very different opinion from that of M. Georget on several of the cases above cited, of which he has given a somewhat vague and slight account in his last work. His remarks on this subject are scarcely worthy of the high and justly merited reputation of the author, and display the influence of strong prejudice. The discussion was taked up in a very different

* It is observed by M. Georget that the judges on this trial evinced reluctance to suffer a clear investigation by physicians of the actual mental state of the accused, and in other respects exerted an unusual influence towards the condemnation. The public sentiment appears to have been against that of the physicians, and M. Georget was treated with ridicule by the journalists of Paris. Yet it is impossible to read the account of this trial, which is given from official documents, without strongly suspecting that the unfortunate woman who was the subject of it acted under the influence of an impulse which resulted from disease.

spirit in this country by the author of an excellent paper in the Edinburgh Law Journal. In this the author, Mr. Simpson, has collected much information on the subject of homicide resulting from insane impulse : and in addition to several of the preceding cases from M. Georget's first publication, has adduced many instances which have occurred in Great Britain. The most striking of them is the case of Howison already alluded to. Howison, like several of the madmen mentioned by Georget, had been a solitary, gloomy recluse ; he had displayed moral insanity in his habits, and had been subject to illusions of the senses. He was condemned. Even after the trial additional facts were brought forward in proof of his insanity, of which persons who had always known him never doubted. The King was petitioned by the Society of Friends ; but mercy and even further inquiry were refused.

On the whole it seems fully manifest that there is a form of insanity, existing independently of any lesion of the intellectual powers, in which, connected in some instances with evident constitutional disorder, in others with affections of the nervous system excited according to well-known laws of the animal economy, a sudden and often irresistible impulse is experienced to commit acts which under a sane condition of mind would be accounted atrocious crimes. Most of the French writers by whom this affection has been recognised, particularly Messrs. Esquirol, Georget, Marc, and Michu, have termed it "*monomanie homicide*," which is assuredly an erroneous designation, unless the sense of *monomania* is to be changed. That term is always used to express *partial illusion*, or intellectual derangement affecting only a certain train of ideas ; whereas, in connection with the homicidal impulse now under consideration, there is confessedly no delusive opinion impressed on the belief, and the intellectual faculties are wholly unaffected.

It must be allowed that instances may and do occur in which the discrimination would be difficult between manifestations of insanity and acts of a criminal nature, and that this difficulty would be increased by the admission of a form of insanity free from hallucination or illusion. The following remarks, taken chiefly from M. Esquirol's essay on this subject, may tend in some instances to lessen the ambiguity,

1. Acts of homicide perpetrated or attempted by insane persons have generally been preceded by other striking peculiarities of action, noted in the conduct of the same individuals ; often by a total change of character.

2. The same individuals have been discovered in many instances to have attempted suicide, to have expressed a wish for death ; sometimes they have begged to be executed as criminals.

3. These acts are without motive ; they are in opposition to the known influences of all human motives. A man murders his wife and children, known to have been tenderly attached to them ; a mother destroys her infant.

4. The subsequent conduct of the unfortunate individual is gen-

erally characteristic of his state. He seeks no escape or flight ;
delivers himself up to justice ; acknowledges the crime laid to his
charge ; describes the state of mind which led to its perpetration :
or he remains stupefied and overcome by a horrible consciousness of
having been the agent in an atrocious deed.

5. The murderer has generally accomplices in vice and crime:
there are assignable inducements which led to its commission, motives
of self-interest, of revenge, displaying wickedness premeditated.
Premeditated are in some instances the acts of the madman ; but his
premeditation is peculiar and characteristic.

To these considerations I may add that presumptions of insanity
in any particular instance are afforded by the previous existence of
that disease or of epilepsy in the same individual. Respecting the
latter, it has been shown by M. Georget that a very large proportion
of epileptics are particularly subject to violent agitations of passion ;
that they are rendered by their physical state morbidly irascible,
impetuous, incapable of restraining the sudden expression and gratification of their desires, while a considerable number of the same
afflicted persons are weakened in their intellect, if not reduced to
dementia or incoherence. In reference to the other point above
alluded to, 1 shall cite the forcible and highly judicious observation
of Mr. Simpson :—" There is so much evil in the very risk that
man's vengeance should follow God's visitation, that all cases of
crimes of violence, I repeat, in which previous mental disease is
unequivocally proved, should have the whole benefit of the presumption that such disease may in a moment run into irresponsible mania,
and the unhappy patient be judged fit for confinement, and not for
punishment."

The difficulties with which administrators of justice have to contend in distinguishing crimes from the result of insane impulse will
never be entirely removed, but they will be rendered much less
important when the good sense of the community shall have produced
the effect of abolishing all capital punishments. That this will sooner
or later happen I entertain no doubt. Many persons have begun
already to hesitate as to the moral rectitude of putting men to death
in cases in which the powerful motive of self-defence cannot be
pleaded, and when it is easy to keep the offending individual out of
the way of committing further mischief. A single private individual
would scarcely think himself justified in taking upon himself the
office of the Almighty, and inflicting moral punishment on a person
whom he knew to have perpetrated a crime. If such an act would
be, not meritorious, but culpable, when executed by one individual,
it does not seem clear how it becomes more righteous when that
person has any given number of accomplices, or in other words,
what invests any number of individuals, say twelve men, over whom
presides a thirteenth, with the right to put to death a fellow-creature
who has incurred guilt. The community is but an aggregate of individuals. How come such an aggregate of individuals to be possessed, morally, of the right to take away life, the plea of self-defence
being precluded by the circumstances of the case ?

SECTION VII.—*Of Suicide.*

The question whether the act of suicide constitutes a proof of insanity was agitated before the parliament of Paris in 1777, but was set aside by some proceedings of form. The prevalent opinion is, that insanity is not always the cause of suicide, though the verdict of lunacy is generally brought in by juries, owing to the extreme barbarity of the law on this subject.

M. Fodéré has expressed long ago the opinion that suicide is always the result of madness. Though every one would wish to be of the same sentiment, it seems difficult to maintain it when we consider the frequent and almost ordinary occurrence of suicide in some countries, as among the Romans, who, as Pliny says, esteemed it " quod homini dedit optimum Deus in tantis vitæ pœnis."*

But in a great proportion of cases suicide is certainly the result of physical disease. The arguments on which this opinion is founded may be summed up briefly under the following heads.

1. The propensity to suicide is very often combined with the impulse to homicide. This has been observed long ago, but the evidence adduced by M. Falret puts the fact beyond all doubt.† These impulses are so often conjoined as to prove clearly that the conditions which give rise to one are in close affinity and conjunction with those from which the other originates.

2. Suicide is in a very marked and striking manner hereditary ; and this is a strong ground for regarding it as constitutional, or depending on disorder in the state of organic structure. Dr. Rush, M. Esquirol, and others have recorded instances of the hereditary transmission of this propensity. M. Falret has collected a variety of observations on the subject, and has concluded that, of all the kinds of insanity, the form distinguished by this tendency is probably that which the most frequently becomes hereditary.

3. Like other forms of madness, suicidal insanity prevails most in certain seasons and temperatures. M. Falret says it is most frequent in the summer and autumn. MM. Fodéré and Duglas observed that at Marseilles suicides were most frequent when the thermometor of Reaumur was 22 degrees above zero.

4. Acts of suicide, like those of homicide, are generally preceded by a morbid change in the character and habits of the agent. Individuals who had been cheerful, active, animated, taking a lively interest in the pursuits of life, in the society of their friends, in their families, become melancholy, torpid, morose, and feel an aversion towards their relatives or most intimate associates, become listless and indifferent. These appearances have often been observed to be the preludes of some attempts at suicide, and have sometimes put the relatives of the individual on their guard, and have led to a prevention of the fatal catastrophe.

---

* Fodéré, Traité de Médecine Légale, t. i. p. 272.   1813.
† De l'Hypochondrie et du Suicide, p. 170 et seq.   Paris, 1822.

5. Suicide is connected in many instances with disease of structure, or with disorders of the functions of physical life, some of which have been detected by necroscopy, others by observations made before death. This general fact is sufficiently established by the observations made on the subject by Awenbrugger, Leroy, Fodéré, and Esquirol, although we must confess that the same obscurity yet involves the physical causes of suicidal as of other forms of insanity.

6. Like the impulse to homicide, this propensity to suicide is simply a moral perversion, and therefore neither of these affections falls within the restricted definition of insanity, which has been the most prevalent one. There is generally no particular illusion impressed on the understanding of the self-destroyer; on the other hand, there is a perversion of the strongest instinct of nature, that of self-preservation. Nature has ordained no law more universal in its influence than the desire which all animated beings display, and which is indeed the governing principle in the greater part of their actions, to preserve their existence, and to secure themselves from the influence of circumstances which bring it into danger. It is the characteristic of moral insanity to pervert the natural instincts or propensities, and suicide displays the most signal of these perversions.

SECTION VIII.—*Of other Manifestations of morbid Propensity.*

There are several modifications of moral insanity, and two most decided examples which require the arrangements suggested by Hoffbauer in some cases of imbecility : I allude to the placing of individuals under *curatela,* or guardianship, for personal security, who do not require confinement. Extreme parsimony has induced persons to starve themselves. When an individual would destroy himself through this propensity. which is in many instances the effect of disease, he is sometimes declared a lunatic and sent to a place of confinement. There is no other way of proceeding by which his life can be saved under the existing regulations. But confinement is unnecessary for such a person, who is in no way dangerous to society. If the management of his property—for such individuals are generally possessed of property—could be so settled as to ensure his having the usual supports of life, this would be sufficient. Another case is that of profuse extravagance, and this is the most common. Individuals whose moral character is perverted by disease often become profusely extravagant, and the apprehension of ruin to their families is the motive which induces the latter to take measures with a view to prevent such a calamity. Confinement is more often requisite with regard to cases of this description than those of an opposite one, on account of other manifestations of disorder which are combined with the leading propensity : but there are probably many individuals who are wholly incompetent, through a habit of thoughtless extravagance resulting from disease, to administer their own estates, or manage their domestic affairs, and in whose condition there is yet nothing that requires confinement in a mad-house. Many of these are examples of extreme difficulty as to the proceedings which ought to be adopted. It will be advantageous, however, to the medical persons who may be consulted in such cases, to be fully in possession of the circumstances connected with them, and aware of the difficulties with which they are surrounded, although these difficulties may be almost insuperable.*

Under the head of *moral insanity* I have adverted to a form of disease of which the principal or sole manifestation is a propensity to break and destroy whatever comes within reach of the individual ; in short, an irresistible impulse to commit injury or do mischief of all kinds. This propensity is observed in cases in which it is impos-

---

* So much space has been already devoted to the subjects treated in the present chapter, that I must only allude to the curious and interesting relations between crimes properly so termed and cases of insanity which have been pointed out by late writers on moral statistics. The following brief statement of some results obtained by M. Quetelet in his " *Recherches Statistiques sur le Royaume des Pays Bas*," which I extract from Professor Fodéré's treatise already cited, will be perused with interest by such of my readers as are yet unacquainted with the works of these writers.

" Afin d'explorer les causes qui agissent pour développer ou pour amortir le penchant au crime, l'auteur a passé en revue l'âge, les sexes, les professions, les saisons, les climats ; après avoir établi d'après des chiffres que dans les deux royaumes de France et des Pays-Bas, le nombre des crimes contre les personnes n'est que d'environ le quart de tous ceux qui ont été jugés par les différentes cours de justice, pendant l'intervalle de trois années (ce qui est la même chose en Angleterre), et que ces crimes ont principalement été commis dans l'âge de la plus grande violence des passions, M. Quetelet nous apprend qu' il a réconnu que le développement du penchant au crime a un rapport trèsdirect avec le développement des forces physiques de l'homme, et celui de sa raison ; que c'est entre 20 et 30 ans que l'homme, poussé par la violence de ses passions, se livre d'abord au viol et aux attentats à la pudeur ; qu'il commence aussi à entrer dans la carrière du vol, qu'il semble suivre comme par instinct jusqu'à son dernier souspir ; qu'il est porté ensuite par le développement complet de ses forces physiques à tous les actes de violence, à l'homicide, à la rebellion, aux vols sur les chemins publics ; que plus tard la reflexion convertit le meurtre en assassinat ou en empoisonnement ; qu' enfin l'homme, en avançant dans la carrière de la vie, et en même tems dans celle du crime, substitue de plus en plus la ruse à la force, et devient faussaire, plus qu'à toute autre époque de sa vie ; que c'est communément l'âge de 40 à 50 ans, qui fournit le plus d'accusés de délits contre les propriétes, et le moins, contre les personnes ; que d'après un article que M. Esquirol a inséré dans les Annales d'Hygiène, du mois d'Avril 1829, les résultats sont les mêmes, quant à l'âge et aux saisons, pour les aliénations mentales par les nombres qu'il a réunis à Charenton, en 1826, 1827, et 1828 ; de l'âge de 10 et de 15 ans, 0 ; de 20 ans 24 à 25 ans, 79 ; à 30 ans, 109 ; à 35 ans, 134 ; à 40 ans, 128 ; à 45 ans, 129 ; à 50 ans, 131 ; à 55 ans, 108 ; à 60 ans, 51 : à 70 ans et plus, 63 ; or y ayant quant à l'âge à peu près les mêmes proportions pour les deux sexes, dans l'échelle criminelle tant contre les personnes que contre les propriétés, il en résulte suivant M. Quetelet, que l'âge exerce la même influence pour faire naître ou diminuer le nombre des aliénations mentales et des crimes contre les personnes, en même tems que le développement intellectuel et moral qui s'opère avec plus de lenteur, favorise le penchant au crime contre les propriétés depuis l'âge de 40 à 50 ans, bien plus, il y aurait un connexion suivant l'auteur, entre les crimes réfléchis, l'aliénation, et l'aptitude à la composition des chefs-d'œuvres dramatiques laquelle n'aurait presque jamais eû lieu qu' à l'âge de 45 à 50 ans."

sible to discover any motive influencing the mind of the person who is the subject of it. No illusive belief, for example, can be detected, that the lunatic is performing a duty in perpetrating that which manifests his disease. There are, indeed, cases of a different description in which such an illusion is the groundwork of the proceeding, but these belong to another class of mental disorders.

Many lunatics, whose disorder was merely a destructive propensity, have set fire to houses or public buildings, and it is not to be doubted that men have been occasionally executed as criminals for such actions, who, if they had been kept in confinement, would have proved to be insane. Until the existence of moral insanity is distinctly recognized, there will always be a danger of this event ensuing on the trials of mischievous lunatics. Popular feeling is generally excited in such instances against the perpetrator of a destructive act, and this circumstance increases by much the probability of a criminal condemnation.

CHAPTER XII.

OF ECSTATIC AFFECTIONS.

Section I.—*General Account—Ordinary phenomena.*

Under the general term of ecstatic affections I purpose to comprise several states of the nervous system more or less analogous to each other, but differing in various particulars. The common characteristic which associates them is a suspension either perfect or incomplete of external sense, while the imagination is in state of activity, and the individual is not conscious of his real condition, but fancies himself to exist under different circumstances from those which actually surround him. Dreaming is one modification of their state, but it does not afford so great a variety of phenomena as somnambulism, or display so many peculiar signs of the real condition of the faculties. Many forms of delirium, catalepsy, trance or ecstacy, and some other conditions which have been regarded as examples of insanity—those for instance in which the patient on recovery is found suddenly to have lost all recollection of what had passed during the period of his disease—belong to the same class of affections.

An inquiry into the real character and pathological relations of dreaming and somnambulism will afford us an opportunity of throwing some light on a variety of obscure phenomena which display themselves in the state of the system above described, and this inquiry will prove the more interesting through its bearing on some speculations which have become of late prevalent, especially in France and in Germany. I allude to animal magnetism, and the various hypotheses to which the practice of that art has given rise. There are likewise curious facts connected with the histories of trance or ecstacy and of febrile delirium, and it is probable that phenomena which appear so recondite and mysterious, may be rendered more comprehensible by a comparison with the more ordinary events of dreaming and somnambulation.

There is an obvious relation between the state of the faculties in somnambulism and that which exists during dreams. It is, indeed, probable that somnambulism is dreaming in a manner so modified, that the will recovers its usual power over muscular motion, and likewise becomes endued with a peculiar control over the organs of sense and perception. This power, which gives rise to the most curious phenomena of somnambulism, is of such a kind, that, while the senses are in general obscured, as in sleep, and all other objects are unperceived, the somnambulator manifests a faculty of seeing, feeling, or otherwise discovering those particular objects of which he is in pursuit, towards which his attention is by inward movement directed, or with which the internal operations of his mind bring him into relation.

The near connexion between somnambulism and dreams is established by the following considerations:—

1. Sleepwalkers, after they have awakened from the slumbers which ushered in and continued after somnambulation, have sometimes remembered the circumstances or adventures of the period, and have correctly related them as the impressions of a dream. This fact has been noticed by Sylvius and by Hoffmann : " Somniantibus et somniorum ratione obvenire hominibus somnambulorum affectum patet ex ipsorum evigilantium relatu, putantium se somniâsse duntaxat, quæ actu fecerunt." A striking instance of this kind is related by Horstius. A young nobleman in the citadel of Brenstein was observed by his brothers, who occupied the same room, to rise in his sleep, put on his cloak, and, having opened the casement, to mount, by the help of a pulley, to the roof of the building. There he was seen to tear in pieces a magpie's nest, and wrap the young birds in his cloak. He returned to his apartment, and went to bed, having placed his cloak by him with the birds in it. In the morning he awoke, and related the adventure as having occurred in a dream, and was greatly surprised when he was led to the roof of the tower and shown the remains of the nest, as well as the magpies concealed in his cloak. A similar observation as to the occasional remembrance of the impressions made on the mind during somnambulism, was made long ago by Muratori, to whose work I shall again have occasion to refer.

2. As in dreams, so likewise in somnambulism the individual is intent on the pursuit of objects towards which his mind had been previously directed in a powerful manner, and his attention strongly roused ; he is in both states impelled by habit, under the influence of which he repeats the routine of his daily observances. A somnambulator is a dreamer who is able to act his dreams.

Many facts may be cited in proof of this remark. A man known to me, who was accustomed to attend a weekly market, rose from his bed, saddled his horse, and actually proceeded on his journey as far as a turnpike, which being closed during the night, he was awakened by the circumstance. Another individual who had been in the habit of frequenting a public promenade, where he used to meet his acquaintances, was seen to rise from his bed at night and walk in his shirt along the same path, which extended for a mile on the brow of a hill, stopping very frequently and greeting different individuals whom he had been accustomed to see in the same place. Hoffmann relates the case of a somnambulator who dreamed that he was going to set out on a journey, rose and put on his clothes, shoes, and spurs, and then striding across the sill of an open window, began to kick with his heels and to exert his voice, supposing that he was exciting his horse to speed. Henricus ab Heer mentions another person, a student at an university in Germany, who, having been very intent on the composition of some verses which he could not complete to his satisfaction, rose in his sleep, and opened his desk, sat down with great earnestness to renew his attempt. At length, having succeeded, he returned to bed, after reciting his composition aloud, and setting his papers in order as before. Martinet gives the case of a man who was accustomed to rise in his sleep and pursue his business as a saddler.

M. Bertrand considers it to be a peculiar feature of somnambulism that the individual, though on waking he is generally found to have lost all recollection of what passed during his sleep, yet recalls, when the periods of this state return, the whole train of obliterated ideas. "Somnambulism," as the same writer observes, "thus constitutes really a new life, returning at unequal intervals, connected together by a new species of memory."* We may observe that something of this kind is perceived in the instance of dreams. A person strongly impressed by a dream, on again falling asleep, experiences not unfrequently a recurrence of the same impressions, and the imagination will even take up the dream at the precise point where it was before interrupted.

These observations seem to prove that somnambulism is a modification of dreaming ; and this conclusion appears so probable, that it will perhaps be admitted without hesitation ; yet there are many writers of great research and ability who maintain a different opinion. Bertrand, who has investigated the circumstances connected with the history of sleep-walking with great pains and accuracy, considers the state in question to be something entirely different from dreaming. The same opinion is expressed in the most positive manner by Professor Heinroth, who says that somnambulists are to be reckoned as awake, since their perceptive powers is in some respects even more acute than during the ordinary waking state ; and that this condition bears no relation to dreaming, inasmuch as dreamers exist in an ideal world, whereas night-wanderers are conversant with actually existing and material objects.† Both of these writers maintain an opinion

* Traité du Somnambulisme, par A. Bertrand. Paris, 1823.
† Lehrbuch der Stoerungen des Seelenlebens und ihrer Behandlung, von Professor J. C. A. Heinroth. Leipsig, 1818, b. ii. p. 270.

which is very prevalent in France and Germany, that somnambulists, as well as persons who have been brought into a state resembling that of sleep-walking by the process of animal magnetism, have the ordinary channels of sensation entirely closed ; that they neither see with their eyes nor hear with their ears, but are endowed with a peculiar mode of sensation, which, in its highest degree, constitutes what is termed *clairvoyance.* This is supposed to be diffused over the whole surface of the body, but to be especially seated in the epigastrium and fingers' ends. It is not exactly sight or hearing, but fulfils all the functions of both these modes of perception.

An opinion so improbable will be thought by some scarcely worthy of consideration. Its extensive reception, however, among a large number of continental writers, together with some other reasons which will become apparent, must prevent my passing it over as an idle speculation. The facts, also, of somnambulism are, as I have above remarked, deserving of further attention on account of their relation to a variety of obscure pathological phenomena, with which I shall have to compare them. For these reasons I deem it advisable to enter into further details of the history of somnambulism ; but in order that my readers may be fully aware of the points connected with this subject which are controverted, and may be prepared to collect from the facts adduced the evidence which they are calculated to afford, I shall in the first place lay before them a brief history of animal magnetism, as I have collected it from the French and German writers who have delivered it.

Section II.—*Of Artificial Somnambulism : History of Animal Magnetism.*

It is well known that the practisers of animal magnetism profess to have the power of calling forth, by the exercise of their art, a state of the system analogous to that of natural somnambulism, or to the ecstasy of cataleptic persons, and that surprising accounts are related of individuals in this state. They are said to become possessed of *clairvoyance,* a sort of second sight, or the power of seeing at an indefinite distance, of foretelling future events, discovering diseases in the interior of their own bodies and in those of others, knowing the unexpressed thoughts of persons by whom they are magnetised, or with whom they are brought into magnetic connection. Such testimonies are treated in this country with the ridicule which they seem at the first view of the subject to deserve ; they are rejected in the mass ; few persons give themselves the trouble to inquire whether there is any basis of truth on which a superstructure of such extraordinary pretensions has been raised. The Germans and French have treated the matter differently. Among the physiologists and other scientific men on the continent, many are persuaded that animal magnetism, though its powers have been greatly exaggerated, is not without a foundation in truth, and even contains in itself the discovery of some hitherto unknown and very important fact or series of facts in the animal economy. M. Cuvier expressed this opinion many years since, and long before the persuasion became so general as it is at present. He says, " We must confess that it is very difficult, in the experiments which have for their object the action that the nervous system of two different individuals can exercise one upon the other, to distinguish the effect of the imagination of the individual upon whom the experiment is tried, from the physical results produced by the person who acts upon him. The effects, however, obtained on persons ignorant of the agency, and upon individuals whom the operation itself has deprived of consciousness, and those which animals present, do not permit us to doubt that the proximity of two animated bodies in certain positions, combined with certain movements, *have a real effect.* independently of all participation of the fancy. It appears also clearly that these effects arise from some communication which is established between their nervous systems." Here we find Baron Cuvier apparently giving a full assent to the fundamental doctrine of the animal magnetists.

M. De la Place, in his work entitled "Théorie Analytique du Calcul des Probabilités," says, " The singular phenomena which result from the extreme sensibility of the nerves of some individuals, have given rise to many opinions upon the existence of a new agent, that has been called animal magnetism. It is natural to suppose that the action of these causes is of a very delicate nature, and very easily disturbed by a number of accidental circumstances; thus, when in many cases it is not manifested, we must not conclude that it does not exist. We are so far from knowing all the agents of nature and their different modes of action, that it would be very unphilosophical to deny the existence of phenomena solely because they are inexplicable in the present state of our knowledge."

In Germany and other northern countries animal magnetism has long had partisans among men celebrated for their attainments in science, and for their rank in the medical profession.

The supporters of animal magnetism carry back its history, as do the historians of freemasonry, to a period of high antiquity. Some of these writers persuade us that it was the great arcanum of the mysteries, the initiations, and secret ceremonies of the pagan world; that the vertigo of the Delphian priestess, the prophetic visions of the sybils, the wonderful powers of magic, the raptures of eastern seers, and, in fact, all that is related of miraculous or portentous in former periods of the world, is to be explained by reference to this power, now for the first time developed and understood. Many passages have been discovered in the writings of the ancients which have appeared to afford some plausible ground for the supposition that animal magnetism was not unknown to the priests who ministered in the temples of Æsculapius, or in those of Apollo. Some of these passages bear allusions more or less obvious or probable to ceremonies not unlike those of the magnetisers. In none is the allusion in this sense more closely applicable than in a passage attributed to Solon, and preserved by Stobæus, which was first pointed out in a work very recently published:—

> " The smallest hurts sometimes increase and rage
> More than all art of physic can assuage.
> Sometimes the fury of the worst disease
> The hand by gentle stroking will appease."*

A passage in Plautus has been cited to the same purpose. The poet means to express, in a humorous manner, "What if I knock him down?" *Quid si illum tractim tangam ut dormiat!* There seems, as it was remarked by Schelling, to be an allusion to some method of setting persons asleep by a particular process of manipulation similar to that of the magnetisers.†

It has been only in periods comparatively recent, and especially in the visionary times of Paracelsus and Van Helmont, that we find theories becoming general which approach very nearly to those of Mesmer, and in fact identify themselves with the very speculations which that singular person actually adopted and made the basis of his art. The doctrine of a subtle fluid universally diffused, which was supposed to be the agent in all the great movements of the heavenly bodies, was very long general, and served to account for the phenomena of electricity and of magnetism at the several periods of their discovery. By the chemical physiologists this fluid was imagined to have its chief seat in organized living bodies. Here a preparation was obviously made for pretensions such as those with which Mesmer began his career.‡

Antony Mesmer was a Switzer by birth, who came to Vienna in low circumstances to study medicine. After being for some years an auditor of Van Swieten and Von Haen's prelections, he took his degree in 1776, and wrote his inaugural dissertation, "*On the Influence of the Planets on the Human Body.*" According to his theory all the phenomena of life depend upon a particular current of the universal magnetic fluid enclosed in each organized body. It can be increased or diminished in intensity by external agencies, and especially by the medium of magnetic instruments. According to Bertrand, Mesmer was a man of very moderate talents, but possessed with an ardent desire to distinguish himself by novelties, and by escaping from the beaten track of his contemporaries. Maximilian Hell, a Jesuit, an astronomer at Vienna, had invented artificial magnets of different forms. Mesmer, in conjunction with Hell, made

* See Mr. Colquhoun's Introduction to the Report on Animal Magnetism by a Committee of the Royal Academy of Medicine of Paris.
† Versuch einer darstellung des Animalischen Magnetismus als Heilsmittel von C. A. F. Kluge. Berlin, 1818.
‡ Kluge has a long catalogue, filling several pages with the titles of works published in various countries on animal magnetism before the time of Mesmer. Van Helmont, Goclenius, Fludd, and Athanasius Kircher, are some of the most celebrated names which occur among the authors of these; and, judging from the titles, one might suppose that many of the modern doctrines as well as practices had been long ago anticipated. In England, Valentine Greatrakes was particularly celebrated. See Mr. Colquhoun's Introduction; Kluge's Derstellung, p. 19; and Dr. Stieglitz, über den thierischen magnetismus,—" *Die Geschichte des Mermerismus vor Mesmer.*"

experiments on the influence of these on the living body, with results as marvellous as those which Perkins obtained in later times by his tractors. The effects of the magnetic remedy were published, but the statements of Mesmer were contradicted by Hell, and only drew on their author ridicule and contempt ; and Mesmer quitted Vienna for Paris, as affording a more ample field. At the latter place he took up his residence in 1778 ; and here he soon became the object of general curiosity. Crowds of persons, of all ages and both sexes, resorted to him, in the hope of obtaining cures for their complaints ; and his fame spread far and wide. He made some attempts to obtain the sanction of the Academy of Sciences and of the Royal Society of Medicine ; but being treated with coldness, he expressed his contempt for such bodies, and declared that he sought patronage from the king, the father of his people, and not that "*d'un tas de petits importans.*" After some interval Mesmer addressed himself to the faculty of medicine, and became intimately associated with M. Deslon, a *docteur régent* of that body, and physician to the Count d'Artois, who strongly espoused his part, notwithstanding the resolution of the faculty to expel any of its associates who refused to enter into a positive renunciation of Mesmer and his pretentions. Mesmer talked of leaving France and carrying his precious discovery into foreign countries : but the multitude of persons who placed a high value on his curative power prevailed upon the government to offer him a stipend of 30,000 livres in order to fix him among them. This he disdainfully refused, and went to Spa, where he was residing when the alarming intelligence was brought him that Deslon had set up for himself, and was magnetising multitudes in Paris, and eclipsing his master. Mesmer returned to Paris, and engaged to communicate his secret to a number of persons, on condition of his receiving payment at the rate of 100 luis-d'or from each. By this arrangement he is said to have obtained the enormous sum of 340,000 livres. His pupils designated themselves as the Society "de l'harmonie." When they had acquired the instructions for which they had paid so considerable a sum, and were preparing to publish the same for the benefit of humanity, Mesmer complained indignantly of their conduct, declared that they were bound to secrecy by an indenture, which appears to have been the fact ; and being yet unable to prevent their proceeding, which interfered with his unbounded hopes of gain, left France, carrying with him the riches which he had acquired, and complaining that he had been cruelly treated and betrayed.*

Animal magnetism was practised very extensively in France. Ladies of the first quality were among its most sanguine votaries, as well as crowds of all descriptions. At length the government interposed, it being evident that either good or mischievous results were likely to ensue from so popular an object of attention. The appointment of the celebrated royal commission to try the merits of Mesmerism is a great event in the history of this art. The commis-

* *Bertrand*, Traité du Magnetisme Animal.

sioners were men of the highest authority in science ; Franklin,. Lavoisier, Bailly, and Jessieu were among the number.   The report of their observations on the practices of animal magnetism, carried on at that time by M. Deslon, is an authentic and important document. It was drawn up by M. Bailly ; and it is well observed by Bertrand, that no unprejudiced person who reads it can fail of partaking in the opinions of the celebrated men who were parties to its adoption.

The following is their description of the method in which Mesmer and his colleagues carried on their proceedings. According to this report, a little wooden tub, of different forms, round, oval, or square, raised one foot or one foot and a half, was placed in the middle of a large room.   This tub was called *" the baquet ;"* its covering was pierced with a certain number of holes, from out of which came branches of iron, jointed and flexible.   The patients were placed in several rows round this *" baquet,"* and each person held the branch of iron, which, by means of the joints, could be applied directly to the part affected ; a cord was placed round the bodies of the patients, which united them one to another.   Sometimes a second chain was formed by communication with the hands, that is to say, by applying the thumb of one between the thumb and first finger of the next person ; the thumb thus held was then pressed, and the impression received on the left was returned by the right, and circulated all around.   A piano-forte was placed in a corner of a room ; different airs were played upon it ; sometimes the sound of the voice in singing was added.   All the magnetisers had in their hands a little rod of iron, ten or twelve inches long.   This rod was looked upon as the conductor of magnetism ; it possessed the advantage of concentrating it in its point, and of rendering the emanations more powerful. Sound, according to the principles of Mesmer, was also a conductor of magnetism : and, in order to communicate the fluid to the piano, it was sufficient to let the rod approach it.   The cord with which the patients were surrounded was destined, as well as the chain of thumbs, to augment the effects by communication.   The inside of the *"baquet"* was said to be so formed that it might concentrate the magnetic fluid: there was nothing, however, in reality, in its formation which could excite or retain magnetism or electricity.

The patients, ranged in great numbers and in several rows round the baquet, received magnetism by all the different ways ; by the iron branches which came out of the tub, by the cord which was entangled round their bodies, by the union of the thumbs, by the sound of the piano, and agreeable voices which mingled with it. They were more directly magnetised by means of the finger and the iron rod, moved before the face, above or behind the head, and upon the diseased parts, always observing the distinction of the poles. They were acted upon by a fixed look, but, above all, they were magnetised by the application of hands and by the pressure of fingers upon the hypochondria, and upon the abdominal region ; an application often continued for a long time, sometimes during several hours. Such was the method of Mesmer, to which was added a multitude of practices, much too long to describe. They magnetised in this manner several natural objects, and among others trees, which hence acquired magnetic virtue ; so that persons who put themselves " en rapport" with them, fell into a crisis. They could likewise magnetise lifeless bodies, such as a bottle, a glass, or a cup.

The effects produced on the subjects of this strange ceremony are thus described :—

" Some remained calm and tranquil, others coughed, spat, felt some slight pain, a local or universal heat, and had sweats ; others were agitated, tormented with convulsions most extraordinary by their force, their number, and their duration ; as soon as one began, another succeeded ; the paroxysms lasted sometimes three hours ; the patients spat a thick, viscous, and sometimes bloody fluid ; the attacks were characterised by precipitate, violent, and involuntary movements of the members or the whole body, by constrictions of the throat, by spasms at the epigastrium and hypochondria, piercing cries, tears, hiccough, and immoderate laughter. Nothing could be more astonishing than the sight of these agitations and various seizures ; the sympathies which established themselves between all these individuals struck us with amazement. We beheld the patients precipitating themselves one towards the other, smiling and talking to each other with affection, and mutually alleviating their agitations. Every thing depended upon the will of the magnetiser ; were they in an apparently deep sleep, his voice, a look, a sign drew them out of it."

" We cannot," say the commissioners of the king, " prevent ourselves from recognising in these constant effects a powerful agent, which acts upon patients, subdues them, and of which the person who magnetises them seems to be the depository."

The commissioners soon discovered that it was very difficult to ascertain to what point the results produced were the effects of imagination, to the excitement of which so many circumstances were adapted, and how far to any peculiar agency. They resorted to private trials of the same manipulations. Some of the most interesting of these experiments were performed at Passy, at the residence of Dr. Franklin, who could not be present at Paris at the public exhibition. Here M. Deslon tried his art in vain upon the obdurate American, as well as upon the members of his family, who, notwithstanding that some of them were ladies in delicate health, were found quite insensible to the whole ceremonial of magnetism. Neither of the other commissioners could perceive any effect in his own person. One of the experiments made at Passy is worthy of a particular recital. It consisted in the magnetising of a tree in Dr. Franklin's garden. M. Deslon affirmed that if this was done by himself and a youth introduced who should be purposely selected as an individual susceptible of the magnetic influence, the result would be manifest on his approaching the particular tree. A boy, aged twelve years, was chosen by M. Deslon, who insisted on the necessity of his presence and co-operation. Care, however, was taken to prevent collusion. The boy was made to approach four trees successively, without know-

ing which was the magnetised one, having his eyes covered with a
bandage, and to embrace each tree for two minutes, according to the
previous arrangement with M. Deslon. That gentleman stood in
the garden, and kept his cane pointed at the magnetised tree, in order
to maintain its magnetism. Under the first tree not magnetised, at
the end of a minute the boy perspired in great drops, coughed,
expectorated, felt a slight pain in his head ; he was then twenty-
seven feet distant from the magnetised tree. Under the second tree
he felt stupor and the same pain in his head. Under the third tree
these symptoms were greatly increased : he believed himself to be
approaching the magnetised tree ; he was, however, then at the distance of not less than thirty-eight feet from it. Under the fourth
tree not magnetised, at the distance of twenty-four feet from the
magnetised tree, the young man fell into a crisis. He lost all consciousness, was carried to a neighbouring grass-plot, where M. Deslon
soon reanimated him. The operator accounted for this untoward
phenomenon by saying that the trees had probably become spontaneously magnetic. " But," rejoined the commissioners, " if trees
are in the dangerous habit of assuming this state of their own accord,
a susceptible person walking in a garden must incur the continual
risk of falling into a crisis."

The commissioners having repeated and varied the experiments in
every way that seemed to afford an opportunity of arriving at the
truth, at length came to the conclusion that the whole proceeding of
the magnetisers was calculated in several ways to do injury ; that it
was devoid of any salutary or useful influence, and that the results
were wholly to be attributed to the imagination and to the feelings
which were excited by the performances. M. Jussieu, however,
refused to coincide in the report.

Notwithstanding the unfavourable nature of this report, and the
retirement of the principal from the scene, Mesmerism continued to
be practised extensively in France. The members of the Society of
Harmony, who where spread through the country, continued their
operations in the provinces. Among them the Marquis de Puységur
was one of the most distinguished, and it was during his proceedings
that the most remarkable phenomenon accompanying these exhibitions was first noticed. We allude to the production of that state
which has been termed the magic or artificial somnambulism. The
commissioners in the report to which we have already alluded, had
remarked that nothing was more astonishing than the spectacle which
they witnessed in the operations of M. Deslon, and that they were
equally surprised at the profound repose of a part of the assembled
groupe, and at the agitation of others. These opposite effects were
produced by the same agency, according to the different predispositions of individuals. But as the method of display was gradually
changed by later operators, the agitations in a great measure ceased
to be observed, while the appearance of a state of somnolency became
much more striking and general ; and in numerous instances, though
by no means in a great proportion of persons, a species of somnam-

bulism displayed itself, of which we shall proceed hereafter to examine the peculiar characters.

The political revolutions in France withdrew the public attention from animal magnetism. Many of the parties interested in this pursuit perished, and others were exiled. It was not till the return of better times that the practice of this art was resumed in France, and its historians declare that on its revival animal magnetism was found to have retained very few features of its ancient character. The mode of treating patients was quite changed ; the theory of the magnetisers was new ; the only circumstances connecting the old magnetism of the age of Mesmer and his immediate disciples with the present method, was the appearance in both of somnolency and somnambulism. These changes in the character of the art are attributed principally to the attention bestowed upon it by the deeply studious and reflective but not incredulous persons who took up the study in Germany.* In that country it has had from an early period advocates among the most distinguished physicians.

I shall trace very rapidly the few remaining events in the history of animal magnetism, and then say a few words on its actual character.

In the year 1813 M. Déleuze, a writer highly respectable for his moral integrity, talents, and good sense, published his critical history of animal magnetism. The appearance of this work occasioned a favourable change in the opinion of many scientific men in respect to the new art, and some who had before concealed their opinions were now emboldened to speak more openly in defence of it. In 1820 M. Husson instituted a series of experiments at the Hôtel Dieu, which were attended by scientific men, and the result was a general conviction that some very powerful influence was brought into operation, though some difference of opinion existed as to the nature of this influence.

A series of experiments at the Salpêtrière was followed by similar effects, and it was now that animal magnetism obtained two highly distinguished proselytes, viz., M. Rostan, the celebrated pathologist, who is the author of the essay on this art in the Dictionnaire de Médecine, and M. Georget, well known as a man of most acute penetration, who adopted with entire sincerity the whole doctrine.

In 1825 a letter was addressed by M. Foissac, an advocate for animal magnetism, to the Royal Academy of Medicine, urging that body to appoint a new commission to inquire into its merits. The proposal met with strong opposition, but was at length carried, and a number of individuals were requested to investigate the subject anew. The report of this body was drawn up by M. Husson, already well known as an advocate for animal magnetism. It is said by M. Bertrand to have produced a strong impression in favour of the art, but as this document has lately been translated and published in

* Kluge's Darstellung. Erster abschnitt.

Scotland, I shall say nothing more on the subject on the present occasion.*

Section III.—Of the Phenomena of Animal Magnetism.

The method of operating, by which the magnetic state is induced, is thus described by M. Rostan :—The person, who is to be subject to this proceeding, is seated in a chair, and the operator places himself opposite in such a manner that their knees and the extremities of their feet may touch ; then the magnetiser takes the thumbs of the subject and holds them till their temperature is brought into equilibrium with that of his own hands. He afterwards places his hands on the shoulders of the patient, and after some minutes draws them down the arms, taking care to direct the extremity of the fingers along the tract of the nerves which are there spread. This manipulation must be repeated several times, after which the hands must be applied to the epigastrium and held there for some instants of time, and then drawn down towards the knees and even to the feet. Afterwards the hands of the operator must be brought back to the head of the patient, care being taken to keep them in returning at a distance from his person ; again they must be drawn down the arms, and as far as the feet. After this practice has been repeated several times, magnetic phenomena begin to display themselves. The patient experiences involuntary drawings of the limbs (tiraillemens), a sense of uneasiness (embarras) in the head, heaviness of the eyelids. After some repetitions of this performance, and sometimes even at the first sitting, he falls into a profound sleep.

M. Rostan adds that the magnetiser must not let his thoughts wander while he is performing the operation ; his attention must be entirely concentrated upon it ; any distraction of mind is incompatible with success. He informs us that the looks and the expression of countenance of the magnetiser powerfully contribute to the effect. We must observe that M. Rostan is one of those who suppose that the volition of the operator, his intense desire to bring about the result, the agency of *his* mind rather than any influence exerted on the mind of his patient, is the first and principal cause of the effects which ensue.

The most systematic account of the various phenomena said to belong to the magnetic state is given by some of the German writers on this subject. Kluge, one of the most accurate of these writers, enumerates six stages or degrees, each of which is characterised by its peculiar traits. The apparent distinctness and systematic arrangement with which the phenomena belonging to these degrees are described, carries with it a most imposing air of correctness and precision, and renders it extremely difficult to suppose that the whole affair can be merely a matter of fancy or misconception. The first

* Report of the Experiments on Animal Magnetism made by a Committee of the Royal Academy of Medicine of Paris, read at the Meetings of the 21st and 28th June, 1831. Translated by J. C. Colquhoun, Esq. Edin. 1833.

degree is termed the waking state of somnambulism ; the second is
that of imperfect or half-sleep ; the third is termed by Kluge the
stage of " Innere Dunkelheit," inward darkness or magnetic stupor.
This is succeeded by "Innere Klarheit," or inward illumination,
which subsists during the fourth, fifth, and sixth stages. The fourth
stage is that of somnambulism ; the fifth is that of Selbstbeschauung
or Clairvoyance ; the sixth is " Allgemeine Klarheit," or universal
clearsightedness : of each of these degrees I shall give from Kluge a
brief description.

First degree. In the first, or *Waking Stage* of magnetisation,
the ordinary phenomena are, a sense in the person magnetized of
strong perflation from the head to the extremities, followed by a
general increase 'of temperature, which is easily perceptible by the
thermometer, increased redness of the skin, which is covered by
transpiration, and a feeling of lightness and comfort in the whole
body, sensation being during this time quite unimpaired.

II. In the second degree, or in that of *Half-sleep*, to the phenomena of the first stage already enumerated, which, however, become more intense, others are superadded. The sense of warmth
increases and extends itself by a sort of radiation from the stomach,
as from a centre, over the whole person, the pulse becomes fuller,
the breathing slower and deeper. The patient feels drowsiness and
a drawing down of the eyelids, which being closed he finds himself
unable to open them again during the process ; by the other senses
he still remains in relation with external things, though often unable
to express himself. The senses undergo partial excitations : luminous appearances are seen before the eyes, pricking is felt in the
ends of the fingers, profuse sweats break out, rigors are experienced
and sometimes spasms, or cramps of the limbs and other nervous
sensations.

III. The third degree is that of *Innere Dunkelheit*, or the magnetic sleep, which is very distinct in its phenomena from the preceding. The patient is now wholly insensible to words and even to the
loudest cries, is buried in a profound sleep, and on waking from it
has no recollection of any thing that may have occurred during the
period. Faintings, cataleptic or apoplectic attacks, and convulsive
shudderings sometimes occur during this stage. It terminates gradually, and the patient indicates by a sigh, the transition into the
second stage as a prelude to complete awakening.

IV. In the fourth degree, which is that of *Somnambulism*, commences that series of remarkable phenomena so often controverted,
but established, as Kluge declares, by the most complete and perfectly authenticated evidence. The patient now recovers his internal consciousness, his outward senses being still closed in sleep, or
at least existing only under a particular modification : he recognizes
himself, but under new relations to surrounding objects. This stage
is considered to bear a near analogy, in the state of the sensorium,
to that of ordinary sleepwalkers, whence it has derived its denomination. The state of waking inwardly, joined with outward sleep,

does not take place suddenly but by degrees. Nasse has described the gradual progress from magnetic sleep to somnambulism. During the first eight evenings a patient, subjected to the magnetic process, fell into a state resembling ordinary sleep ; it was not till the ninth day that the first signs of the inward awakening began to display themselves in the altered aspect of the features. It was now manifest that the individual was not really asleep. On the succeeding days the phenomena began gradually to be perceived which characterise what the German writers term *Innere Klarheit*, and of which *magnetic somnambulism* is only the commencement. The somnambulist can merely distinguish, by means of the eyes, strong light from darkness ; and according to Treviranus, when the eyelids are open, which seldom happens, the pupils are either turned up as if spasmodically, or are dilated and insensible, all power of moving them being suspended. At the same time the sense of feeling becomes metamorphosed into something equivalent to perfect sight, so that the individual perceives by means of it the finest of those modifications which are generally only perceptible to the visual sense ; she recognizes,—for the subjects of these observations are generally females,—not only the circumferences and surfaces, but also the colours of objects. She can distinguish the position of the hands of a watch held before her, and by merely touching, or sometimes without coming into contact with it : she can read writing and write without any aid from her eyes ! The epigastrium is the chief seat or medium of this new species of vision, and somnambulists distinguish the hour on a watch held close to the region of the stomach, and as Gmelin positively declares, know the cards of a pack from each other when they are so placed, without, any possibility of their having been seen by the eyes. A somnambulist, mentioned by Tardy, read a piece of writing in characters strange and unknown to her, by pressing it on her stomach, her eyes having been securely closed. At first, according to these writers, a strong effort is required on the part of the percipient to exercise this new species of vision with accuracy, but by degrees and long practice it acquires greater perfection. At length, according to the grave and serious declaration of a host of magnetisers, the patient is enabled to perceive through opaque media, and not only without actual contact but at considerable distances and in a most unaccountable way. A young lady, mentioned in Wienholt's Miszellen, was able to read a letter which was at the time folded up and lodged in the pocket of Count von Lützelburg. Mouilleseaux brought a somnambulist into magnetic relation with a stranger who had his hand in his pocket, and asked her of what colour was an object which he held ; she replied, after some effort, that it was *red*. That is true—but what is it ? After a stronger exertion she said, it is a small pocket-book of red morocco. The answer was correct, and none of the reporters seem to have suspected that the reply was the result of any thing else than some extraordinary perception. A damsel, whose case is given in the Strasburg Zeitung, was able to read, not only letters folded up and placed within a cover over her stomach, but a book in another chamber, on a leaf of which a man had placed his open hand, while with the other he held the hand of a third person, the latter holding in like manner a fourth, and a chain being thus formed, as in electrical experiments, the last holding his open hand upon the stomach of the somnambulist. Some of these facts are reported as having occurred to individuals who fell spontaneously into the magnetic state without the manipulatory process ; but it has been well observed that they were all collected in places where the practice of the art was rife and a matter of public interest. How far the cases of sleep-walking which have occurred under opposite circumstances are similar to these or different from them I shall endeavour in the sequel to determine. It is assumed by the historians of animal magnetism that there is a strict analogy in all the phenomena of natural and artificial somnambulism, and this is one of the grounds on which they attempt to render the facts which they report less incredible by connecting them with a series of phenomena frequently observed.

In a still higher degree of intensity the new species of vision without eyes becomes capable of displaying objects too fine for the ordinary ken of mankind. Fischer and Tardy report that their patients saw during the process of magnetising, a halo of light surrounding both themselves and the operators, and rays issuing from the points of their fingers. Nasse has reported a series of experiments on this magnetic light. His somnambulist saw the breath of her magnetiser issuing from his mouth like flames of fire !

The sense of hearing undergoes strange modifications. Pétetin discovered accidentally that a young woman, whose ears were insensible to noises, heard plainly and replied to questions uttered close to the epigastrium. A suspicion occurs that the sound reached the ears of the patient. This was obviated by Petzold, who spoke to his somnambulist with so slight a whisper, close to the pit of her stomach, that it was impossible for her ears to be affected. In general magnetised persons are insensible of loud sounds, and hear nothing when addressed by persons who are not in magnetic connection with them, though they reply readily when the operator speaks to them, or when accosted by a third person with whom the magnetiser brings them into relation. This I have myself observed, when I had an opportunity of witnessing the performance of a celebrated magnetiser in Paris ; and I must confess that, however obvious the suspicion, there was every appearance of good faith and sincerity in the parties, and not the slightest indication of collusion.

F. Hufeland and many others have instituted numerous experiments on the effects of electrical and magnetic substances on persons under the state induced by animal magnetism. The application of magnets, particularly of the mineral magnet, produces pain. Hufeland supposes that this differs according as different poles are applied. The application of the north-pole of a magnet to the hand occasioned pain felt as far as the fore-arm ; the south-pole gave pain only to the part touched. As animal magnetism has been referred to electrical agency, Gmelin, Heinecken, and Nasse, instituted experiments on this subject, but could detect no trace of electricity excited in any period of the process.

When a patient awakes from the magnetic sleep, all traces of what had occurred to her during the period of somnambulism are in general obliterated ; but it was observed by Nasse, that ideas which have excited lively interest and emotion have sometimes recurred to the individual in dreams. It is a more ordinary observation that all the impressions of the magnetic state, though obliterated during the waking period, are renewed when somnambulism is restored.

V. The fifth and sixth stages of the magnetic state retain all the characteristics of the fourth, or of somnambulism, and only differ from it in the addition of new phenomena. The fifth stage does not follow the fourth quickly and without effort, but requires frequent and strong exertions on the part of the magnetiser and the mag-netised, to direct the attention of the latter and concentrate it powerfully in inward consciousness and the contemplation of his internal bodily state, before he can become possessed of that faculty which is termed *Selbstbeschauung*, self-inspection or self-contem-plation, and by the French *Clairvoyance*. In this state patients view the whole interior of their own bodies, and are able to describe minutely all the internal organs with as much accuracy as an anatomist who sees them laid open by the knife. Heinecken's patient said, " I see the interior of my body ; all parts of it seem to me equally transparent, and penetrated by light and warmth. I see the blood flow in my veins, remark accurately the irregularities which exist in this or in another part, and direct my attention to the means by which they may be removed. It then seems to me as if some body counsels me,—this or that measure must you adopt." In this state of things the clairvoyant has the instinct of remedies, and is capable of prescribing for himself. Often when he is unac-quainted with the names of particular drugs, he describes them in such a way as they can be recognised by physicians. This last assertion, absurd as it is, has a host of magnetical witnesses in its favour.

It is a still more curious fact that the Insichhineingehen, or power of self-penetration, is not limited to the body of the *clairvoyant* himself ; it extends also to the bodies of other persons who are brought into magnetic *rapport* with the illuminated individual. Some amusing anecdotes in illustration of this fact are related by Fischer. When the magnetiser puts pepper or salt into the mouth, the magnetised person tastes it immediately by sympathy. Gmelin once magnetised when he had a diarrhœa, and the patient on the following day suffered great uneasiness. The sympathy between persons in magnetic relation is so great that they partake of all the corporeal feelings of each other, and each has the power of inspecting internally the body of his fellow as exactly as his own ; if one has a disease the other participates in its symptoms : and among Nadler's patients, if one was deaf the other became hard of hearing.

VI. *Sixth degree—Allgemeine Klarheit.*—In passing from the fifth to the sixth stage, the luminous perspective of the clairvoyant which had been confined to the interior of his body, penetrates the outward veil and obtains an insight into all nature: things hidden in futurity or in distance of space are subjected to his survey. Weinholt's patient ascertained the illness of her brother separated from her at the distance of some hundred miles. In the Strasburg hospital a patient, being in relation with a stranger, told him that his indisposition arose from a fall on horseback, which had really occurred fifteen years before. A clairvoyante in this degree can foretell the complaints which not only herself but others brought into relation with her are destined to undergo at almost any future period of time. She requires now only the will of the magnetiser to bring her into rapport with any absent person to such a degree that she can absolutely see through him, and tell not only what he is doing at the present time, but what will become of him hereafter. In fact, the examples of this state recorded by Kluge and other German writers approach very nearly to the stories of *second sight,* which were formerly so commonly related in Scotland.

Section IV.—*Theory of Animal Magnetism.*

How does the proceeding of the magnetisers operate in giving rise to these effects? The theory generally adopted by the partisans of this art is as follows. The instrument which is set in action is a peculiar vital fluid, to which the nerves perform the office of conductors. This fluid, which presides over all the movements of the body, is in an especial manner under the direction of the will, and may, through its influence, be propelled, or directed towards, and accumulated upon, any external body living or inert. If this theory is not clearly developed in the writings of all the magnetisers, it is at least implicitly adopted by them. The characteristic peculiarity of their doctrine is the admission of an influence, residing in the will of the magnetiser, on the emanation of the fluid alleged to exist, and on the consequent production of magnetic phenomena—an influence so great, according to the prevailing theory, that all magnetic action is regarded as subordinate to the exertion of will which sets the fluid in activity.

The doctrine thus stated, which has been with some trifling modifications adopted by MM. Georget, Rostan, Husson, and the generality of those who maintain the efficacy of animal magnetism in France, must, in the actual state of our knowledge, be considered as a very wild speculation. It soars so far above the region of observation and experiment, that it cannot be subjected to proof, and it is at the same time impossible to determine whether, if conceded or established, it would be sufficient to account for the phenomena of which an explanation is sought. A different opinion has been maintained by M. Bertrand, who, after surveying with discrimination the whole history of magnetism, and witnessing the proceedings of the operators in this art, and practising them himself with considerable effect, has come to the conclusion that all the results of these operations are brought about through the influence of the mind ; not by the will of the magnetiser, radiating forth his own vital spirit, and operating through this material or immaterial instrument on the vital spirits of other men, who are the passive recipients, but by the energy with which the feelings and imagination of the latter act upon themselves.

A strong confirmation of this opinion is derived by Bertrand, from the manner in which the Abbe Faria performed magnetisation, in which he brought about all the results of this agency in the persons subjected to his attempts without the instrumental methods used by Mesmer's earlier or later followers, and in a way which seems to preclude any other influence than that merely of the mind. Abbe Faria made no attempt to avoid the imputation of quackery, and actually received sums of money for his exhibitions. Yet, according to M. Bertrand, he entertained much more correct notions of the real principles of magnetic phenomena than most of its partisans. Having been taught by a long course of experiments that the cause of somnambulism, or, as he termed it, the *lucid sleep*, as well as of all the other magnetic phenomena, is connected with the state of the individual who is the subject of treatment, he varied his proceedings in such a manner as to render them expeditious. He sometimes placed the patient in an arm-chair, and after telling him to shut his eyes and collect himself, suddenly pronounced, in a strong voice and imperative tone, the word " dormez," which generally produced an impression sufficiently strong to give a slight shock, and occasion warmth, transpiration, and sometimes somnambulism. If the first attempt failed, he tried the experiment a second, third, and even a fourth time, after which he declared the individual incapable of entering into the state of lucid sleep. Abbe Faria used to boast that he had put more than five thousand persons into somnambulism ; and though in this there may be some exaggeration, yet it is incontestible, as M. Bertrand observes, that he very often succeeded. A very considerable number of persons, removed from all suspicion of connivance, have experienced the influence. The complete identity of the phenomena produced by a method which operated confessedly through the imagination, with those which display themselves under the ordinary treatment of the magnetisers, affords a strong reason for concluding that the results in other instances depend upon a similar principle. The state of crisis or insensibility produced in Dr. Franklin's garden, in the experiment before described, is sufficient of itself to prove that the influence ascribed to the imagination is not greater than the reality. We have here a cause proved to be sufficient for the phenomena, with which it is more philosophical to rest satisfied than to resort to the visionary hypothesis of the magnetic fluid radiated forth by the will of the operator upon surrounding persons and objects, or to confess the strange doctrine, that the volition of a human body is capable of exerting an immediate influence on other minds and bodies than his own. The generality of magnetisers insist, indeed, in the assertion that the manipulations of the performer have no effect upon the subject, unless accompanied by a powerful agency of the will, by continued, strong, intense volition to produce the result. This is denied by M. Bertrand, who declares that in trials made by himself, precisely the same results followed, whether he WILLED to produce them or not, provided that the patient was inwardly persuaded that the whole ritual was duly observed.

The theory of animal magnetism has been investigated in a most elaborate manner by Dr. Johann Stieglitz of Hanover. According to this writer* there are three different hypotheses, each of which deserves the attentive consideration of those who wish to comprehend the mysteries of the magnetic art. These are, ?, the theory of sympathy and antipathy ; 2, the assumed existence of a sort of polarity in every individual, forming a medium of communication between the operator and the subject ; and, 3, the more lately prevalent doctrine of a "Gemeingefühl," coenæsthesis, or common feeling, maintained by Autenrieth and Reil, and connected with the imagined elevation of the nervous system of the abdominal ganglions to the function of sensorial nerves.

According to this hypothesis the operations of the brain and the system of cerebral and spinal nerves being suspended during the magnetic somnambulism, the nervous structure connected with the ganglions, and appropriated generally to the functions of physical life, assumes vicariously the office of the brain, and becomes a new sensorium. Specific sensation through the organs of sense ceases to exist, but the " Gemeingefühl," or common feeling, taking its centre in the epigastrium near the gastric system of nerves, becomes capable through its exaltation of all that belongs naturally to the cerebral structures, and in many instances in a higher and more intense degree. Attempts have been made to support this speculation by a variety of cases of somnambulism which took place without the magnetising process, and in which analogous phenomena are said to have been observed. The most remarkable of these, as I have already observed, were published by M. Pétetin, a physician of Lyons. In a work on what he entitled "Animal Electricity," this writer detailed experiments made by him on eight cataleptic females,—a surprising number as occurring in the practice of one physician within a short space of time,—in which, according to the statement, the seat of sensation was transferred to the epigastrium. Young females, quite deaf to sounds in the ordinary way, heard plainly when M. Pétetin whispered to them close to the epigastrium. M. Bertrand also refers to the Annales de Chimie et de Physique, and to the Gazette de Santé, for December, 1807, for the account of another female who saw with her fingers' ends ; and to a publication in Germany, by Baron Strombeck, describing the case of a

* Dr. J. Stieglitz, über den thierischen Magnetismus. Hannover, 1814.

young woman, who had the still more admirable faculty of seeing
through floors and walls, and even of discovering objects in an upper
story of the house where she dwelt, and far removed from her own
apartment. With respect to these cases, I have already observed
that they have been brought forward by professed supporters of
animal magnetism, and that they occurred in places where that
practice was at the time an object of interest. I have therefore considered these cases as belonging properly to the history of animal
magnetism, and as forming a part of the same aggregate of facts.
My readers will be disposed to allow the fairness of such a proceeding when they shall have observed how different are all these relations from those of real somnambulism as collected from different
sources.

It would be altogether beside my present purpose to make any
attempt at estimating the evidence brought forward by the supporters of animal magnetism. I have given a brief outline of the
alleged facts, principally with a view of illustrating somnambulism,
and suggesting some inquiries important as to our conception of
that state.

I shall now return to the history of somnambulism properly so
termed, and independent of any magnetic proceedings, in analysing
the most remarkable of the facts upon record in connexion with this
subject, shall endeavour to discover whether they afford any proof
of that change in the state of the nervous system which the writers
above cited imagine to take place. The state of the sensorium in somnambulism is very curious, and the facts related are sufficiently surprising. I shall select some of the most characteristic cases, and learn
from them whether the organs of sense are entirely without action,
and whether in reality the nerves of physical life assume the function
which belongs to the brain and its derivatives or connexions.

SECTION V.—*Phenomena of real Somnambulism: Ordinary
and Cataleptic Somnambulism, or Ecstasis: Comparison of
the Phenomena of Somnambulism with those of the State
induced by Animal Magnetism.*

I shall now call the attention of my readers to some of the most
remarkable of the cases of somnambulism which have been recorded
in different countries, and which are occasionally appealed to as
affording evidence on controverted points.

Somnambulism was known to Hippocrates and Aristotle, and to
Galen by his own experience, but is briefly mentioned by them.
Diogenes Laertius has recorded two cases of this affection. One
was that of a stoic philosopher, who in this state used to compose
works, read, and correct them. Such actions, as M. Bertrand observes,
under the ordinary circumstances would imply the possession of
sight; still this writer is inclined to maintain that somnambulists
have rather a new faculty which supplies the place of vision,
though he admits that the supposition should not be adopted without

incontestible proof.* Gassendi has related in a more detailed manner several cases of somnambulism. These are extracted by Muratori in his work on "The Imagination," in which are also to be found some of the most interesting facts on record connected with this and other mental phenomena.† One of Gassendi's somnambulists used to rise and dress himself in his sleep, go down to the cellar and draw wine from a cask : he appeared to see in the dark as well as in a clear day ; but when he awoke, either in the street or cellar, he was obliged to grope and feel his way back to his bed. He always answered his wife as if awake, but in the morning recollected nothing of what had passed. It often seemed to him as if there was not light enough, and he thought he had risen before day. He then struck fire, and lighted a candle. Another sleepwalker, a countryman of Gassendi, passed on stilts over a swollen torrent in the night, but on waking was afraid to return before daylight, or until the water had subsided. Two of the most curious and best related cases on record are those of Signor Augustin Forari and John Baptist Negretti : both of these are given by Muratori, from whom I shall take a brief extract of them.

"Signor Augustin was an Italian nobleman, dark, thin, melancholic, and cold-blooded, addicted to the study of the abstract sciences. His attacks occurred at the waning of the moon, and were stronger in autumn and winter than in the summer. An eye-witness, Vigneul Marville, gave the following description of them.

"One evening towards the end of October, we played at various games after dinner ; Signor Augustin took a part in them along with the rest of the company, and afterwards retired to repose. At eleven o'clock his servant told us that his master would walk that night, and that we might come and watch him. I examined him after some time with a candle in my hand. He was lying upon his back, and sleeping with open, staring, unmoved eyes. We were told that this was a sure sign that he would walk in his sleep. I felt his hands and found them extremely cold, and his pulse beat so slowly that his blood appeared not to circulate. We played at trictrac until the spectacle began. It was about midnight, when Signor Augustin drew aside the bed-curtains with violence, arose, and put on his clothes. I went up to him and held the light under his eyes. He took no notice of it, although his eyes were open and staring. Before he put on his hat, he fastened on his sword-belt, which hung on the bed-post : the sword had been removed. Signor Augustin then went in and out of several rooms, approached the fire, warmed himself in an arm-chair, and went thence into a closet where was his wardrobe. He sought something in it, put all the things into disorder, and having set them right again locked the door and put

* Bertrand, Traité du Somnambulisme.

† L. Á. Muratori, della forza della Fantasia Umana, Venez. 1766. It is singular that this treatise has not been translated into either French or English. The German translation is a very valuable work, containing various notes and additions by the editor, Richertz of Göttingen.

the key into his pocket. He went to the door of the chamber, opened it, and stepped out on the staircase. When he came below, one of us made a noise by accident : he appeared frightened, and hastened his steps. His servant desired us to move softly and not speak, or he would become out of his mind ; and sometimes he ran as if he were pursued, if the least noise was made by those standing round him. He then went into a large court and to the stable, stroked his horse, bridled it, and looked for the saddle to put on it. As he did not find it in the accustomed place, he appeared confused. He then mounted his horse, and galloped to the house door. He found this shut ; dismounted, and knocked with a stone which he picked up, several times at the door. After many unsuccessful efforts he remounted, and led his horse to the watering-place, which was at the other end of the court, let him drink, tied him to a post, and went quietly to the house. Upon hearing a noise which the servants made in the kitchen, he listened attentively, went to the door, and held his ear to the keyhole. After some time he went to the other side, and into a parlour in which was a billiard-table. He walked round it several times, and acted the motions of a player. He then went to a harpsicord on which he was accustomed to prac- tice, and played a few irregular airs. After having moved about for two hours, he went to his room and threw himself upon his bed clothed as he was, and the next morning we found him in the same state ; for as often as his attack came on, he slept afterwards from eight to ten hours. The servants declared that they could only put an end to his paroxysms either by tickling him under the soles of his feet, or by blowing a trumpet in his ears."

The history of Negretti was published separately by two physi- cians, Righellini and Pigatti, who were both eye-witnesses of the curious facts which they relate. The former corresponded with Muratori, and gave replies to his questions as to particular circum- stances. Negretti was about twenty-four years old, was a sleep- walker from his eleventh year, but his attacks only occurred in the Month of March, lasting at farthest till the month of April. He was a servant of Marquis Luigi Sale. On the evening of the 16th of March 1740, after going to sleep on a bench in the kitchen, he began first to talk, then walked about, went to the dining-room and spread a table for dinner, placed himself behind a chair with a plate in his hand, as if waiting on his master. After waiting until he thought his master had dined, he uncovered the table, put away all the materials in a basket, which he locked in a cupboard. He after- wards warmed a bed, locked up the house, and prepared for his nightly rest. Being then awakened and asked if he remembered what he had been doing, he answered no. This, however, was not always : he often recollected what he had been doing. Pigatti says that he would awake when water was thrown into his face, or when his eyes were forcibly opened. According to Maffei he then re- mained some time faint and stupid. Righellini assured Muratori that his eyes were firmly closed during the paroxysm, and that, when a candle was put near to him, he took no notice of it. Sometimes he struck himself against the wall, and even hurt himself severely. Hence it would seem that he was directed in his movements by habit, and had no actual perception of external objects. This is confirmed by the assurance that if any body pushed him he got out of the way, and moved his arms rapidly about on every side, and that when he was in a place of which he had no distinct knowledge, he felt with his hands all the objects about him, and displayed much inaccuracy in his proceedings; but in places to which he had been accustomed, he was under no confusion, but went through his business very cleverly. Pigatti shut a door through which he had just passed : he struck himself against it on returning. The writer last mentioned was confident that Negretti could not see. He sometimes carried about him a candle, as if to give him light in his employment ; but on a bottle being substituted, took it and carried it, fancying that it was a candle. He once said during his sleep that he must go and hold a light to his master in his coach. Righellini followed him closely, and marked that he stood still at the corners of the streets with his torch in his hand not lighted, and waited a while in order that the coach which he supposed to be following might pass through the place where lights was required. On the 18th of March he went through nearly the same process as before, in laying a table, &c. and then went to the kitchen and sat down to supper. Signor Righellini observed him in company with many other cavalieri very curious to see him eat. At once he said, as recollecting himself, " How can I so forget? To-day is Friday, and I must not dine." He then locked up every thing and went to bed. On another occasion he ate several cakes of bread and some salad, which he had just before demanded of the cook. He then went with a lighted candle into the cellar and drew wine, which he drank. All these acts he performed as usual, and carried a tray upon which were wine-glasses and knives, turning it obliquely on passing through a narrow doorway, but avoiding any accident.

My limits prevent me from extracting the further details which relate to the history of this night-wanderer. The preceding relations, to which I shall incidentally add a few other particulars from the same sources, furnish a body of facts sufficient for displaying, as far as these individual cases are concerned, the state of the faculties in somnambulism. In the analysis of these I shall now attempt to discover some general principle which may serve as a clue to the variety of analogous phenomena on record. To begin with the inferior senses : Pigatti says that Negretti sat down to eat a bowl of salad which he had prepared. It was taken from him, and some strongly seasoned cabbage put in its place ; this he ate without perceiving the difference, as he did also some pudding which was presently substituted. At another time, having asked for wine, he drank water which was given him. He sniffed ground coffee instead of snuff, which he had demanded. Other sleepwalkers are well known to have detected similar deceptions, as it will appear from a

case hereafter to be related. The difference appears to be in the
degree of attention : a more lively perception as to the qualities of
the object desired existed in one case than in the other, the mind
being more directed to particular sensations in the one case, and
more distracted or diverted from them in the others.

The sense of hearing presents similar variations. In general
somnambulists do not hear persons who talk aloud in their presence.
It has often been observed that very loud noises are unperceived by
them,—that a trumpet must be sounded in their ears before their
attention can be forcibly withdrawn from reverie to the perception
of the real world, and to the waking state. At other times they
converse and hear the lowest sounds. Signor Augustin repeatedly
listened and heard slight noises at a distance. The difference seems
here to depend upon the same principle as in the preceding instances
which refer to smell and taste. When attention is by a voluntary
act directed to the particular operations of sense, the perceptive
faculty of the sleeper is perfect, even remarkably acute. But when
his mind is distracted, his reverie presenting different objects, even
loud sounds are imperceptible to him. Perhaps from the same consideration we shall obtain a clue to unravel the perplexing varieties
of phenomena connected with the state of vision in some cases
which will be presently mentioned. Negretti, as it seems, had his
eyes shut and saw not. Habit guided him in places with which he
was familiar, and in other places he frequently showed the want of
accurate perception, and assisted himself by feeling and groping
about. Etmuller observed that sleepwalkers go about " oculis
clausis," but he adds that some have acted " oculis conniventibus."
Haller says decidedly, that they get out of their beds fast asleep,
their eyes being either firmly closed or otherwise sightless, since a
strong light is unperceived, though held near.* The fact is doubtless, yet why may we not avail ourselves of the analogy presented
by the sense of hearing, and allow the insensibility to light under
the ordinary circumstances of sleep-walking to be compatible with
the use of the same faculty in other instances where we can find no
other explanation of the phenomena ? Such cases will presently
come under our notice. Negretti and Augustin did not see, and
Richertz well observes that the want of vision seems to have been
supplied by various means. Habit, as we have observed, is the
principal guide. The sense of feeling, when under the guidance of
attention, and even that of hearing in similar circumstances, appear
to be remarkably acute. Then as to the hypothesis to which in the
sequel we shall have further to advert, viz. that somnambulists have
a new kind of sight independent of the eyes ;—although we are not
called upon to disprove such a position, yet many facts may be
found in the history above related which would enable us to do so.
The defect was not supplied in such a degree and manner as the
hypothesis implies. Negretti stood behind his master's chair sup-

posing him to be at dinner ; he fancied that the torch which he held to guide his coach was lighted when it was not. In a variety of cases he displayed the total want of any sensation analogous to sight ; he stumbled when he walked in places to which he had not been accustomed, felt his way on various sides, struck himself against a wall. In attempting to pass through a closed door, he hurt himself. Other histories of somnambulists supply parallel remarks. Galen mentions of himself that he once walked about a whole night in his sleep till he was awakened by striking himself against a stone which happened to be in his way.*

These are facts which prove that even the sense of feeling, which is the principal guiding faculty in somnambulism, is limited in its sphere of action, and exists under a modification similar to that which affects the other perceptive powers, and which, according to the opinion above stated, explains the anomalies of their operation. Negretti seems not to have distinguished accurately even objects of feeling *when they were not particularly the objects of attention.* When struck a blow by a stick on the leg, he fancied that a dog had touched him, and scolded it. Being again struck, he threw a bit of bread, calling the hound by name. A muff was thrown at him, which he again took for the dog.†

In other instances somnambulists have been known to write, and even to correct their compositions, and to do other acts which could not possibly be performed without sight.

Castelli, a sleepwalker whose case is one of the most remarkable, was a pupil of Porati, an Italian apothecary. His history has been published by Francesco Soave, a physician, who personally observed him. He was found one night in the act of translating from Italian into French, and looked for words in a dictionary as usual, being asleep. His candle being extinguished, he found himself to be in the dark, groped for the candle, and went to light it again at the kitchen fire. Bertrand thinks that Castelli did not really experience the want of light, because the room was, as we are informed, actually illumined at the time by other candles. This is a most improbable supposition, and seems irreconcilable with the fact just related, that he perceived his candle to become extinguished. There, are, indeed, many circumstances related of this somnambulist which prove to our entire conviction that he not only saw, but had his other organs of sense in a state capable of perception whenever his attention was excited, and he wished to avail himself of their operation. He used to leave his bed, go down to the shop and weigh out medicines to supposed customers, to whom he talked. When any one conversed with him on a subject on which his mind was bent, he gave rational answers. He had been reading Macquer's Chemistry, and somebody altered his marks to try if he would notice it. This puzzled him, and he said, " Bel piacere di sempre togliermi i segni."

---

* De Motu Musculorum, lib. ii. cap. 5. Bertrand, ouv. cit.
† *Muratori*, ubi supra, p. 323.

He found his place and read aloud, but his voice growing fainter, his master told him to raise it, which he did. Yet he perceived none of the persons standing round him, and "though he heard," says Soave, "any conversation which was in conformity with the train of his ideas, he heard nothing of the discourse which those persons held on other subjects." His eyes seemed to be very sensible to objects relating to his thoughts, but appeared to have no life in them, and so fixed were they that when he read he was observed not to move his eyes but his whole head, from one side of the page to the other.*

Facts which appear even still more strongly to evince the possession of accurate sight are related in a very curious case of somnambulism, which was published in the French Encyclopædia. The account has been copied by Bertrand, who endeavours to turn aside the evidences afforded by it, or to reconcile it with his own hypothesis. I shall conclude this part of my inquiry with an abstract of the most remarkable facts contained in the narrative, and request my readers to bear in mind the explanation of the phenomena which I have proposed.

This somnambulist was a young priest in a Catholic seminary ; the witness and reporter of the facts, the archbishop of Bordeaux, who used to go into his chamber after the priest was gone to sleep, and observe his proceedings. He sometimes arose from bed, took paper, and wrote sermons. After finishing a page, he read (if the act was properly reading) the whole aloud ; and, if necessary, erased words and wrote his corrections over the line with great accuracy. " I have seen the beginning of one of his sermons, which he had written when asleep ; it was well composed, but one correction surprised me : having written at first the words ' ce divin enfant,' he had afterwards effaced the word *divin*, and written over it *adorable*. Then perceiving that *ce* could not stand before the last word, he had dexterously inserted a *t*, so as to make the word *cet*." The witness, in order to ascertain whether he made use of his eyes, put a card under his chin, so as to intercept the sight of the paper which was on the table ; but he continued to write without perceiving it. Wishing to know by what means he judged of the presence of objects which were under his eyes, the witness took from him the paper on which he was writing, and substituted others repeatedly. He always perceived this by the difference of size, for when a paper of exactly the same shape was given to him, he took it for his own, and wrote his corrections on places corresponding to those on the paper which had been taken away from him. The most astonishing thing is that he would write music with great exactness, tracing on it at equal distances the five lines, and putting upon them the clef, flats, and sharps. Afterwards he marked the notes, at first white, and then blackened those which were to be black ; the words were

* Riflessioni sopra il Somnambolismo; di Francesco Soave. Many of the particulars relating to this case of Castelli have been inserted by Mr. P. B. Dunean, fellow of New College, in a very ingenious essay on somnambulism.

written under, and once happening to make them too long, he quickly perceived that they were not exactly under the corresponding notes ; he corrected this inaccuracy by rubbing out what he had written, and putting the line below with the greatest precision.

On one occasion, in the midst of winter, he fancied himself to be walking on the bank of a river, and to see a child fall into it, in danger of drowning. He leaped into the river, as he thought, in order to rescue the child, and actually threw himself upon his bed with the action of a man swimming. He imitated the movements of a swimmer for some time, and at length feeling in a corner of the bed a bundle of the clothes, fancied that he had seized the child, held it in one hand, and with the other swam, as he supposed, to the bank of the river ; he there put down the bundle, and came out shivering and chattering with his teeth, as if he really had just emerged from a cold stream. He said to the persons near him that it was freezing, and that he was almost dead with cold, and asked for a glass of brandy to warm him ; as there was none at hand they gave him water, but he knew the deception, and again demanded brandy, mentioning the risk which he incurred. He drank a glass of strong liquor, and seemed refreshed, but without awaking, lay down, and continued to sleep soundly.

The reporters of this curious story suggest, by way of comment, the following queries :—" 1. How is it possible for a man buried in profound sleep, to hear, speak, write, see, and in short enjoy the use of his senses, and perform correctly different movements ? To facilitate the solution of this problem, we shall add," says the writers, " that the somnambulist sees only those objects which he seeks, or which are present to his imagination. This individual composed sermons, saw his paper, his ink, pens, could distinguish whether they marked or not the paper. For the rest he did not suspect that any person was in his room, neither seeing nor hearing any body, unless when he had asked for any thing.

" 2. How any person can experience sensation without the assistance of the organs of sense ? The somnambulist above-mentioned appeared evidently to see those objects which had relation to his own ideas. When he traced the notes of music, he knew exactly those which ought to be black and those that were to be left white, and without mistake blackened the former and omitted the others, and if the lines were not dry, he took the precaution to avoid blotting them. There is no reason to suspect that the other channels of sensation were less interrupted than the ordinary one of vision. This might have been ascertained by stopping his ears, &c.

" 3. How did it happen that during the paroxysm of somnambulism he remembered what had occurred during former paroxysms, although, when awake, he lost all traces of such matters ?

" How is it possible that, without any real cause, he was strongly affected by agents of which he had only imagined the existence, as by the coldness of the water, in which he supposed himself to be immersed ?"

I shall leave these inquiries to the consideration of my readers, and now proceed to another division of the subject.

Cataleptic somnambulism.

A morbid affection analogous in many of its phenomena to sleep-walking, but occurring under different circumstances, has been well known to medical writers since the time of Sauvages and Lorry, who first described it. Sauvages gave it the designation of cataleptic somnambulism. According to this writer the attack is ushered in and followed by a complete fit of catalepsy. This happened in the case described by him, but in other instances the preceding symptoms are not so strongly marked : coma, or insensibility in various degrees, may, however, be considered as universally present. The most correct idea of the phenomena of this affection will be conveyed by some examples. The following is the first case published by Sauvages :—" In the month of April 1737, a female who had been for some time affected with fits of hysterical catalepsy, experienced in conjunction with these attacks other symptoms, of which she had more than fifty returns. The fits were divided into three periods : the beginning and termination had perfectly the character of catalepsy ; the intermediate period, which sometimes lasted from the morning till the evening, was occupied by what the girls in the house called the *live fit*, while they termed the catalepsy the *dead fit*. I shall now describe the phenomena," says Sauvages, " which I should certainly have believed to be feigned if I had not become convinced of the contrary by numerous proofs. What I shall say respecting one attack may be understood to apply, with the variation of some circumstances, to all the rest. On the 5th of April 1737, visiting the hospital at ten o'clock in the morning, I found the patient in bed, which she kept on account of her debility and the pain in her head : the fit of catalepsy had just seized her, and it quitted her after five or six minutes ; this was perceived by her yawning and raising herself into a sitting posture, the prelude to the following scene. She began to talk with a degree of animation and *esprit* never observed in her except when in this state. She sometimes changed her subject, and appeared to converse with some friends whom she saw around her bed. Her discourse had relation to what she had said during her attack on the preceding day. She repeated word for word an instruction in the form of a catechism, which she had heard on the evening before, and she made pointed applications of it to persons in the house, whom she took care to designate by invented names, accompanying the whole with gestures and movements of her eyes, which *she kept open*, and alluding to the circumstances and actions of the preceding evening. Yet she was all this time in deep sleep ; a fact which was strongly averred, but which I should never have ventured to declare if I had not obtained satisfactory proof by a series of experiments on the organs of sense : when she began to talk, a blow of the hand inflicted smartly on her face, a finger moved rapidly towards her eyes, a lighted candle brought so near to the organ of vision as even to burn the hair of her eyebrows, a person unseen uttering suddenly a loud cry into her ear, and making a stunning noise with a stone struck forcibly against her bedstead, brandy and a solution of ammoniacal salt placed under her eyes and introduced into her mouth, the feather of a pen, and afterwards the extremity of a finger applied on the cornea, Spanish snuff blown into the nostrils, pricking by pins, twisting her fingers ; all these means were tried without producing the least sign of feeling or perception. Soon afterwards she rose, and I expected to see her strike herself against the neighbouring beds; but she passed between them and turned corners with the greatest exactness, avoiding chairs and other furniture that happened to be in her way, and having walked about the ward, returned between the beds without feeling her way, lay down, covered herself, and in a few minutes became again cataleptic. She afterwards awoke as if from a deep sleep, and perceiving by the looks of those about her that she had been in her fits, she became very confused and wept all the rest of the day, not having the least idea of what had passed during the paroxysm." Sauvages adds that this patient recovered ; her fits became less frequent ; she had some relapses, but the disorder at length entirely left her.[*]

Lorry has described the phenomena of two remarkable cases of ecstasis, of which he was an eye-witness. A woman in a state resembling somnambulism used to converse aloud with absent persons, supposing them to be present. She was so insensible to external impressions that she could not be excited by pricking or pinching her body, yet she perceived objects to which the current of her thoughts directed her, or to which they had relation. Her arms and fingers retained the positions in which they were placed till they were changed by a voluntary movement of the limb. After the paroxysm she had lost all recollection of what had passed. The other case given by Lorry was that of a female who had deficient catamenia. During her paroxysms she used to address herself to some individual actually present, whom she evidently saw, while all that she said to him turned upon the subject of her reverie. In the mean time she appeared unconscious of the presence of others, and could not be made to hear them or perceive them. " This fact," says Lorry, " I witnessed with the utmost astonishment, but many other persons are living who can attest it. The mother of this female died unexpectedly ; after which the daughter used to hold conversations with her as if she were present."

A remarkable circumstance in these cases is the fact that while

---

[*] Histoire de l'Academie des Sciences, an 1742. Traité du Somnambulisme, par A. Bertrand. Paris, 1823. A very curious and remarkable case of ecstatic somnambulism is to be found in the German translation of Muratori. It was extracted by Richertz from the Breslau Sammlungen. See Muratori über die Einbildungskraft, band. i. p. 361.

the individual is insensible to all other impressions in a wonderful
degree, he retains perception of all objects which fall in with the
course of his ideas, or connect themselves with the thoughts and
feelings which occupy his attention for the time being. This feature
is common to the cases of ecstasy and somnambulism. It was observed in an example of the former kind, of which an account was
published several years ago in my work, "On Disorders of the
Nervous System." A boy, about thirteen or fourteen years of age,
suddenly exclaimed that somebody was beating him on his head,
and fell into a state of insensibility ; he became subject afterwards
to similar attacks. He first perceived a mist or darkness before his
eyes, and would say that he was then going off. He became unconscious of external impressions ; had his eyes open, but did not perceive objects ; used to hold conversations with absent persons, repeat
his lessons, supposing himself to be at school, and play on a flute,
during which action he sometimes perceived that other boys accompanied him, and evidently directed his attention to them. He
recovered from this state by starting as if from sleep, and never
retained the slightest trace of any occurrence during the paroxysm.
The circumstance above indicated, in reference to the state of the
perceptive faculty, is important as illustrating the character of these
affections, and as accounting for the phenomena.

The fact mentioned by Lorry, which he witnessed with so much
astonishment, is likewise interesting by its bearing on the phenomena of animal magnetism. In Lorry's account, written long
before the time of magnetism, it appears that a female in somnambulism held conversation with one individual with whom her feelings and ideas brought her into relation, while she was unaware of
the presence of any other individual and unconscious of her state.

Another striking characteristic of this affection is the instanta-
neous change which it occasions in the thoughts and state of consciousness, and in the whole catastasis of the mind, the total suspension of present ideas which takes place during an indefinite
period, and the equally sudden and remarkable restoration of the
former state of mind after the termination of the paroxysm.

I shall close this series of cases by adducing the facts of one not
long since recorded by Dr. Dyce of Aberdeen, and published in the
Edinburgh Philosophical Transactions.* This case is one of singular interest : in some respects it resembles that of Negretti, but it
will be thought, unless I am mistaken, to be quite conclusive on the
question whether somnambulism involves or not a suspension of
specific sense, or of sense through the ordinary channels, and a
transference of external feeling to the nervous system of physical
life.

The subject of this relation was a girl sixteen years of age, and
the phenomena ceased when the uterine functions were established.

* Report of a communication from Dr. Dyce of Aberdeen to the Royal Society
of Edinburgh. Edinb. Phil. Trans. 1822, vol. ix.

The first symptom was a propensity to fall asleep in the evening : this was followed by the habit of talking on these occasions, but not incoherently, as sleep-talkers are wont to do. She repeated the occurrences of the day, and sang musical airs, sacred and profane. Falling one evening asleep she imagined herself to be going to Epsom races, placed herself on a kitchen stool, and rode into a room with a clattering noise. Afterwards she became able to answer questions put to her in this state without being awakened. The fits occurred more frequently, and came on at different times. She dressed the children of the family, still " dead asleep," as her mistress termed her state, and once set in order a breakfast-table with her eyes shut.

Some of the phenomena of this case are astonishing, and would be almost incredible, if the testimony were not fully supported by the analogy of other circumstances. When taken to church, she heard and was affected by a sermon, particularly by an account of an execution of three young men, and of their progress in depravity, which was related by the preacher. On returning home, when questioned, after the fit had passed, she denied that she had been at the church, but in a subsequent paroxysm, repeated the text and substance of the sermon. The following fact is still more remarkable. " Another young woman, a depraved fellow servant of the patient, understanding that she wholly forgot every transaction that occurred during the fit, clandestinely introduced a young man into the house, who treated her with the utmost rudeness, while her fellow servant stopped her breath with the bed-clothes, and otherwise overpowered a vigorous resistance, which was made by her even while under the influence of her complaint. Next day she had not the slightest recollection of even that transaction, nor did any person interested in her welfare know it for several days, till she was in one of her paroxysms, when she related the whole facts to her mother. Some particulars are given by Dr. Dyce in Latin, and others were told him which he does not think it necessary at all to detail."

This relation renders the account recently given of a lady in Paris who underwent an operation during a fit of magnetic somnambulism without being roused from it, less incredible than, taken by itself, it would appear to be.* The phenomena of divided consciousness, as Dr. Dewar has termed them, were very remarkable. During the paroxysms, the girl, whose case is reported by Dr. Dyce, remembered things which had excited her attention in former paroxysms, but had been entirely forgotten during the intervals, and on recovering from an attack recurred to the impressions which had last been made upon her mind previously to a fit. Facts nearly parallel to these are recorded in the history of a case given by Dr. Silliman in the American Journal of Science. The subject of the

* Sir M. Colquhon's Translation of the Report of a Committee of the Royal Academy of Medicine.

relation was a lady in New England, who was subject to sudden fits of ecstasis. After awakening from a paroxysm she used to continue the conversation in which she had been engaged previously to the fit, and even to take up an unfinished story, or sentence, or word; and during the next paroxysm she pursued in like manner the discourse of the preceding one, so that, as the writer observes, she might be fancied to have two souls, each active, and each dormant in alternation.

In a strongly marked case of ecstatic somnambulism, the phenomena of which are so accurately and satisfactorily recorded, as are those related by Dr. Dyce, it is interesting to observe the facts which relate to the state of the senses, with a reference to the pathology of somnambulism in general, and particularly to the question whether magnetised persons as well as spontaneous sleepwalkers, have the ordinary channels of sensation closed, and perceive by a new medium.

It appears evident that hearing took place in the natural and ordinary way. The patient heard a sermon at church, and replied to questions put to her by other persons apparently in the usual way. We find no hint of M. Pétetin's new process of hearing through the epigastrium.

The state of vision is a matter of more difficult determination; but it seems on the whole evident that she saw by means of her eyes. "It was remarked, that while under the paroxysm she knew a person better by looking at the shadow than at the body; that is, she perceived those objects best which were presented merely in outline, or even very dimly illuminated." Dr. Dyce examined her eyes during a paroxysm: "Her eyelids appeared shut; but when he stooped and looked to them from below, he found them not entirely closed. When he raised the upper eyelid a little, it seemed to give her pain. When desired to point out different objects, she could not do it when the light of a candle shone fully on them, but did it accurately when they were in the shade. He then found the pupils greatly contracted, though in his previous examinations they had been dilated, and did not even contract when turned towards the direct rays of the sun. On one occasion *her stare* during a fit was accompanied by something resembling a squint of the eye. One day, during a fit, she walked over a single plank between two vessels on a quay, and danced on it. After the paroxysm she denied this circumstance, but remembered it again under the fit. She evidently saw when she directed her attention, and one day read the text in a book which she had not before seen, though it was on that occasion that her iris appeared dilated and insensible. There seems to be no doubt that her vision took place through the usual organs, though their state was in some respects singular. The condition of the organ of sight appears to have been very similar in the cases of Signor Augustin, Negretti, and Castelli, as before described.

If we now advert to the bearing which the history of real somnambulists has upon the state of persons who fall under the operations of animal magnetism into torpor and the temporary loss of external sense, we shall conclude that this acquired state is in many respects very similar to natural somnambulism, that some of its phenomena are illustrated and rendered more credible by the comparison ; but that other changes supposed to take place in the artificial process become still more improbable. The dipsychical phenomena, if I may invent such a term, are placed within the sphere of analogy and probability; but the notion that the ordinary specific sensation is lost, and a new sense acquired, is rendered extremely improbable, by the consideration that no such change appears to have taken place in the most strongly marked and best authenticated cases of real somnambulism.

SECTION VI.—*Of Maniacal Ecstacy or Ecstatic Madness.*

There are two modifications of cataleptic or ecstatic somnambulism which give rise to some remarkable phenomena. In one of these the mind of the individual is, during the paroxysm, in a condition different from that which the preceding relations display; it is more nearly in the state of mania or of incoherence : such cases may be termed examples of ecstatic madness, or of maniacal ecstacy. In the other modification the peculiarity consists in the subsequent recollection retained by the patient of the reverie which had occupied his mind during the paroxysm, and which afterwards appears to him as a vivid and impressive dream, or as an ideal scene, which he can scarcely distinguish from reality. This last affection is termed a trance, or ecstatic vision. I shall consider the former of these affections in the first instance.

I observed, when entering on this subject, that somnambulism bears a near relation to ordinary dreaming. I must now remark that there is a difference between these affections in regard to the state of the mind. In general the reverie which occupies the mind of the somnambulist is connected or coherent, his purposes are defined, his conceptions apparently clear, and his ideas consequent or relevant to the pursuit in which he is engaged ; they do not come into his mind in irregular groupes or make those sudden and casual changes and reverses which render ordinary dreams so absurd and confused. In the internal operations of his mind, the somnambulist is in this respect more like a person awake than a dreamer. Volition is more alive, the will more active, in the somnambulist than in the dreamer, not only with respect to bodily action, but also in the influence exerted over the train of thoughts. But there are some instances in which the case is different, the thoughts are confused and incoherent or imperfectly connected, and the active exertions to which volition gives rise are consequently like those of a maniac or a demented person. Such instances of ecstasis or somnambulism appear to have been taken for cases of madness. They differ from madness in the circumstance that the individual falls suddenly into a new state of consciousness, if such an expression may be allowed, or if ideal existence, and after being aroused from it, or passing out of it, is found to have lost the recollection of ideas which had passed through his mind in the interval. In these particulars the affection resembles somnambulism ; and it only differs from somnambulism as to the state of the mind and of the sensorium displayed during the paroxysm.

Dr. Haslam has recorded a case which fully exemplifies these remarks. The phenomena of the disease were during its continuance those of a maniacal attack ; by the complete obliteration of all the ideas which had occupied the mind of the patient, and which in real mania are more or less remembered, this affection was assimilated to ecstasis.

Two of the cases already referred to in the American Journal of Science, published by Dr. Silliman of Yale College, appear to have been similar to the preceding. I have remarked in a former section that one of them was an example of ecstasis properly so termed, the state of the mind during the paroxysm having been, not that of madness, but of consistent reverie. Both of the individuals now adverted to remained a long time under the affection : one of them, a lady in New York, about seven years, the other, who was a farmer, several years. Both recurred, immediately after the paroxysm ceased, to the ideas which had occupied the mind in the moments preceding the attack. I have copied both of these cases from Dr. Silliman's Journal, in the article *Somnambulism* in the " Cyclopædia of Practical Medicine," and omit them here for the sake of brevity.

Section VII.—*Of Ecstatic Visions or Trances.*

I now proceed to the consideration of cases in which the impressions of the paroxysms are retained in the memory of the person affected, and give rise to a variety of singular phenomena.

The expression " day-dream" is a familiar one, and answers to the French word reverie, which our language has almost adopted : it means a voluntary abandonment of the mind to the leading of fancy, which differs from the state of ecstacy, or trance. The ideas of reverie have not in retrospect the appearance of reality. A person who falls into ecstacy believes his impressions to be real, and could not at the time convince himself of their unreal nature. Sleep-walkers, properly so termed, occasionally retain, as I have shown, a recollection of the visionary scenes presented to them during their paroxysms. When this reminiscence occurs after a paroxysm of ecstacies, into which a person has fallen when awake, it produces the result above described.

There are instances in which the impressions retained after a paroxysm of ecstacy are so connected with external events or objects, and so blended with realities, as to make up a most singular and puzzling combination, and this is perhaps the true rationale of many a strange and mysterious tale.

I know the relatives of a clergyman who had been for some time in indifferent health, when standing one day at the corner of a street he saw a funeral procession approaching him. He waited till it came near to him, saw all the train pass him with black nodding plumes and read his own name on the coffin, which was carried by and entered with the whole procession into the house where he resided. This was the commencement of an illness which put an end to his life in a few days.

The following is a very striking case, with which my readers will not fail to be interested.

A gentleman, about thirty-five years of age, of active habits and good constitution, living in the neighbourhood of London, had complained for about five weeks of slight headach. He was feverish, inattentive to his occupations, and negligent of his family. He had been cupped and had taken some purgative medicine, when he was visited by Dr. Arnould, of Camberwell, who has favoured me with the following history. By that gentleman's advice he was sent to a private asylum, where he remained about two years ; his delusions very gradually subsided, and he was afterwards restored to his family.

The account which he gave of himself was almost verbatim as follows. I insert the statement as I received it from his physician. "One afternoon in the month of May, feeling himself a little unsettled and not inclined to business, he thought he would take a walk into the city to amuse his mind ; and having strolled into St. Paul's Church-yard, he stopped at the shop-window of Carrington and Bowles, and looked at the pictures, among which was one of the cathedral. He had not been long there before a short grave-looking elderly gentleman, dressed in dark brown clothes, came up and began to examine the prints, and occasionally casting a glance at him, very soon entered into conversation with him, and praising the view of St. Paul's which was exhibited at the window, told him many anecdotes of Sir Christopher Wren, the architect, and asked him at the same time if he had ever ascended to the top of the dome. He replied in the negative. The stranger then inquired if he had dined, and proposed that they should go to an eating-house in the neighbourhood, and said that after dinner he would accompany him up St. Paul's; 'it was a glorious afternoon for a view, and he was so familiar with the place that he could point out every object worthy of attention.' The kindness of the old gentleman's manner induced him to comply with the invitation, and they went to a tavern in some dark alley, the name of which he did not know. They dined, and very soon left the table, and ascended to the ball just below the cross, which they entered alone. They had not been there many minutes, when, while he was gazing on the extensive prospect, and delighted with the splendid scene below him, the grave gentleman pulled out from an inside coat-pocket something like a compass, having round the edges some curious figures ; then having muttered some unintelligible words, he placed it in the centre

of the ball. He felt a great trembling and a sort of horror come
over him, which was increased by his companion asking him if he
should like to see any friend at a distance, and to know what he
was at that moment doing, for if so, the latter could show him any
such person. It happened that his father had been for a long time
in bad health, and for some weeks past he had not visited him. A
sudden thought came into his mind, so powerful that it overcame
his terror, that he should like to see his father. He had no sooner
expressed the wish than the exact person of his father was immediately presented to his sight on the mirror, reclining in his arm-chair,
and taking his afternoon sleep. Not having fully believed in the
power of the stranger to make good his offer, he became overwhelmed
with terror at the clearness and truth of the vision presented to
him ; and he entreated his mysterious companion that they might
immediately descend, as he felt himself very ill. The request was
complied with ; and on parting under the portico of the northern
entrance, the stranger said to him, ' Remember, you are the slave
of the man of the mirror !' He returned in the evening to his house,
he does not know exactly at what hour ; felt himself unquiet, depressed, gloomy, apprehensive, and haunted with thoughts of the
stranger. For the last three months he has been conscious of the
power of the latter over him." Dr. Arnould adds, " I inquired in
what way his power was exercised ? He cast on me a look of suspicion mingled with confidence, took my arm, and after leading me
through two or three rooms, and then into the garden, exclaimed,
' It is of no use—there is no concealment from him, for all places
are alike open to him—he sees us and he hears us *now*.' I asked
him where this being was who saw and heard us? He replied, in
a voice of deep agitation, 'Have I not told you that he lives in the
ball below the cross on the top of St. Paul's, and that he only comes
down to take a walk in the church-yard, and get his dinner at the
house in the dark alley. Since that fatal interview with the necroman-
cer,' he continued, ' for such I believe him to be, he is continually
dragging me before him on his mirror, and he not only sees me every
moment of the day, but he reads all my thoughts, and I have a
dreadful consciousness that no action of my life is free from his inspection, and no place can afford me security from his power.' On
my replying that the darkness of the night would afford him protection from these machinations, he said, 'I know what you mean,
but you are quite mistaken. I have only told you of the mirror,
but in some part of the building which we passed in coming away,
he showed me what he called a great bell, and I heard sounds which
came from it, and which went to it ; sounds of laughter, and of
anger, and of pain ; there was a dreadful confusion of sounds, and as
I listened with wonder and affright, he said, 'This is my organ of
hearing ; this great bell is in communication with all other bells
within the circle of hieroglyphics, by which every word spoken by
those under my control is made audible to me.' Seeing me look
surprised at him, he said, ' I have not yet told you all ; for he prac-

tises his spells by hieroglyphics on walls and houses, and wields his power, like a detestable tyrant as he is, over the minds of those whom he has enchanted, and who are the objects of his constant spite, within the circle of the hieroglyphics.' I asked him what these hieroglyphics were, and how he perceived them? He replied, ' Signs and symbols which you in your ignorance of their true meaning have taken for letters and words, and read as you have thought, ' *Day and Martin* and *Warren's blacking*.' Oh! that is all nonsense! they are only the mysterious characters which he traces to mark the boundary of his dominion, and by which he prevents all escape from his tremendous power. How have I toiled and laboured to get beyond the limits of his influence! Once I walked for three days and three nights, till I fell down under a wall exhausted by fatigue, and dropped asleep; but on awaking I saw the dreadful signs before my eyes, and I felt myself as completely under his infernal spells at the end as at the beginning of my journey.'"

It is probable that this gentleman had actually ascended to the top of St. Paul's, and that impressions there received being afterwards renewed in his mind when in a state of vivid excitement, in a dream or ecstatic reverie, became so blended with the creations of fancy as to form one mysterious vision, in which the true and imaginary were afterwards inseparable.

SECTION VIII.—*Further Observations on the Pathology of Ecstatic Affections.*

Richertz has observed that the tendency to somnambulism is to be reckoned among morbid conditions of the system, and he founds his opinion on the following reasons :—First, the relation of this affection to various diseases. He says that when somnambulism has continued long, with frequent and severe returns, it is apt to pass into epilepsy, apoplexy, hypochondriasis, melancholy, and madness, to which last he thinks it has a near relation.* I shall presently consider the reasons for this opinion.

Secondly, he regards somnambulism as a disease, inasmuch as it is a phenomenon contrary to nature, which ordains sleep as a state of repose and refreshment from labour, whereas with night-wanderers it becomes an occasion of additional weariness and more than ordinary fatigue. Paroxysms of somnambulism are generally followed by long and heavy sleep, and by a feeling of debility and lassitude on the ensuing day.

Among the predisponent causes of somnambulism, the most important, as may be observed with respect to other diseases of the nervous system, is a peculiarity of constitution. This appears from the fact that the disease is hereditary. Negretti's son was subject to it from early boyhood. Dr. Willis knew a family in which the

* Zusätze des herausgebers von Muratori über die Einbildingskraft, th. i. p. 326, &c.

father and all the sons were afflicted with this troublesome complaint: the sons in their nightly discursions ran against and awakened each other.

Intemperance is said to be among the causes of somnambulism, and the analogy of facts prevents our doubting the assertion. Scipio Maffei, a correspondent of Mead, and one of the eye-witnesses of Negretti's adventures, attributed the disorder of that person to his immoderate fondness for wine.

Age and sex are to be taken into the account by those who investigate the etiology of any constitutional disease. According to Richertz, somnambulism is chiefly incident to the male sex and to the early period of manhood. It seldom appears in a strongly marked form in early youth, and generally lessens or ceases with the commencement of old age.

A plethoric state of the constitution, and whatever causes tend to induce fulness in the vessels of the head, increase the disposition to this disorder. Signor Pozzi, body-physician to his holiness Pope Benedict XIV. assured Muratori, that he was obliged to have his hair cut at least every second month, in order to prevent his becoming a somnambulist.

Richertz was certainly correct in his opinion as to the pathological relations of somnambulism both to comatose and to maniacal diseases, and this is a consideration of some interest. In the first place, the symptoms which usher in and terminate the paroxysms of somnambulism, and the transitions from one disease to another, mark the connection between sleep-walking and comatose affections. These facts may be noticed in many of the cases above mentioned. There are frequent conversions of one of these diseases into the other. Ecstatic somnambulism, as being the most severe affection, has been most frequently connected with other disorders of the brain. In females it is often conjoined with catalepsy and hysteria, and in males with epilepsy. Dr. Darwin has related a case of ecstasis occurring in a boy, which was supposed to proceed from worms. It began with an epileptic aura, and terminated in stupor. Another instance recorded by the same writer was that of a female, and it was combined with uterine epilepsy, or perhaps with hysteria. In its phenomena it appears to have resembled the example related by Sauvages. Two cases are described by Martinet, in both of which epileptic fits formed a part of the disease. In one of these somnambulism was vicarious of epilepsy : in the other, fits of ecstasis were ushered in by the usual symptoms of epilepsy.

The relation of ecstasis to insanity is in several of its phenomena still more apparent than that which it bears to comatose diseases.

SUPPLEMENTARY NOTE

ON

Peculiar Configurations of the Skull connected with Mental Derangement, with Observations on the Evidence of Phrenology, and on Opinions respecting the Functions of the Brain.

In that part of my work which relates to the congenital predisposition to insanity, I have referred to a supplementary note some further remarks on peculiarities of external form, which are connected with, and give indications of, defects or disorders of the mind. A consideration of this subject seemed requisite, in order to render complete the history of mental derangement; and in any other place than that which I have assigned to it, it would have occasioned too long a digression from the matter in hand. I shall now subjoin some observations on the subject referred to, which appear to be necessary for its illustration.

The attention of medical writers has long been directed to peculiarities in the form of the skull as connected with mental derangement, Plattner, in 1767, reported instances in which the forehead, and others in which the occiput, was flattened. Dr. Greding observed that the size of the head is generally natural in deranged persons. He says that, in one hundred lunatics, there were four whose heads were larger, and only two with heads much smaller than the general size. In twenty-six epileptic madmen there were four, and in sixteen epileptic idiots two, with small heads. In thirty idiots six had large heads, and only two very small ones. These remarks refer to size or dimension: with respect to the shape of the head, Greding says that it is in most lunatics natural: sixteen only had small and contracted foreheads, compressed temples, and large and expanded occiputs. A few had the head too long and compressed at the sides. Some had their heads almost round, or of a square shape; these were epileptic idiots. Two epileptic madmen had small heads of a circular form.*

M. Pinel instituted an inquiry into the forms of the head occurring in lunatics and idiots. The result, as he declares, proved to him that there are certain peculiarities in the shape of the skull which are frequently connected with mental diseases, particularly with dementia and idiotism. He reduced these forms to two prevalent varieties, which are a laterally compressed shape of the head, giving a very long diameter from the forehead to the occiput, and a short and almost spheroidal form, the line above described being shorter than usual. He adds that he could never detect any mental conditions or peculiarities in the state of the intellectual faculties that corresponded with these opposite forms of the head.†

M. Georget, in his work on insanity, has given the result of observations on the form of the head in lunatics, which were made chiefly in the collection of M. Esquirol, containing at that time more than five hundred heads carefully prepared. The following are the most important of M. Georget's remarks.

" The observations which I have made, have led me to this one result; one-half of the skulls had nothing remarkable; they appeared as regular and as well-formed as in other circumstances of life. The other half present peculiarities in the form, the regularity of the bony case, in the thickness, the density, the organization of the bones which compose it. We remark some skulls un-

---

* Observations on Insanity, by Dr. Greding, of Waldheim.—Crichton on Insanity.
† Pinel, Traité Philosophico-Médicale sur l'Aliénation.

equally developed, one of the sides being larger and more arched than the other; it is the right side that I have generally found with this disposition. Some skulls are as if they were twisted in such a manner that one side of the head is too forward, and the other too much behind. There are some which have not the antero-posterior diameter more extended than the lateral; the cavity of these is elevated very much, especially in the posterior part. The cavities of the base of the skull present likewise inequalities; those of one side are sometimes larger than those of the other."*

It has often been observed that lunatics who have very contracted heads, fall more easily than others into dementia: such cases of insanity are less curable than others, owing to a predisposition, as it would appear, to a decay of the faculties. Hence it happens that a contracted size and deformity in the shape of the head are so frequent in demented persons.

Of the Form of the Head in Idiots.

Idiots have faults in the conformation of the head much more frequently than insane persons; there are comparatively few who have not some defect or anomaly in the shape of the skull. M. Belhomme, in a thesis published in Paris in 1824, remarked that, out of one hundred idiots and imbecile persons in the Salpêtrière, only fourteen had heads of a natural form, and these were imbeciles and not complete idiots. Pinel has given descriptions, with drawings of the heads of two idiots laterally flattened, with the fronto-occipital diameter very long. I have seen some idiots with very small heads, wanting a great part of the space which usually contains the anterior lobes of the brain, and likewise of that belonging to the cerebellum. M. Esquirol observes that the skulls of idiots are either too large or too small: the anomalies of form which he particularly mentions, are a flattening of the head laterally or behind. In the former case the fronto-occipital diameter is lengthened, and the parietal bones flattened down towards the plane of the sagittal suture, giving a short transverse diameter. Sometimes, as M. Esquirol observes, the two sides of the cranium are unequal: this happens more frequently in imbecile and deranged persons than in others, though it is not peculiar to the former. M. Georget has enumerated the varieties of form observed by him in the heads of idiots, and among them are included almost all the anomalies of which the figure of the human cranium is susceptible.

An inquiry will here suggest itself to many of my readers, whether the peculiarities in the shape of the head said to exist in deranged persons, correspond with the observations or opinions of Dr. Gall and the school of phrenologists. I have had my attention directed to this inquiry for many years, and have omitted no opportunity that has presented itself of gaining information on the subject. Before I state the results which I have obtained, I think it necessary to introduce some remarks on the general credibility and evidence of Dr. Gall's system. This doctrine has been so much discussed in connection with disorders of the mind, and phrenology, if founded in truth, has so extensive a bearing on the nature of the human faculties and on all the morbid affections to which they are liable, that it cannot be well passed over in a treatise on mental disorders. By many it will be expected that I should state my reasons for having hitherto omitted all reference to this subject.

Phrenology has obtained many zealous advocates in different countries, and some of them have been men of distinguished talents and extensive knowledge, though in general they have not been among the most cautious reasoners. Few opinions, however, on physical subjects which have gained so many proselytes have been without some foundation in truth. Even animal magnetism, as we have seen, wild and visionary as it appears when taken as a whole, has yet brought with it the discovery of some curious and interesting facts. Phrenology appeals for proof to facts and observations, and therefore a number of voices in its favour may be deemed a presumptive proof that it rests on some foundation

* M. Georget, de la Folie, 8vo. Paris.

of evidence. This conclusion may, however, be questioned, if it is true, as I believe it to be, that the real ground on which so many have become converts to phrenology has not been the evidence of facts, but the plausible and specious nature of the theory, and the ready explanation which it *seems to afford* of a great number of phenomena in natural history and psychology.

About the period when Dr. Gall began to advance his new speculations, the prevailing notions repecting the mental faculties were almost everywhere such as had been founded on Mr. Locke's doctrine of the human understanding. The followers of Hartley, of Condillac, and Helvetius were not satisfied with the denial of innate ideas and innate speculative principles; some of them went on so far as to call in question the natural diversity of mental powers, or the endowment by nature of particular individuals with peculiar moral or intellectual qualities. Under the persuasion that the human understanding is, like a white surface previously unmarked, capable of receiving any impressions that might be stamped upon it, metaphysicians amused themselves by attempting to account for the formation of peculiar powers or tendencies of mind by tracing some early bias given to the thoughts and inclinations of children in the cradle. The perception of the beautiful in the forms of external nature was suggested to the infant by the winding surface of his mother's breast. Many a puerile conceit passed current under the name of a philosophical speculation. Few in the meantime were perfectly satisfied with such inadequate attempts to explain phenomena, though they were supported by the authority of learned names. Facts daily observed afforded convincing proofs that the real constitution of the human mind is far other than it was thus represented to be, that not only the powers of the understanding are given naturally in different proportions, but that peculiar moral dispositions and propensities belong in different degrees, by original distribution, to different individuals. The first writer who should reduce these observations into a connected form was sure to make many proselytes. This, in fact, was done by Dr. Gall, who stated in a more distinct and systematic way than any preceding writer, the doctrine of the innateness of particular talents and intellectual and moral propensities. The chief peculiarity, however, of Dr. Gall's *psychological theory* was the attempt to draw a parallel between the animal qualities displayed by the lower tribes, and the individual varieties discovered among men. By tracing the phenomena of action, feeling, appetency, so strikingly diversified in the various tribes of animals, he endeavoured to illustrate and render more probable a diversity of talents and innate propensities in the human mind.

The point of view in which Dr. Gall and the phrenologists have contemplated the mental faculties may be termed that of *comparative psychology*. It is founded on the principle that the innate or original faculties are common to man and the lower tribes of animals, to those at least which bear to man a general analogy in their organization, and especially in the structure of their nervous system: it discovers analogies in psychical phenomena between the brute tribes, and traces in them the rudiments of those properties which in the highest degree of development and taken collectively form the human character, and which in lower degrees and various relations constitute the distinctive nature of each of the inferior kinds. This is a new view of the mind and its powers, founded on a principle analogous to that which comparative anatomy applies to the structure of the body.

It was a novel and amusing speculation to trace the fundamental laws of political society, not in the higher principles where Aristotle or where Hooker have sought them, but in analogies with the economy of the ant or of the bee. By some it may be objected to such attempts that they are unworthy of so dignified a theme, and tend to lower rather than to ennoble the philosophy of the human mind. But perhaps this is only one of the *idola tribûs*. There is sound reason in the observation that the Author of man's existence formed also the inferior orders of the creation, and that extensive analogies may and do exist in the different departments of his works, the development of which may lead in this, as it has done in other instances, to the discovery of important principles.

The second department of Dr. Gall's doctrine is *Organology*. A comparison having been instituted between the psychical endowments of different tribes, the inquiry is next suggested, in what part of the constitution of men and of animals are these properties inherent?—of what are they the attributes or powers? If the question had referred only to the nature of man, the reply would probably have been,—as Dr. Gall with most of his countrymen appears to admit the existence of such an entity,—that the phenomena of which we are conscious, the properties of the mind, of feeling, of desire and will, belong to the soul or immaterial part of our compound nature. But the inferior animals are not commonly reputed to be, like men, of a compounded nature, and it would have appeared paradoxical to assume that they have souls or immaterial essences. The idea that a psychical principle, or a principle in its nature distinct from organized body, exists in all sentient beings,* has not been generally recognised, otherwise it would have occurred to many that such an entity, if it exists at all, must have attributes of its own, and the psychical manifestations of animals would have been considered as in some manner their result.

As it did not enter into the view of the phrenologists to assume the existence of a psychical principle coextensive with conscious or sentient being, the only resource left was to connect the series of animal properties developed by their system of comparative psychology, with some part of the corporeal organization that should be found common to mankind and the lower animals. Here the brain and the nervous system came in as having the best claim. This, in vertebrated animals, from which the comparative observations of the phrenologists were principally deduced, bears such a degree of correspondence in its structure through different tribes, as readily to fall in with the ideas of those who sought to connect with it a series of analogous psychical manifestations, and who were desirous of tracing a coincidence between varieties in those manifestations and diversities to be pointed out in the structure with which they were to be connected. Accordingly, where one tribe differed from another in the phenomena of instinct or feeling, it was often found that a parallel variety might be traced or imagined between the cerebral structures of the respective species. There was no great hiatus, or remarkable and sudden difference in the powers of sense, in instinct, or other animal properties, or, on the other hand, in the series of gradations by which the organic type of tribes higher in the scale of intelligence gradually deviates into a lower stage of development. On this groundwork, accordingly, the school of Dr. Gall have chosen to erect their system of organology.

I shall not insist on the assertion that the above is precisely the train of reflections which led Dr. Gall in his first speculations, but it is nearly that in which they were set forth by his amiable and ingenious follower and coadjutor, Dr. Spurzheim; and I doubt not that it is the way in which most of the converts to phrenology have been led to adopt their persuasion of its truth. In this they have chiefly been confirmed by the ready solution which this doctrine affords of so many phenomena. In the first place, the various appetites, propensities, or active impulses, of which the operation holds so large a place in the sphere of human action, were regarded as original and constituent principles of our nature. The attempts to account for them in various accidents of education, in early impressions and associations, which had been for the most part unsatisfactory, were rejected, and these properties were laid down as innate and distinct principles. The originally distinct nature of these properties was rendered somewhat more probable by tracing phenomena apparently or really analogous to them in other departments of the creation. Then came in organology, with its train of asserted relations or universal correspondences between psychical endowments and proportional developments in various parts of the nervous structure. The whole series of these speculations was calculated to excite great interest. They opened new views of both psychical and organic nature, and so extensive a field could scarcely be cultivated without bringing to light some valuable discoveries.

* On the considerations connected with this subject I beg to refer the reader to my treatise on the "Doctrine of a Vital Principle."

I shall now state briefly some of the objections which have probably occurred to the minds of many persons, and have prevented their admitting the truth of those assumed principles on which the phrenologists build their system. I have but a few words to offer on the scheme of comparative psychology in addition to what has been said already on this subject.

The attempt to illustrate the phenomena of the human mind, and, viewed externally, of human action, by comparison with the powers, habits, and propensities of the inferior orders of the creation, is extremely ingenious, and seems to hold out the prospect of discovering curious and interesting relations. The only question that occurs to us as a preliminary one, or as requiring a solution before we are at liberty to embark in the enterprise,—the only impediment we have to remove before we get fairly into the new field of inquiry without leaping over the fence forbidden to cautious reasoners, is, whether the analogies to be found between human actions and sentiments and the characteristic habitudes of the brute tribes are real and complete, or only apparent and superficial. Has it not been tacitly assumed as a preliminary step to this comparison, that the supposed distinction between instinct and reason is unreal, and that the active principles are of the same kind in the higher and lower beings in the creation? Perhaps metaphysical writers have been mistaken in laying down so broad a line of difference as they have established. We must, then, either elevate the brutes or lower the superiority of mankind. Shall we say, after tracing the operations of a constructive instinct so wonderfully displayed by the beaver, or in the cells in which the bee lays up its honey, that an impulse to action precisely similar gave origin to the pyramids of Egypt or to the building of Constantinople? Shall we venture to affirm that the tunnel under the Thames owes its existence to a burrowing propensity resembling that of the rabbit or the mole? Shall we conclude that Parry and Franklin sought the regions of the north impelled by the instinct of the migratory rat, and that Magellan and De Gama traversed the southern oceans directed by an influence analogous to that which moves the flight of swallows? Or may we, with greater probability, determine that the lower tribes act under the guidance, not of blind instinct, but of enlightened reason,—that metaphysicians were mistaken when they laid down the principle, "Dens est anima brutorum,"—that the birds of passage have some acquaintance with physical geography, and know the quarter where tropical warmth exists and genial breezes blow;—that the bee has studied the exact sciences, and knows by calculation the form most advisable for its cells?—in short, that there is a real analogy and correspondence between the mental faculties of man and the psychical endowments of those creatures whom he conceitedly regards as his inferiors? If either of these positions can be maintained, there will be a sound foundation for the comparative psychology of Dr. Gall and his followers: but if they should be rejected as improbable, we must admit that the analogies pointed out are remote, the things compared are different in kind, they agree only in outward appearances, and we shall be brought to the conclusion that it has pleased the Author of nature to bring about corresponding results, in the rational and irrational departments of the creation, by very dissimilar means.

I shall now proceed to make a few remarks on the remaining part of the phrenological theory, which may be distinguished by the term organology.

We have seen that the basis of this doctrine is a supposed universal connection between psychical powers and particular modifications of the cerebral structure, the varities of one kind being thought to bear every-where perceptible relations to corresponding varieties in the other. The proof held forth is an alleged universal coincidence in point of fact, or the actual correspondence between the two things in degrees and modifications. The nervous fabric being, throughout certain departments of the animal kingdom, analogous to its general form and type, this circumstance is thought to be the groundwork of that general resemblance in psychical endowments which is traced or imagined through all of them, and slighter variations in this type are only maintained to be connected with such psychical varieties on the alleged ground that they do, in point of fact, universally correspond with them.

If the evidence brought in support of the organological system depends so entirely on universal coincidence between psychical properties and corresponding variations in the structure of the nervous fabric, it must be important to determine whether there are any departments of the animal kingdom in which instincts and motive habitudes, and an entire psychical nature are displayed analogous to those of vertebrated animals, while yet in these departments there is no structure which can be said to bear resemblance to the complicated cerebral system of the so-termed higher animals. In all the vertebrated kinds, as I have observed, the organisation of the nervous fabric is on one principle, and the same fundamental type with different degrees of development is traced in man and in all other mammifers, in birds, reptiles, and fishes; but here the resemblance terminates, and the nervous system of molluscous animals and insects presents but few and remote analogies to that which belongs to the first great branch of the animal creation. It is indeed to be presumed that the nervous system, taken as a whole, fulfils, in the tribes last mentioned, the same offices as in those animals who have it enclosed in a bony case. Still, nothing exists at all resembling the complicated formation of the brain with its lobes and convolutions. It is so much the more surprising to find the higher instincts, which had almost disappeared in fishes, display themselves with new splendour and variety in the brainless insects, creatures which, in the wonderful imitations of intelligence that govern their motive habits, rival, if they do not even exceed, the sagacity of the animals which most approximate to man.

The psychical phenomena displayed by the insect tribes have been the favourite theme of many popular writers, but I know of no author who has placed the relation which they bear to the active principles of vertebrated animals, and particularly to those of mammifers, in so striking a point of view as Jacobi, whose observations on this subject I shall venture to insert, with some abridgment.

"It is a fact," as he remarks, "that among insects, if we take collectively the different tribes, manifestations of all the psychical qualities which we observe in mammifers and birds, regarding as a whole the properties divided between different departments, may be recognised in the most strict analogy. Attention, memory, the faculty of combining means to obtain ends, cunning, the desire of revenge, care of offspring, and all the other psychical qualities which have been traced in the former classes of animals, are likewise to be discovered in the latter as typical or characteristic phenomena, sometimes in one, sometimes in another combination, or in different groupes, sometimes more strongly, at others more feebly expressed.

"Nor can it be maintained on any solid ground that phenomena so analogous depend on different causes, or that the lower tribes of animals, and these exclusively, act under merely mechanical impulses, while their activity displays effects parallel to the manifestations of animal life in the higher orders. For what essential difference can be pointed out in the principle of action, when we observe the young bee, in its first flight from the maternal hive, hasten straightways to the nearest meadow, or sunny bank, and return home laden with wax and honey; and when the colt of the river-horse, foaled upon the land, after his mother has been killed, rushes from the spot, and betakes himself to the water which he has never seen; or when the young goat in the first hours of his life hides himself in the clefts of rocks, which nature already points out to him as his dwelling-place? Does psychical life display itself under a more limited or doubtful character in the flights of grasshoppers or dragon flies, than in the marches of lemmings, so closely bound by the impulse which directs the course of their wanderings, that they even attempt to gnaw through rocks which lie in their way rather than go round them, and follow each other troop by troop to their certain destruction, into the deepest rivers or widest lakes? Does not the earth-worm secure himself against the pursuit of the mole, provided with a well-formed brain, by making his way along the surface of the soil, where the latter cannot further trace him, with as much cunning as the fox and the beaver display in acts which are typical or characteristic of their kinds? I will ask again, what difference is there between the skill with which the insect ichneumon and the ant-eater procure for themselves the same food, between that of the diving-spider or the corpse-beetle, and the arts displayed by so many birds and mammifers impelled to similar pursuits? Are not like phenomena repeated in the economy of the beaver or of the Alpine marmot? And if we must refer to manifestations of a higher and freer sphere of agency, in what tribe of sucking animals does such a power display itself more wonderfully than in the wars of conquest carried on by different races of termites, in which the subdued become vassals to the victorious tribes, and serve their lords, in laying up for them their stores and watching and protecting their young?

" If we look but cursorily through the works of writers who have investigated the instincts, the habits, and the economy of insect tribes, we may well ask ourselves, while contemplating this wonderful panorama, where psychical life even in the same directions in which we trace it in mammifers, in fishes, and in birds, has taken a higher development, or when its phenomena are surveyed collectively, displays itself in richer and more varied forms. In the interesting work of Kirby and Spence we find collected examples of parental attachment and provident care which different tribes of insects evince towards their off-spring:—how the cymea griseus, like the hen, leads about her young brood, gathers them together, and exerts herself to defend them—how the earwig sits upon her eggs, when they are scattered collects them again under her, and after the young are hatched watches over them with equal care—how the aranea saccata watches over the sac in which she has enclosed her eggs, pines away with sorrow if she is robbed of it, and on the other hand evinces the liveliest joy if she succeeds in regaining it when lost—how she sustains the most valorous conflict for it against other insects, and even sacrifices her own life in its defence —how an ant, when cut through, yet ceased not to evince care for the eggs of her nest exposed to jeopardy, and although mutilated, rescued ten of them from the peril—how a throng of drones exerted themselves with energy, courage, and self-devotedness, when their young had been placed by Huber in a situation of apparent danger—with what astonishing endeavours and apparent calculations of means, and with what varied art and contrivances the apis papaveris and apis centuncularis furnish their dwellings—how many water-insects make use of the materials which accident seems to throw in their way to construct for themselves dens in which they dwell in the water.—And in order to become aware that psychical life displays its other manifestations among animals of all departments in ways nearly alike, we may read how wasps, as soon as new external condi-tions take place which produce an essential change in the state of their organi-zation, exert themselves with rage to destroy the very brood which they had till then watched over with the greatest care—how the working bees are at first so eager after the eggs that are laid by the female bees that they consume them as fast as they can obtain possession of them, until the eggs, after a few hours, be-come changed in such a manner that the instinct of appropriation takes another direction, and they now tend these eggs and the larvæ springing from them with the most inviolable fidelity—how some spiders, like some beasts of prey, cannot approach each other even for coupling without danger, since amidst their appa-rent caresses they are sometimes so powerfully impelled by a different direction of organic tendencies, that they fall suddenly one upon another, and the one entangles its mate in its nest, and unexpectedly devours it."

Now if it should be established that all those properties of animal life, approximating to intelligence or bearing analogies as striking to the manifesta-tions of mind, which in one great division of the animal kingdom are assumed to be essentially connected with and depending upon a particular system of organization, exist in another department, and display themselves in all the same various profusion, while the creatures belonging to this latter department are yet destitute of that system of organization and of any thing that bears resemblance to it, the advocates of phrenology will be obliged to abandon that broad ground on which they have attempted to fortify their position. Within the more confined field which the vertebrated tribes alone present, it will be more easy to maintain such an assumed connexion of physical properties with a peculiar structure, or, rather, it is more difficult to disprove it when assumed. The general analogy which prevails throughout these tribes in the organization of their cerebral and nervous system, affords no room for so decisive a contradiction to the relation which the phrenologists would establish.

Yet even within this field great and striking facts display themselves which are adverse to the hypothesis. Birds and reptiles, as Jacobi has observed, are nearly if not wholly destitute of many cerebral parts, which in mammifers are held as of high importance for the manifestation of physical properties, and yet they display physical phenomena similar to those of mammifers. Wherever an undoubted and tangible fact can be laid hold of in the different proportional development of cerebral parts, which can be brought into comparison with the relative differences of animal instinct or of psychical properties in general, there is, if I am not mistaken, a manifest failure of correspondence between the two series of observations. This has been shown by Rudolphi in a striking manner with respect to the cerebellum. The cerebellum, as this writer has observed, is found to lessen in its proportional development as we descend in the scale of organized beings, without any corresponding diminution and even with increase of the propensity which Gall connects with it. How remarkably powerful is this instinct in birds, and yet how small is the cerebellum in the feathered tribes compared with its size in mammifers; and even in the latter, when we consider the magnitude which it attains in the human species! We observe those tribes in which the cerebellum nearly or entirely ceases to exist, obeying, nevertheless, the impulsation of instinct as blindly or devotedly as other kinds which have the organ in question remarkably developed. When we consider the great amplitude which the cerebellum attains in man in comparison with its size in lower animals, we are obliged, if we really attach any importance to such a system of correspondences, to acknowledge some relation between this circumstance and the transcendant superiority of the human intellect compared with the psychical power of brutes. Other paths of observation lead us to a similar conclusion. Cretins, in whom the cerebellum is very defective, display in different degrees idiotism or deficiency of intellect, but no correspondent weakness in the sexual instinct, which on the contrary often exists in such unhappy beings in the greatest intensity, and impels them to violent excesses. Again, injuries of the posterior part of the head are observed to be followed by stupor and loss of memory, indicating the function of the cerebellum to be connected with the exercise of the mental faculties rather than with that of animal propensity. As for the assertion made by Gall, that the cerebellum undergoes a change in the rutting season, it is entirely without proof, for the swelling of the neck which is observed at that period has no connexion with the state of the brain, and is a phenomenon of quite a different kind. On the whole, it would perhaps be scarcely too much to say that not only positive evidence is wanting to support the opinion of Gall, respecting the cerebellum, but that whatever evidence on the negative side of the question the nature of the subject is likely to admit has actually been adduced. The only structures in animal bodies the development and condition of which is manifestly associated with the phenomena of instinct so strangely referred to the cerebellum, are those immediately connected with the process of reproduction. With the temporary as well as the more permanent conditions of these particular structures the state of animal instinct is immediately connected. In like manner is the appetite for food related to the condition of the digestive organs. In these as in many other instances nature has associated appetites or tendencies to action with conditions of structure in such wise that modifications in the former keep pace with changes in the latter, but on a system, as it would appear, more comprehensive and less subject to exceptions than that suggested by the theory of the phrenologist.

The facts which suggest themselves as we follow these trains of reflection are scarcely to be reconciled with the phrenological theory : they seem, in the first place, to show that the relations which in it are assumed to prevail through all nature are subject to vast exceptions, and as one great proof of the doctrine is the assumed universality of such relations, or the endowment of psychical properties in co-extension with certain peculiarities of structure in cerebral parts, the exceptions endanger at least the outworks of the whole doctrine. When, in a more limited survey, we confine our observation to the sphere of vertebrated animals, and discover that variations in psychical phenomena take place without any evidence of corresponding changes in the structure of cerebral parts, and that these changes, on the other hand, occur without such alterations as we are led to anticipate in psychical properties, the system of organology seems to be shaken to its very centre.

Still the advocates of this doctrine will rest on the alleged experience of uniform coincidences in the human species between the relative exaltation of particular mental powers and a corresponding development of cerebral parts, and within this sphere the phenomena would establish the inference if they were decidedly in its favour. If relative amplitude in a given region of the brain were always coincident with a proportional display of one particular faculty or quality of mind, the constant coincidence would prove a connection between the two phenomena. The phrenologist needs not to go beyond the limits of the human species in order to establish his doctrine on the basis of experience, but then this experience must be uniform and unquestionable. It is not enough to have a few chosen coincidences brought forward by zealous partizans who go about in search of facts to support their doctrine, and pass by or really cannot perceive the evidence that ought to be placed in the opposite scale. The principles of the system ought to be applicable in every instance. The phrenologists, however, aware of numerous and striking exceptions, elude their evidence by asserting that when a certain portion of the cranium and of the brain is greatly developed, while the faculty there lodged has never been remarkably distinguished, it nevertheless existed naturally, though the innate talent, for want of proper cultivation, has never been displayed : the predominant organic power was never discovered by the owner, though, according to the principles of the doctrine, with this organic power a proportional impulse to exertion or an instinctive energy is combined, which communicates of itself a strong and irresistible tendency to particular pursuits. When, again, a strongly marked propensity or a decided talent has been manifested without any corresponding amplitude of structure, it is in like manner pleaded that by sedulous exercise and culture, a natural deficiency has been overcome. Thus the phrenologist avails himself of a double method of elusion—his position, like the cave of Philoctetes, affords him an escape on either side, and in one direction or another he contrives to baffle all the address of his opponents.

If, however, the testimony of facts on a great scale should be found adverse to the alleged coincidences or to the correspondence of given mental qualities with certain conditions of the brain, phrenology will not continue to make proselytes, and it will be ultimately discarded as an hypothesis without foundation. At present most inquisitive persons seem to be in doubt on this subject, and to be looking out for evidence. I have taken every opportunity that has occurred to me for many years of making inquiries of persons who had a great field of observation within their reach, what had been the result of their experience on this subject. Many of these persons have been physicians, who were superintendents of extensive lunatic establishments. Some of them have been men who had addicted themselves to the study of phrenology, and were predisposed to imbibe the opinions of its authors ; some have been persons distinguished by their researches in the anatomy and physiology of the brain and nervous system. Among them I do not remember to have found one who could say that his own observation had afforded any evidence favourable to the doctrine. Yet we should imagine that a man who lives amidst hundreds of monomaniacs must have constantly before his eyes facts so obvious that he could not be mistaken in their bearing. Some hundreds and even thousands of such persons have passed a part of their lives under the inspection of M. Esquirol, who possesses most extensive resources for elucidating almost every subject connected with the history of mental diseases, and has neglected no inquiry which could further the attainment of that object. The result of his observations will be allowed to be of some weight on the decision of this question, in which the appeal is principally to facts of the precise description of those with which he has been chiefly conversant. At his establishment at Ivry he has a large assemblage of crania and casts from the heads of lunatics, collected by him during the long course of his attendance at the Salpêtrière and at the Royal Hospital at Charenton, which is under his superintendence. While inspecting this collection, I was assured by M. Esquirol, that the testimony of his experience is entirely adverse to the doctrine of the phrenologists; it has convinced him that there is no foundation whatever in facts for the system of correspondence which lay down between given measurements of the head and the existence of particular mental endowments. This observation by M. Esquirol was made in the presence of M. Mitivié, physician to the Salpêtrière, and received his assent and confirmation. M. Foville, physician to the extensive lunatic asylum at St. Yon, gave me a similar assurance. There are few individuals in Europe whose sphere of observation has been so extensive as that of M. Esquirol and M. Foville, and certainly there are none whose science and habits of observation better qualify them to be witnesses in such a subject of inquiry; but testimonies to the same result may be collected from unbiassed witnesses, whose evidence taken collectively may have nearly equal weight. Among these there are men unscientific, though capable of correct and unprejudiced observation, as well as anatomists and physiologists. In the number of this latter is Rudolphi, who declares that he has examined many hundreds of brains without finding any thing that appeared to him favourable to the phrenological theory.

I have endeavoured to survey, in what appears to myself to be the true point of view, the foundations and the system of inferences which constitute phrenology. I believe that the majority of those who have taken the trouble to consider this subject attentively, coincide with me in the opinion that whatever merit may belong to the founders of this system,—and that they have great merit, especially on the ground of ingenuity and diligence of research, all must allow,—still there is a great defect in the evidence by which their doctrines are supported, and this becomes sufficiently apparent to those who take a near and accurate view of them. I entertain a strong persuasion that the time is not far distant when the whole theory will be abandoned. This persuasion is founded on the prospect of more substantial and secure discoveries in the real physiology of the brain and nervous system. As yet this subject has been the " terra incognita" of physiology, a region into which every bold adventurer has been at liberty to make conjectural incursions. We have now reason to hope that it will, ere long, be satisfactorily explored. Much attention of late has been devoted to the functions of the brain and of its parts, particularly by physiologists on the continent; and although a want of agreement is still to be found among them in essential respects, which may prevent our adopting with full security the conclusions which any party among them have drawn, we have yet sufficient insight into the subject, if I am not greatly mistaken, to perceive that some of those who are engaged in this research are proceeding on the track which is likely to conduct them to the ultimate object.

It is well known to all those who have paid attention to the recent progress of physiology. that attempts have been made to ascertain the functions of different parts of the brain and its appendages, by removing successively parts of those living organs from animals, and noticing the changes which ensued in their actions when thus mutilated. The most celebrated of these was the series of experiments instituted by M. Flourens, of which a report was made by Baron Cuvier to the Academy of Sciences. MM. Magendie and Serres, and more lately Fodéra and Bouillaud, have occupied themselves with similar researches. The results which they have obtained, though differing considerably in some particulars, are yet on the whole somewhat analogous. Very different conclusions have, however, been deduced from inquiries instituted and pursued for several years on a different path, chiefly by M. Foville and M. Pinel Grandchamp. These writers, particularly M. Foville, are disposed to distrust all the results of vivisection, or experiments performed by cutting away the brains of living animals. The method of inquiry which they have pursued is that of minute and accurate observation of pathological facts. I shall take a very brief survey of the conclusions to which both parties have arrived.

The proceeding of M. Flourens was by cutting away gradually thin slices of the brain and noting the effects produced on the animals subjected to the operation. Entire removal of the cerebrum occasioned profound coma, or stupor and loss of the power of voluntary motion: hence it was concluded that perception, memory, volition, have their seat in the cerebrum. These conclusions are in a great measure disproved by the later observations of M. Bouillaud, who demonstrated that animals wholly deprived of the cerebrum retain sensation, that they give the plainest evidences of feeling when struck or exposed to causes of pain. Even the iris remains, under such circumstances, sensible to the stimulus of light; nor is the power of locomotion wholly lost, for animals, after being deprived of their brains, made efforts to escape from irritation, and performed various movements of body similar to those of habit and instinct. A power of effecting regular and combined movements on external stimulation evidently survived the destruction of the hemispheres of the brain.*

M. Flourens made similar experiments on the cerebellum. Pigeons, from which the whole of the cerebellum had been cut away in successive slices, retained sensation, and made attempts at locomotion, but had lost the power of rendering the muscles obedient to the will. It was hence concluded by M. Flourens, and in this opinion M. Bouillaud concurred, though he differed from that physiologist in regard to the functions of the cerebrum, that the office of the cerebellum is "to balance, regulate, and combine the action of muscles and limbs, so as to bring about those complex movements depending upon simultaneous and conspiring efforts of many muscles, which are necessary to the different kinds of progressive motion." Strange and unaccountable modifications of these results have been obtained by other experimenters. M. Magendie found that a duck, after he had removed its cerebellum, could only swim backwards, and M. Fodéra discovered that a similar retrograde action was produced in all cases by removing a considerable part of the same organ. Magendie found that division of the crura cerebelli was followed by incessant rotation. After the right crus of the cerebellum had been cut through, the animal subjected to the experiment whirled himself round incessantly from left to right, and continued to do so for twenty-four hours. If both crura were divided, no movement whatever was observed.

Objections have been urged with much force against the conclusiveness of all these experiments by M. Foville, whose researches into the structure and the morbid changes of the brain and nervous system place him in the very highest rank among the anatomists and pathological observers of the present day. I have already cited at length his account of the morbid changes traced by him in the brain in cases of insanity. His general views of the structure of the brain, in which he is at issue with the followers of Dr. Gall, are briefly given in a memoir under the head "Encephale," in the "Dictionnaire Pratique de Médecine et de Chirurgie," and the author is now occupied in preparing a fuller exposition of them. M. Foville, as I have said, has expressed his distrust in the physiological results which are obtained from the mutilation of cats, puppies, ducks, and rabbits, and from the observation of their movements under torture, and in the unnatural and agitated condition in which they are placed by vivisectors. Another source of fallacy which he has pointed out in all these experiments lies in the fact that the influence of the brain, as the common centre of the nervous system, is so much the more important in man than in the lower animals, as its fabric is more developed in proportion to other parts of the system, and the powers which belong to the whole of that system in the animal economy are more concentrated in it. Hence it is that injuries to the brain, which are sustained with comparatively little inconvenience in other animals, are immediately fatal to man; and if we find some functions of the nervous system surviving in frogs, or even in pigeons, on a total removal of the brain, we are scarcely entitled to infer that in man such functions are altogether independent of that organ.

The doctrine maintained by M. Foville respecting the functions of different parts of the encephalon appears to have been suggested by the great discovery of Sir Charles Bell, that nerves arising from the posterior division of the medulla spinalis are nerves of sensation, while those which proceed from the anterior por-

* An analysis of the researches of M. Flourens was given in the Edinburgh Medical and Surgical Journal. A critical account of them may be seen in Dr. Bostock's Physiology. See also a very able report on the result of these and similar experiments by Dr. Henry, in the second volume of the Transactions of the British Association.

tion are destined to supply the muscles of locomotion, whence arose the obvious inference that the posterior and anterior fasciculi in the medulla spinalis itself are respectively appropriated to sensation and voluntary motion From this secure ground, it appears to be no unwarrantable transition if we go on to the conclusion, at any rate a highly probable conjecture, that those portions of the encephalon where such fasciculi of the spinal marrow take respectively their origin, or with which they are anatomically connected, are likewise connected with them in function. It has been discovered that the posterior fasciculi of the medulla, related to sensibility, are prolonged into the cerebellum, which may be regarded as an appendicle to or development of their structure, while the anterior, belonging to motion, after crossing at the pyramids, proceed thence to the cerebrum, into the substance of which they deeply penetrate. The opinion which M. Foville founds partly on this consideration, is that the cerebellum is the organ of sensation, and the cerebrum of motion.

In support of this position, assumed not on mere conjecture, but as an inference from the anatomical relations of the respective organs, M. Foville adduces a great number of pathological facts. With respect to the cerebrum, he considers his conclusions fully established by this latter species of evidence, but holds it to be much less certain with respect to the cerebellum. The facts which relate to the cerebrum are of daily occurrence, and the inference seems, indeed, to be indisputable. In those parts of the brain which are most distinctly connected with the crura cerebri, or the prolongations of the medulla oblongata into the cerebrum, viz. the corpora striata and the optic thalami, it is well known that the cause of hemiplegia is most frequently found, that effusions and other diseases in these parts are followed by loss of the motive power. In these parts of the human encephalon—I use that term to include both brains and the medulla—which, as we have seen, are so nearly related by continuity of structure to the anterior or motive part of the spinal marrow, we find the function of voluntary motion to be seated, the facts presented by pathology following out and confirming the anticipation. We are by all these circumstances led to place the more confidence in the other part of the doctrine relating to the cerebellum; and although it is not fully proved, yet many pathological facts are adduced in its support. M. Foville observes that morbid changes of sensation, paralysis of feeling in some parts, and increased intensity in others, have been found connected with diseases of the cerebellum. I have myself witnessed facts which coincide with this observation. We must wait for a further accumulation of evidence that may lead to some positive conclusions on this subject, and in the meantime we may perhaps consider the opinion of Foville as the most probable in the present state of our knowledge. His conclusion is, that the cerebral lobes are the primary organs of motion, and the cerebellum the seat of sensation.

I shall not attempt to follow M. Foville into the further details of his theory. In 1823 he published, in conjunction with M. Pinel Grandchamp, a series of clinical observations, in which he endeavoured to prove that the locomotive powers of the muscles of the upper and lower extremities originate from different parts of the cerebrum. The fibrous structure of the anterior lobe of the brain is, according to these observations, the source of the motive power by which the lower limbs are moved, while the fibrous structure of the middle and the posterior lobes of the brain is the organ of movement for the upper extremity. These opinions have been controverted by many writers, and indeed there are very obvious considerations which seem at first sight to forbid our placing any confidence in them. Such an one arises from the fact, that where injury received in one side of the brain causes, as it often does, paralysis of the opposite side, it is comparatively rare to find the arm affected without the leg, or the leg without the arm. From this fact we might conclude that the cerebral structure on which the motive power related to these limbs depends is in one and the same part. To this and other objections urged against his doctrine, M. Foville has made replies which are more satisfactory than we might have anticipated, and he has brought a strong evidence of facts to bear out his conclusions. The hypothesis which he advanced in 1821, in conjunction with Dr. Delaye, founded in part on the phenomena of general paralysis, that the cortical or cineritious part of the cerebral hemispheres is the seat of operations subservient to intellect, is in like manner open to theoretical objections. It is most probable that if the cerebellum is the organ of sensation and perception, it is likewise the local seat of those processes by which impressions once made are preserved or repeated, that memory and imagination,—which appear so nearly related to the impressions of sense that one of these phenomena, in certain states of our consciousness, is often mistaken for another—do not belong to an entirely different part of the organized system. But on this and other subjects we must wait for the elucidations which M. Foville will probably afford us, when we shall have obtained the more extensive work which he has promised.

In the present state of these researches, it would be a rash attempt to draw inferences with any degree of confidence, but I may be allowed to remark that the general bearing of facts seems to direct us towards the conclusion, that the two great organs enclosed within the skulls of vertebrated animals belong respectively to the two principal functions of animal life, which are, first, sensation, conscious perception, and the psychical phenomena related to intelligence; and, secondly, those of voluntary motion. This, however, can only be considered as a probable opinion. Such it has long been thought by many physiologists, and though the grounds on which this conclusion rests appear to be more secure than they formerly were, the proof is still defective. Pathological investigations may hereafter supply the evidence that is wanting. If the examples of accurate research into the anatomy of the different parts of the brain, connected with physiological and pathological inquiries, of which Dr. Abercrombie, Dr. Bright, and Dr. Hodgkin have set examples in this country, should be followed, they cannot fail of leading to a full elucidation of this and many other subjects hitherto involved in doubt.

POSTSCRIPTUM.

Since the preceding observations were sent to the press, I have been informed by Dr. Hodgkin, that Dr. Foville's opinions respecting the functions of different organs in the encephalon were not originally suggested by the discoveries of Sir Charles Bell, though he has appealed to these discoveries as affording a probable evidence in their support. They were communicated to Dr. Hodgkin during the winter 1822—23, as the result of inquiries in which Dr. Foville, then a student at the Salpêtrière, had been for some time engaged. Sir Charles Bell's discoveries were not at that time as yet matured, nor had the first notice of them been given to the Institute by M. Magendie, who, in Dr. Hodgkin's hearing, first announced them to that scientific body as the discoveries of Bell.

THE END

MENTAL ILLNESS AND SOCIAL POLICY
THE AMERICAN EXPERIENCE

AN ARNO PRESS COLLECTION

Barr, Martin W. Mental Defectives: Their History, Treatment and Training. 1904.

The Beginnings of American Psychiatric Thought and Practice: Five Accounts, 1811-1830. 1973

The Beginnings of Mental Hygiene in America: Three Selected Essays, 1833-1850. 1973

Briggs, L. Vernon, et al. History of the Psychopathic Hospital, Boston, Massachusetts. 1922

Briggs, L. Vernon. Occupation as a Substitute for Restraint in the Treatment of the Mentally Ill. 1923

Brigham, Amariah. An Inquiry Concerning the Diseases and Functions of the Brain, the Spinal Cord, and the Nerves. 1840

Brigham, Amariah. Observations on the Influence of Religion upon the Health and Physical Welfare of Mankind. 1835

Brill, A. A. Fundamental Conceptions of Psychoanalysis. 1921

Bucknill, John Charles. Notes on Asylums for the Insane in America. 1876

Conolly, John. The Treatment of the Insane Without Mechanical Restraints. 1856

Coriat, Isador H. What is Psychoanalysis? 1917

Deutsch, Albert. The Shame of the States. 1948

Dewey, Richard. Recollections of Richard Dewey: Pioneer in American Psychiatry. 1936

Earle, Pliny. Memoirs of Pliny Earle, M. D. with Extracts from his Diary and Letters (1830-1892) and Selections from his Professional Writings (1839-1891). 1898

Galt, John M. The Treatment of Insanity. 1846

Goddard, Henry Herbert. Feeble-mindedness: Its Causes and Consequences. 1926

Hammond, William A. A Treatise on Insanity in Its Medical Relations. 1883

Hazard, Thomas R. Report on the Poor and Insane in Rhode-Island. 1851

Hurd, Henry M., editor. The Institutional Care of the Insane in the United States and Canada. 1916/1917. Four volumes.

Kirkbride, Thomas S. On the Construction, Organization, and General Arrangements of Hospitals for the Insane. 1880

Meyer, Adolf. The Commonsense Psychiatry of Dr. Adolf Meyer: Fifty-two Selected Papers. 1948

Mitchell, S. Weir. Wear and Tear, or Hints for the Overworked. 1887

Morton, Thomas G. The History of the Pennsylvania Hospital, 1751-1895. 1895

Ordronaux, John. Jurisprudence in Medicine in Relation to the Law. 1869

The Origins of the State Mental Hospital in America: Six Documentary Studies, 1837-1856. 1973

Packard, Mrs. E. P. W. Modern Persecution, or Insane Asylums Unveiled, As Demonstrated by the Report of the Investigating Committee of the Legislature of Illinois. 1875. Two volumes in one

Prichard, James C. A Treatise on Insanity and Other Disorders Affecting the Mind. 1837

Prince, Morton. The Unconscious: The Fundamentals of Human Personality Normal and Abnormal. 1921

Putnam, James Jackson. Human Motives. 1915

Russell, William Logie. The New York Hospital: A History of the Psychiatric Service, 1771-1936. 1945

Sidis, Boris. The Psychology of Suggestion: A Research into the Subconscious Nature of Man and Society. 1899

Southard, Elmer E. Shell-Shock and Other Neuropsychiatric Problems Presented in Five Hundred and Eighty-Nine Case Histories from the War Literature, 1914-1918. 1919

Southard, E[lmer] E. and Mary C. Jarrett. The Kingdom of Evils. 1922

Southard, E[lmer] E. and H[arry] C. Solomon. Neurosyphilis: Modern Systematic Diagnosis and Treatment Presented in One Hundred and Thirty-seven Case Histories. 1917

Spitzka, E[dward] C. Insanity: Its Classification, Diagnosis and Treatment. 1887

Supreme Court Holding a Criminal Term, No. 14056. The United States vs. Charles J. Guiteau. 1881/1882. Two volumes

Trezevant, Daniel H. Letters to his Excellency Governor Manning on the Lunatic Asylum. 1854

Tuke, D[aniel] Hack. The Insane in the United States and Canada. 1885

Upham, Thomas C. Outlines of Imperfect and Disordered Mental Action. 1868

White, William A[lanson]. Twentieth Century Psychiatry: Its Contribution to Man's Knowledge of Himself. 1936

Willard, Sylvester D. Report on the Condition of the Insane Poor in the County Poor Houses of New York. 1865